BASIC AND CLINICAL SCIENCE COURSE

Refractive Surgery

Section 13

2008–2009

AMERICAN ACADEMY OF OPHTHALMOLOGY
The Eye M.D. Association

LEO
LIFELONG EDUCATION FOR THE OPHTHALMOLOGIST®

The Basic and Clinical Science Course is one component of the Lifelong Education for the Ophthalmologist (LEO) framework, which assists members in planning their continuing medical education. LEO includes an array of clinical education products that members may select to form individualized, self-directed learning plans for updating their clinical knowledge. Active members or fellows who use LEO components may accumulate sufficient CME credits to earn the LEO Award. Contact the Academy's Clinical Education Division for further information on LEO.

The American Academy of Ophthalmology is accredited by the Accreditation Council for Continuing Medical Education to provide continuing medical education for physicians.

The American Academy of Ophthalmology designates this educational activity for a maximum of 30 *AMA PRA Category 1 Credits*™. Physicians should only claim credit commensurate with the extent of their participation in the activity.

The Academy provides this material for educational purposes only. It is not intended to represent the only or best method or procedure in every case, nor to replace a physician's own judgment or give specific advice for case management. Including all indications, contraindications, side effects, and alternative agents for each drug or treatment is beyond the scope of this material. All information and recommendations should be verified, prior to use, with current information included in the manufacturers' package inserts or other independent sources, and considered in light of the patient's condition and history. Reference to certain drugs, instruments, and other products in this course is made for illustrative purposes only and is not intended to constitute an endorsement of such. Some material may include information on applications that are not considered community standard, that reflect indications not included in approved FDA labeling, or that are approved for use only in restricted research settings. **The FDA has stated that it is the responsibility of the physician to determine the FDA status of each drug or device he or she wishes to use, and to use them with appropriate, informed patient consent in compliance with applicable law.** The Academy specifically disclaims any and all liability for injury or other damages of any kind, from negligence or otherwise, for any and all claims that may arise from the use of any recommendations or other information contained herein.

Printed in Singapore

Basic and Clinical Science Course

Gregory L. Skuta, MD, Oklahoma City, Oklahoma, *Senior Secretary for Clinical Education*
Louis B. Cantor, MD, Indianapolis, Indiana, *Secretary for Ophthalmic Knowledge*
Jayne S. Weiss, MD, Detroit, Michigan, *BCSC Course Chair*

Section 13

Faculty Responsible for This Edition

Christopher J. Rapuano, MD, *Chair,* Philadelphia, Pennsylvania
Michael W. Belin, MD, Slingerlands, New York
Brian S. Boxer Wachler, MD, Beverly Hills, California
Eric D. Donnenfeld, MD, Rockville Centre, New York
Robert S. Feder, MD, Chicago, Illinois
Steven I. Rosenfeld, MD, Delray Beach, Florida
William S. Clifford, MD, Garden City, Kansas
Practicing Ophthalmologists Advisory Committee for Education
Donald Tan MD, *Consultant,* Singapore
Jayne S. Weiss, MD, *Consultant,* Detroit, Michigan
Helen K. Wu, MD, *Consultant,* Chestnut Hill, Massachusetts

The authors state the following financial relationships:

Dr Belin: Alcon, lecture/honoraria recipient; Allergan, lecturer/honoraria recipient; Oculus Optikgeraete GmbH, consultant, lecturer/honoraria recipient

Dr Boxer Wachler: Advanced Medical Optics, consultant; Alcon, consultant; Addition Technology, consultant; STAAR, consultant

Dr Donnenfeld: Advanced Medical Optics, consultant, grant and lecture/honoraria recipient; Advanced Vision Research, consultant, grant and lecture/honoraria recipient; Alcon, consultant, grant and lecture/honoraria recipient; Allergan, consultant, grant and lecture/honoraria recipient; Bausch & Lomb, consultant, grant and lecture/honoraria recipient; TLC Laser, equity holder, lecture/honoraria recipient; Eyeimaginations, consultant; Insite Pharmaceuticals, consultant

Dr Feder: Alcon, lecture/honoraria recipient

Dr Rosenfeld: Allergan, lecture/honoraria recipient

Dr Weiss: Alcon, lecture/honoraria recipient

Dr Wu: Alcon, consultant, lecture/honoraria recipient; BD Medical Ophthalmic Systems, consultant; Eyeonics, lecture/honoraria recipient; Refractec, lecture/honoraria recipient

The other authors state that they have no significant financial interest or other relationship with the manufacturer of any commercial product discussed in the chapters that they contributed to this course or with the manufacturer of any competing commercial product.

Recent Past Faculty

Dimitri T. Azar, MD
Steven C. Schallhorn, MD
Roger F. Steinert, MD

In addition, the Academy gratefully acknowledges the contributions of numerous past faculty and advisory committee members who have played an important role in the development of previous editions of the Basic and Clinical Science Course.

American Academy of Ophthalmology Staff

Richard A. Zorab, *Vice President, Ophthalmic Knowledge*
Hal Straus, *Director, Publications Department*
Carol L. Dondrea, *Publications Manager*
Christine Arturo, *Acquisitions Manager*
Nicole DuCharme, *Production Manager*
Stephanie Tanaka, *Medical Editor*
Steven Huebner, *Administrative Coordinator*

American Academy of Ophthalmology
The Eye M.D. Association

655 Beach Street
Box 7424
San Francisco, CA 94120-7424

Contents

General Introduction xiii

Objectives 1

PART I Underlying Concepts of Refractive Surgery 3

1 The Science of Refractive Surgery 5

Contribution of the Corneal Layers and Shape to the Optics of the Eye 5
Computerized Corneal Topography 6
Axial Power and Curvature 6
Instantaneous Power and Curvature 7
Corneal Shape 7
Other Features 8
Indications for Corneal Topography in Refractive Surgery 8
Corneal Topography and Irregular Astigmatism 10
Limitations of Corneal Topography 12
Clinical Situations Illustrating the Role of Corneal Topography in Refractive Surgery 12
Wavefront Analysis 14
Wavefront Analysis and Irregular Astigmatism 14
Measurement of Wavefront Aberrations and Graphical Representations 14
Lower-Order Aberrations 16
Higher-Order Aberrations 17
Biomechanics of the Cornea 19
Effects of Keratorefractive Surgery 20
Corneal Wound Healing 27
Laser Biophysics 29
Laser–Tissue Interactions 29
Types of Photoablating Lasers 29
Wavefront-Optimized and Wavefront-Guided Laser Ablations. 30

2 The Role of the FDA in Refractive Surgery 33

The FDA 33
Device Classification 33
Collection of Clinical Data for an Unapproved Device 36
Pathways to Market 36
Premarket Notification 510(k) 36
Humanitarian Device Exemption 37
Premarket Approval 37

Ophthalmic Devices Panel 37
Labeling 38
Delays in FDA Approval 38
Reporting of Medical Device–Related Adverse Events 39

3 Patient Evaluation 41
Patient History 41
Patient Expectations 41
Social History 42
Medical History 43
Pertinent Ocular History 43
Patient Age, Presbyopia, and Monovision 44
Examination 45
Uncorrected Visual Acuity and Manifest and Cycloplegic Refraction Acuity 45
Pupillary Examination 45
Ocular Motility, Confrontation Fields, and Ocular Anatomy 46
Intraocular Pressure 46
Slit-Lamp Examination 47
Dilated Fundus Examination 49
Ancillary Tests 49
Corneal Topography 49
Pachymetry 50
Wavefront Analysis 51
Calculation of Residual Stromal Bed Thickness After LASIK 51
Discussion of Findings and Informed Consent 52
APPENDIX 3-1: Example Informed Consent Form for LASIK 54

PART II Specific Procedures in Refractive Surgery 59

4 Incisional Corneal Surgery 61
Incisional Correction of Myopia 61
Radial Keratotomy in the United States 61
Patient Selection 62
Surgical Technique 62
Outcomes 62
Complications 65
Ocular Surgery After Radial Keratotomy 65
Incisional Correction of Astigmatism 67
Coupling 67
Arcuate Keratotomy and Limbal Relaxing Incisions 68
Instrumentation 69
Surgical Techniques 70
Outcomes 70
Complications 71
Ocular Surgery After Arcuate Keratotomy and Limbal Relaxing Incisions 71

5 Onlays and Inlays 73
Keratophakia. 73
Homoplastic Corneal Inlays 73
Alloplastic Corneal Inlays 74
Epikeratoplasty 75
Background 75
Technique 75
Outcomes 76
Complications 76
Alloplastic Corneal Onlays 76
Intrastromal Corneal Ring Segments 77
Background 77
Patient Selection for Myopia 78
Instrumentation 79
Technique 79
Outcomes 80
Intacs and Keratoconus 81
Complications 83
Uses for Intrastromal Corneal Ring Segments After LASIK 85
Orthokeratology 86
Conclusion 87

6 Photoablation 89
Background 89
Surface Ablation: Photorefractive Keratectomy, Laser Subepithelial Keratomileusis, and Epithelial Laser in Situ Keratomileusis. 92
Patient Selection 92
Surgical Technique 93
Laser Treatment. 98
Outcomes 100
Complications 103
Conclusion. 108
Laser in Situ Keratomileusis 109
Background 109
Instrumentation 110
Patient Selection 114
Surgical Technique 116
Outcomes 124
Complications 129
Conclusion. 145
Wavefront-Guided Surface Ablation and LASIK. 146
Background 146
Instrumentation 147
Preoperative Preparation 147

7 Collagen Shrinkage Procedures 149
History 149
Laser Thermokeratoplasty 150

Conductive Keratoplasty 150
Patient Selection and Results 152
Safety 153
Other Applications 154

8 Intraocular Surgery 157
Phakic Intraocular Lenses 157
Background 157
Advantages 158
Disadvantages 158
Patient Selection 161
Surgical Technique 162
Outcomes 165
Complications 168
Bioptics 171
Outcomes 172
Clear Lens Extraction (Refractive Lens Exchange) 172
Patient Selection 172
Surgical Planning and Technique 174
IOL Calculations in Refractive Lensectomy 176
Complications 177
Advantages 177
Disadvantages 177
Toric Intraocular Lenses 177
Instrumentation 177
Patient Selection 178
Planning and Surgical Technique 179
Outcomes 179
Complications 179
Multifocal Intraocular Lenses 180
Instrumentation 180
Patient Selection 180
Surgical Technique 181
Outcomes 181
Side Effects and Complications 182
Accommodating Intraocular Lenses 182
Single-Optic IOLs 182
Dual-Optic IOLs 183
Deformable IOLs 183
Wavefront-Designed Intraocular Lenses 184
Light-Adjustable Intraocular Lenses 184

9 Accommodative and Nonaccommodative Treatment of Presbyopia 187
Introduction 187
Theories of Accommodation 187
Nonaccommodative Treatment of Presbyopia 191
Monovision 191
Conductive Keratoplasty 192

IOL Implants 192
Custom or Multifocal Ablations 194
Corneal Inlays 195
Accommodative Treatment of Presbyopia 196
Scleral Surgery 196
Accommodating IOLs 198
Other IOL Innovations on the Horizon 200

PART III Refractive Surgery in the Setting of Other Conditions 201

10 Refractive Surgery in Ocular and Systemic Disease. 203
Introduction 203
Ocular Conditions 204
Dry Eye 204
Herpesvirus 205
Keratoconus 207
Post–Penetrating Keratoplasty 208
Ocular Hypertension and Glaucoma 211
Retinal Disease 214
Amblyopia and Strabismus in the Adult and Child 216
Systemic Conditions 219
Human Immunodeficiency Virus 219
Diabetes Mellitus 221
Connective Tissue and Autoimmune Diseases. 222

11 Considerations After Refractive Surgery. 223
IOL Calculations After Refractive Surgery 223
With Pre–Refractive Surgery Refraction and Keratometry and Post–Refractive Surgery Refraction 224
With Pre–Refractive Surgery Refraction and Keratometry 224
With Pre–Refractive Surgery Refraction and Post–Refractive Surgery Refraction 224
With Pre–Refractive Surgery Refraction Only. 225
With No Preoperative Information 225
Conclusion. 226
Retinal Detachment Repair After LASIK. 227
Corneal Transplantation After Refractive Surgery 227
Contact Lens Use After Refractive Surgery 228
Indications 228
General Principles. 229
Contact Lenses After Radial Keratotomy 229
Contact Lenses After Surface Ablation 230
Contact Lenses After LASIK 231
Contact Lens–Assisted, Pharmacologically Induced Keratosteepening . 232
Glaucoma After Refractive Surgery 232

12 International Perspectives in Refractive Surgery 235
Introduction 235
Global Estimates of Refractive Surgery. 235
Variation in Global Prevalence of Refractive Errors 237
International Trends in Refractive Surgery 237
International Regulation of Refractive Surgery Practices and Devices . . . 240
Summary 241

Basic Texts. 243
Related Academy Materials 245
Credit Reporting Form 247
Study Questions 251
Answers. 260
Index 267

General Introduction

The Basic and Clinical Science Course (BCSC) is designed to meet the needs of residents and practitioners for a comprehensive yet concise curriculum of the field of ophthalmology. The BCSC has developed from its original brief outline format, which relied heavily on outside readings, to a more convenient and educationally useful self-contained text. The Academy updates and revises the course annually, with the goals of integrating the basic science and clinical practice of ophthalmology and of keeping ophthalmologists current with new developments in the various subspecialties.

The BCSC incorporates the effort and expertise of more than 80 ophthalmologists, organized into 13 Section faculties, working with Academy editorial staff. In addition, the course continues to benefit from many lasting contributions made by the faculties of previous editions. Members of the Academy's Practicing Ophthalmologists Advisory Committee for Education serve on each faculty and, as a group, review every volume before and after major revisions.

Organization of the Course

The Basic and Clinical Science Course comprises 13 volumes, incorporating fundamental ophthalmic knowledge, subspecialty areas, and special topics:

1 Update on General Medicine
2 Fundamentals and Principles of Ophthalmology
3 Clinical Optics
4 Ophthalmic Pathology and Intraocular Tumors
5 Neuro-Ophthalmology
6 Pediatric Ophthalmology and Strabismus
7 Orbit, Eyelids, and Lacrimal System
8 External Disease and Cornea
9 Intraocular Inflammation and Uveitis
10 Glaucoma
11 Lens and Cataract
12 Retina and Vitreous
13 Refractive Surgery

In addition, a comprehensive Master Index allows the reader to easily locate subjects throughout the entire series.

References

Readers who wish to explore specific topics in greater detail may consult the references cited within each chapter and listed in the Basic Texts section at the back of the book. These references are intended to be selective rather than exhaustive, chosen by the BCSC faculty as being important, current, and readily available to residents and practitioners.

Related Academy educational materials are also listed in the appropriate sections. They include books, online and audiovisual materials, self-assessment programs, clinical modules, and interactive programs.

Study Questions and CME Credit

Each volume of the BCSC is designed as an independent study activity for ophthalmology residents and practitioners. The learning objectives for this volume are given on page 1. The text, illustrations, and references provide the information necessary to achieve the objectives; the study questions allow readers to test their understanding of the material and their mastery of the objectives. Physicians who wish to claim CME credit for this educational activity may do so by mail, by fax, or online. The necessary forms and instructions are given at the end of the book.

Conclusion

The Basic and Clinical Science Course has expanded greatly over the years, with the addition of much new text and numerous illustrations. Recent editions have sought to place a greater emphasis on clinical applicability while maintaining a solid foundation in basic science. As with any educational program, it reflects the experience of its authors. As its faculties change and as medicine progresses, new viewpoints are always emerging on controversial subjects and techniques. Not all alternate approaches can be included in this series; as with any educational endeavor, the learner should seek additional sources, including such carefully balanced opinions as the Academy's Preferred Practice Patterns.

The BCSC faculty and staff are continuously striving to improve the educational usefulness of the course; you, the reader, can contribute to this ongoing process. If you have any suggestions or questions about the series, please do not hesitate to contact the faculty or the editors.

The authors, editors, and reviewers hope that your study of the BCSC will be of lasting value and that each Section will serve as a practical resource for quality patient care.

Objectives

Upon completion of BCSC Section 13, *Refractive Surgery,* the reader should be able to

- explain the contribution of the cornea's shape and tissue layers to the optics of the eye and how these components are affected biomechanically by different types of keratorefractive procedures
- outline the basic concepts of wavefront analysis and its relationship to different types of optical aberrations
- review the general types of lasers used in refractive surgeries
- describe the role of the FDA in the development and approval of ophthalmic devices used in refractive surgery
- outline the steps—including medical and social history, ocular examination, and ancillary testing—in evaluating whether a patient is an appropriate candidate for refractive surgery
- for incisional keratorefractive surgery (radial keratotomy, transverse keratotomy, arcuate keratotomy, and limbal relaxing incisions), review the history, patient selection, surgical techniques, outcomes, and complications
- list the various types of corneal onlays and inlays that have been used for refractive correction
- for surface ablation procedures, review patient selection, epithelial removal and laser calibration techniques, refractive outcomes, and complications
- review patient selection, surgical techniques, outcomes, and complications for laser in situ keratomileusis (LASIK)

- describe the different methods for creating a LASIK flap using a microkeratome or a femtosecond laser as well as the instrumentation and possible complications associated with each
- explain recent developments in the application of wavefront technology to surface ablation and LASIK
- for conductive keratoplasty, provide a brief overview of history, patient selection, and safety issues
- discuss how intraocular surgical procedures, including clear lens extraction with IOL implantation or phakic IOL implantation, can be used in refractive correction, with or without corneal intervention
- discuss the different types of IOLs used for refractive correction
- explain the leading theories of accommodation and how they relate to potential treatment of presbyopia
- describe nonaccommodative and accommodative approaches to the treatment of presbyopia
- discuss considerations for, and possible contraindications to, refractive surgery in the setting of preexisting ocular and systemic disease
- list some of the effects of prior refractive procedures on later IOL calculations, contact lens wear, and ocular surgery

PART I

Underlying Concepts of Refractive Surgery

CHAPTER 1

The Science of Refractive Surgery

Refractive surgical procedures can be categorized as *corneal* or *lenticular.* Keratorefractive (corneal) procedures can be classified as incisional surgery, laser ablation procedures, lamellar procedures, corneal implants, and corneal shrinkage procedures. Incisional procedures include radial keratotomy (RK) and astigmatic keratotomy (AK; arcuate keratotomy, limbal relaxing incisions [LRIs], and transverse keratotomy). Laser procedures include surface ablation, including photorefractive keratectomy (PRK), laser subepithelial keratomileusis (LASEK), and epi-LASIK. Laser in situ keratomileusis (LASIK) is a lamellar procedure using laser ablation. Epikeratoplasty, automated lamellar keratoplasty, and myopic keratomileusis are lamellar procedures that are no longer performed. Corneal implantation procedures include plastic intrastromal corneal ring segments (ICRS). Corneal shrinkage procedures include laser thermal keratoplasty (LTK) and conductive, or radiofrequency, keratoplasty (CK). Lenticular refractive procedures include phakic intraocular lens (IOL) implantation, cataract surgery and clear lens extraction with or without IOL implantation, accommodative and pseudoaccommodative IOL implantation, and piggyback IOL implantation. Each of these techniques has its advantages and disadvantages. In this chapter, we review the optical principles discussed in BCSC Section 3, *Clinical Optics,* as they apply to refractive surgery.

Contribution of the Corneal Layers and Shape to the Optics of the Eye

The air–tear-film interface provides the major optical power of the eye. The tear film itself has a relatively small optical effect unless an abnormality is present. For instance, in patients with epiphora, the tear meniscus may partially cover the pupil and cause blurred vision. In addition, an uneven tear film may result in deterioration of vision quality.

The optical power of the eye derives primarily from the anterior corneal curvature, which produces approximately two thirds of the eye's refractive power, accounting for approximately +48.00 diopters (D). The overall corneal power is less (approximately +43.00 D) as a result of the negative power (–5.80 D) of the posterior corneal surface. Standard keratometers and Placido-based corneal topography instruments measure the anterior corneal radius of curvature. Because the back corneal surface curvature and the exact refractive index are not measured, these instruments *estimate* total corneal power from front surface measurements. The normal cornea flattens from the center to the periphery by up to 4.00 D and is flatter nasally than temporally. A mirror image symmetry often exists in topographic maps between the 2 eyes. In adulthood, the vertical meridian is about 0.50 D steeper than the horizontal meridian, resulting in with-the-rule astigmatism. This difference diminishes with age.

By altering corneal shape, keratorefractive surgical procedures change the refractive status of the eye. The tolerances involved in altering corneal dimensions are relatively small. For instance, changing the refractive status of the eye by 2.00 D may require a shape change of less than 30 μm. Thus, achieving predictable results is sometimes problematic because minuscule changes in the shape of the cornea may produce large changes in refraction.

Another factor in corneal shape is the asphericity of the central cornea. The aspheric shape of the cornea generally reduces spherical aberration, minimizing refractive error fluctuations as the pupil changes size. When the central cornea is steeper than its periphery, the corneal shape is *prolate.* When the central cornea is flatter than its periphery, the corneal shape is *oblate.* Prolate corneas reduce spherical aberrations; oblate corneas increase spherical aberrations.

Another consideration relating to corneal shape after conventional keratorefractive surgery is that, although the surgery may reduce spherical refractive error and regular astigmatism, it often does so at the cost of increasing corneal surface irregularities. This can be seen as irregular astigmatism by topography and as higher-order aberrations by wavefront analysis. Such irregular astigmatism causes many of the optical complications that follow keratorefractive surgery.

Computerized Corneal Topography

Corneal topography can be determined using keratoscopic images or corneal elevation data. Keratoscopy images can be digitally captured and analyzed. Placido disk–based computerized topographers are the most commonly used. A Placido-based system is referenced from the line that the instrument makes to the corneal surface (vertex normal). This line is not necessarily the patient's line of sight or the visual axis, which may lead to confusion in interpreting topographic maps. Elevation-based topography instruments determine the initial shape using triangulation or other methods and then calculate the power map from the shape. Some topographers provide information regarding posterior corneal curvature, which may be especially useful in identifying patients with keratoconus and in the follow-up of patients with, or at risk of developing, corneal ectasia after excimer laser surgery. For a more extensive discussion of other uses of computerized corneal topography, refer to BCSC Section 3, *Clinical Optics,* and Section 8, *External Disease and Cornea.*

Axial Power and Curvature

Axial power provides a "smoother" picture of the cornea because the instrument used assumes a radius of curvature that intersects with the instrument axis. The curvature and power of the central 1–2 mm of the cornea can be closely approximated by the axial power and curvature indices (formerly called "sagittal curvature"); however, the central measurements are extrapolated and thus are potentially inaccurate. These indices also fail to describe the true shape and power of the peripheral cornea. Topographic maps displaying axial power and curvature provide an intuitive sense of the physiologic flattening of the cornea but do not represent the true refractive power or the true curvature of peripheral regions of the cornea.

Instantaneous Power and Curvature

A second method of describing the corneal curvature on Placido disk–based topography is to use the *instantaneous radius of curvature* (also called *meridional* or *tangential power*). The potential benefit of this method's increased sensitivity is balanced by its tendency to document excessive detail ("noise"), which may not be clinically relevant. The instantaneous radius of curvature is determined by taking a perpendicular path through the point in question from a plane that intersects the point and the visual axis but allowing the radius to be the length necessary to correspond to a sphere with the same curvature at that point. With curvature given in diopters, it is estimated by the difference between the corneal index of refraction and 1.000, divided by this tangentially determined radius. A tangential map typically shows better sensitivity to peripheral changes with less "smoothing" of the curvature than an axial map (Fig 1-1). (In these maps, diopters are relative units of curvature and are not the equivalent of diopters of corneal power.)

Corneal Shape

Corneal shape can be indirectly described by Placido disk–based topography. A more direct approach is to derive corneal shape by means of scanning slits, Scheimpflug images, or rectangular grids. Corneal power can then be derived from the shape.

To represent shape directly, color maps may be used to display a *z-height* from an arbitrary plane (iris plane, limbal plane, or frontal plane). Just as viewing the earth from a distance

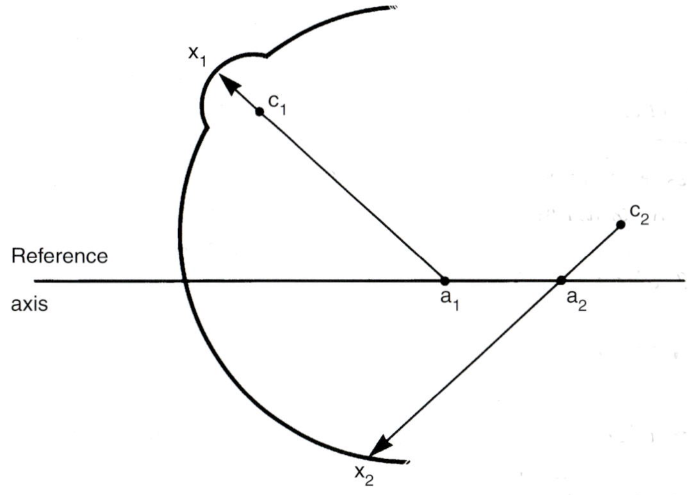

Figure 1-1 Axial and instantaneous corneal power (2 dimensional). Axial curvature at points x_1 and x_2 is based on axial distances x_1 to a_1 and x_2 to a_2. Instantaneous curvature at points x_1 and x_2 is based on radii of curvature from x_1 to c_1 and x_2 to c_2. *(Illustration by Christine Gralapp.)*

does not allow the details of mountains and basins to be seen, so *z* maps, or elevation maps, do not allow clinically important variations to be seen. Geographic maps show land elevation relative to sea level. Similarly, corneal surface maps are plotted to show differences from best-fit spheres or other objects that closely mimic the normal corneal shape (Fig 1-2).

Elevation-based topography is especially helpful in refractive surgery for depicting the anterior and posterior surface shapes of the cornea and lens. Ray tracing can be used to plot an accurate refractive map of the corneal and lens surfaces. With such information, alterations to the shape of the ocular structures can be determined with greater accuracy.

Other Features

In addition to power and elevation maps, computerized topographic systems may display other data: pupil size and location, indices estimating regular and irregular astigmatism, estimates of the probability of having keratoconus, simulated keratometry, and corneal asphericity. Other topography systems may integrate wavefront aberrometry data with topographic data.

The asphericity of the cornea can be quantified by determining the Q value, with $Q = 0$ for spherical corneas, $Q < 0$ for prolate corneas, and $Q > 0$ for oblate corneas. A normal cornea is prolate, with an asphericity Q of –0.26. Prolate corneas minimize the problem of spherical aberrations by virtue of their relatively flat peripheral curve. Conversely, oblate corneal contours, in which the peripheral cornea is steeper than the center, increase the problem of spherical aberrations. Following conventional refractive surgery for myopia, corneal asphericity increases in the oblate direction, which may cause degradation of the optics of the eye.

Indications for Corneal Topography in Refractive Surgery

Corneal topography is essential in the preoperative evaluation of refractive surgery candidates. About two thirds of patients with normal corneas have a symmetric astigmatism pattern that is round, oval, or bow tie–shaped (Fig 1-3). Asymmetric patterns include inferior steepening, superior steepening, asymmetric bow tie pattern, or other nonspecific irregularities.

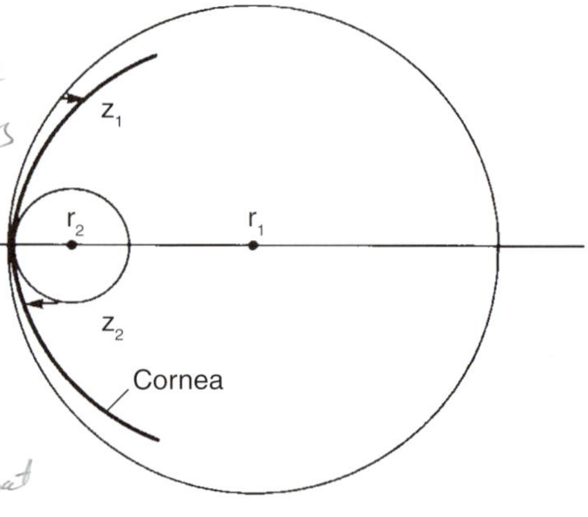

Figure 1-2 Height map (typically in µm). The height is relative to the reference sphere; z_1 is below a flat sphere of radius r_1; z_2 is above a steep sphere of radius r_2. *(Illustration by Christine Gralapp.)*

Quantitative indices to diagnose Keratoconus :- [1] Central steepening >47.2 D
[2] inferior-superior asymmetry index > 1.2 D

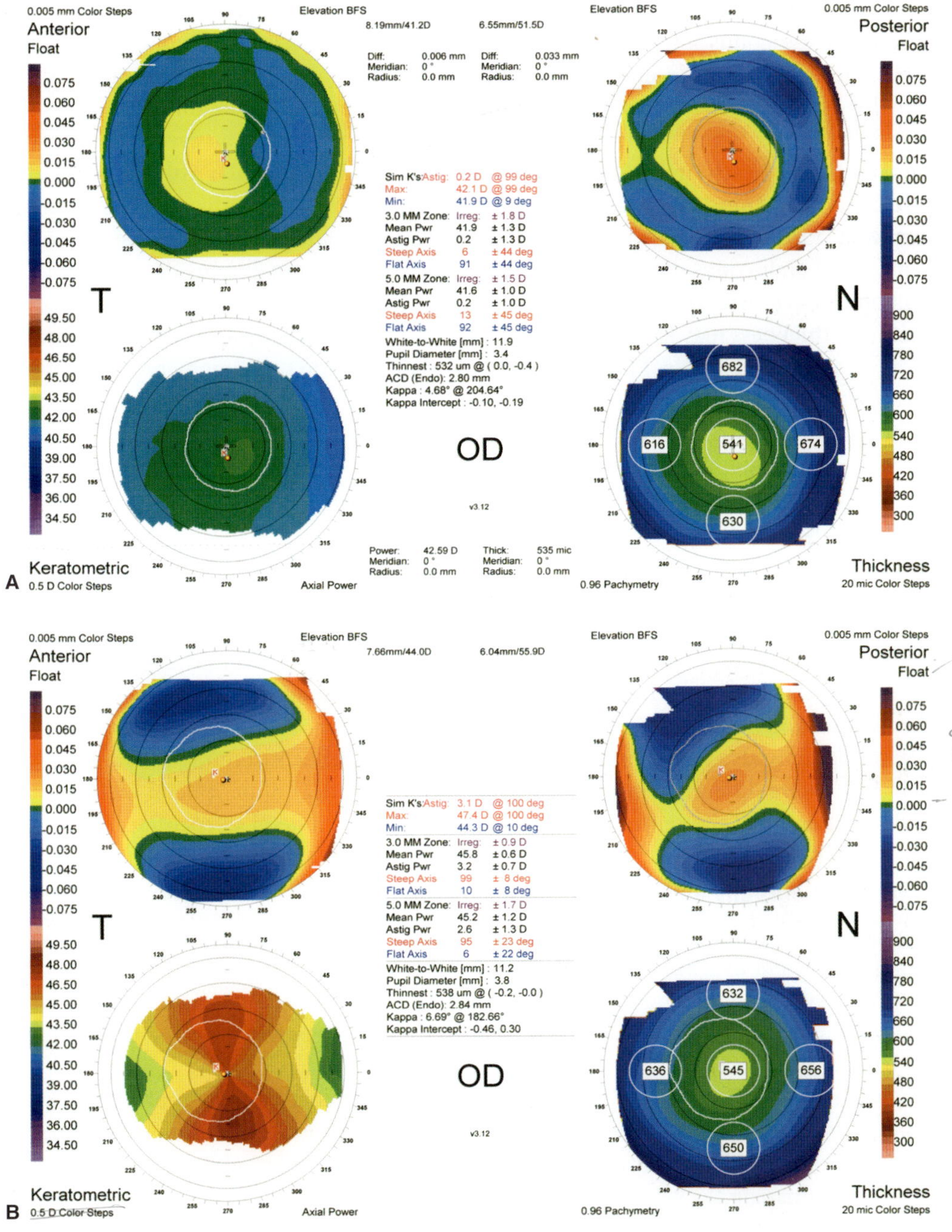

Figure 1-3 **A,** Corneal topography of normal cornea without astigmatism. **B,** Corneal topography of normal cornea with regular bow-tie astigmatism. *(Courtesy of Helen K. Wu, MD.)*

Anterior float = plots elevations of the anterior surface above & below a best-fit sphere

Posterior float = plots elevations of the posterior surface above & below a best-fit sphere

Corneal topography detects irregular astigmatism, which may result from contact lens warpage, keratoconus and other thinning disorders, corneal surgery, trauma, scarring, and postinflammatory and degenerative conditions. Repeated topographic examinations may be helpful in clarifying the underlying etiology. Different values obtained at subsequent examinations can signal a change in corneal contour (assuming the eye and the instrument are aligned each time). Patients with corneal warpage (irregular astigmatism and/or peripheral steepening, distorted keratoscopic mires) benefit from discontinuing contact lens wear prior to refractive surgery so the corneal map and refraction can stabilize. Patients with keratoconus or other ectatic disorders are not routinely considered for ablative keratorefractive surgery, because the thin cornea has an unpredictable response and reducing its thickness may lead to progression of the condition. Forme fruste, or subclinical, keratoconus recognized by Placido disk–based and elevation topography requires caution on the part of the ophthalmologist and is now considered a potential contraindication to certain refractive surgical procedures (eg, LASIK). Further discussion of this subject may be found in Chapter 3. Studies are under way to determine the suitability of other keratorefractive procedures as alternative therapeutic modalities for these patients. (2)

Corneal topography can also be used to demonstrate the effects of keratorefractive procedures. Pre- and postoperative maps may be compared to determine the achieved refractive effect (difference map). Corneal mapping may help to explain unexpected results, including undercorrections, aberrations, induced astigmatism, and glare and halos, by detecting decentered surgery or inadequate surgery, such as shallow incisions in radial keratotomy. Successive difference maps obtained postoperatively can reveal patterns of irregular wound healing, which may lead to the appearance of decentration (Fig 1-4). Corneal topography also confirms the expected physiologic effects of refractive surgery, such as in RK, where difference maps may demonstrate the effect of peripheral incisions that lead to flattening of the central cornea associated with peripheral steepening (Fig 1-5).

Corneal Topography and Irregular Astigmatism

Regular astigmatism can be corrected with spherocylindrical lenses. The traditional definition of *irregular astigmatism* is "a form of astigmatism that cannot be corrected by spherocylindrical lenses." Irregular astigmatism can decrease the patient's best-corrected visual acuity (BCVA) and may cause contrast sensitivity loss. Depending on the magnitude of the irregularities, patients may have only vague complaints.

Irregular astigmatism can be diagnosed clinically, by corneal topography, or by wavefront analysis. Unlike glasses, which can correct only regular astigmatism, gas-permeable and hard contact lenses can correct visual acuity reductions resulting from corneal irregular astigmatism.

Clinically, one important sign of postsurgical irregular astigmatism is a refraction inconsistent with the uncorrected acuity. Another clinical sign is when the refractionist is unable to determine the axis of astigmatism in a patient with a large cylinder. In contrast to patients with regular astigmatism, in whom the axis can be easily and accurately determined, patients with irregular astigmatism following keratorefractive surgery may achieve nearly the same acuity with large powers of cylinder at markedly different axes.

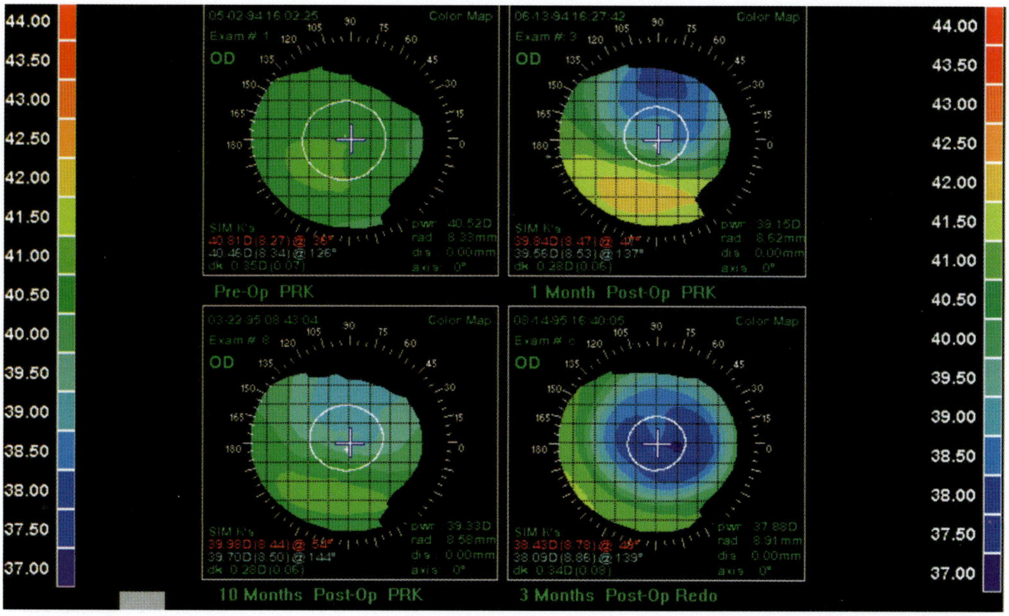

Figure 1-4 Successive corneal topographies after PRK reveal pseudodecentration secondary to uneven anterior stromal healing. The bottom right image illustrates a well-centered ablation after repeat PRK. *(Reproduced with permission from Wu HK, Demers PE. Photorefractive keratectomy for myopia.* Ophthalmic Surg Lasers. *1996;27:29–44.)*

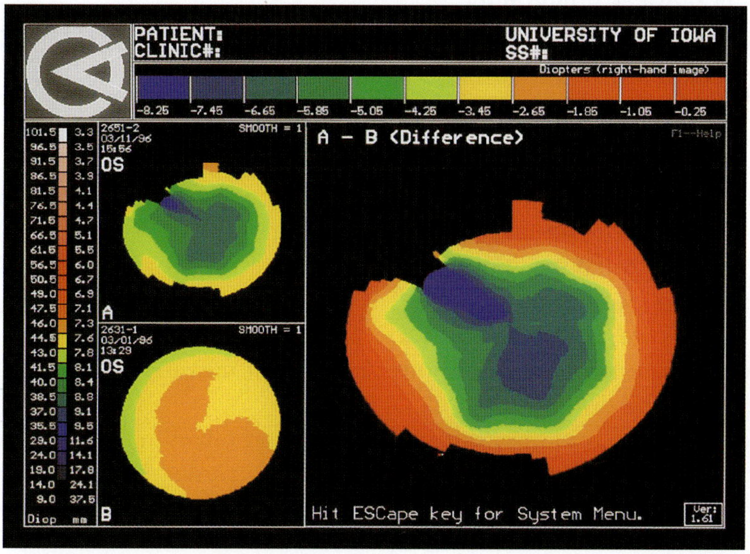

Figure 1-5 Difference map in radial keratotomy. Both central flattening and peripheral steepening are seen in the postoperative image **(A)** and in the difference map on the right. **B** is the preoperative image.

Corneal topography is very helpful in evaluating eyes with irregular astigmatism. Topographic changes include nonorthogonality of the steep and flat axes. Asymmetry between the superior and inferior or nasal and temporal halves of the cornea may also be seen on corneal topography, although these patterns are not necessarily indicative of corneal pathology. Wavefront analysis (discussed later in the chapter) often confirms the topographic findings in patients with irregular astigmatism, showing evidence of higher-order aberrations (such as coma, trefoil, tetrafoil, or secondary astigmatism). Wavefront analysis has the advantage of measuring various forms of higher-order aberration, thus allowing the clinician to quantitate irregular astigmatism in much the same way that we quantitate regular astigmatism.

The ability to differentiate regular and irregular astigmatism has clinical significance. Conventional excimer laser ablation patterns that treat spherocylindrical errors do not effectively treat irregular astigmatism. Customized ablations, either wavefront- or topography-guided, may be useful in the setting of irregular astigmatism. In addition, astigmatic enhancements (such as by astigmatic keratotomy or conventional LASIK) are rather unpredictable in patients with irregular astigmatism. Although it is tempting to perform astigmatic enhancement on patients who had little preexisting astigmatism but have significant postoperative astigmatism, it may be prudent to wait until the refraction stabilizes and then attempt a customized excimer ablation if a treatable wavefront map can be obtained. This is especially important after incisional surgery, where astigmatic enhancements may cause the axis to change dramatically (without much change in cylinder power) and may potentially worsen the uncorrected visual acuity (UCVA).

Limitations of Corneal Topography

In addition to the limitations of the specific algorithms and the variations in terminology among manufacturers, the accuracy of corneal topography may be affected by other potential problems:

- tear-film effects
- misalignment (misaligned corneal topography may give a false impression of corneal apex decentration suggestive of keratoconus)
- stability (test-to-test variation)
- sensitivity to focus errors
- area of coverage (central and limbal)
- decreased accuracy of corneal power simulation measurements (Sim K) after refractive surgical procedures
- decreased accuracy of posterior surface elevation values in the presence of corneal opacities, or often after refractive surgery (with scanning-slit technology)

Clinical Situations Illustrating the Role of Corneal Topography in Refractive Surgery

Keratoconus

Keratoconus (KC) is a progressive condition in which corneal thinning occurs in the central or paracentral cornea, resulting in asymmetric corneal steepening and reduced spectacle-corrected visual acuity. The topography of keratoconic eyes typically shows 2 principal and unrelated shapes: a steep inferonasal or inferotemporal ectatic area that is disease-dependent and a flatter superior paralimbal surface that appears to be pulled flat by the herniating lower cornea. Refractive surgery is typically contraindicated in KC, although ICRS have been FDA approved in the United States for use in select patients with KC to improve contact lens tolerance or as an alternative to penetrating keratoplasty (PKP). For further discussion of ICRS, see Chapter 5.

It is the patient who will ultimately develop KC but has no obvious clinical signs of it who poses the greatest difficulty in refractive surgery preoperative evaluations. Corneal topography may reveal subtle abnormalities that should alert the surgeon to this problem. Newer screening indices take into account a variety of topographic factors that may indicate a higher likelihood of subclinical keratoconus. Historically, I–S (inferior–superior) values have been used to determine this likelihood. The difference between inferior and superior corneal curvature can be measured by comparing the curvature of a defined set of points above and below the horizontal. This I–S number has a high incidence of false positives. The I–S number (normal <1.4 D; KC >1.9 D), central power (normal <47.2 D; KC >48.7 D), and corneal thinning, especially if the cornea is thin in the steep area on corneal topography, are helpful in estimating the likelihood of KC. Significant displacement of the thinnest area of the cornea from the center is also suggestive of KC. Corneas that are not thicker in the periphery compared to the center are suggestive of an ectatic disorder as well. Some clinicians obtain posterior float measurements to quantitate the extent of anterior bulging of the endothelial surface and use a measurement above 50–75 μm (using scanning-slit technology) as suggestive of KC. Excimer laser surgery, especially LASIK, when performed in patients with topographic features of KC, carries the risk of progressive corneal ectasia, which may be detrimental to visual outcomes after surgery.

Pellucid marginal degeneration

Pellucid marginal degeneration is an uncommon, nonhereditary, bilateral disease in which clear, inferior, peripheral corneal thinning is found in the absence of inflammation. Protrusion of the cornea occurs above the band of thinning. At times, a clear distinction between pellucid marginal degeneration and keratoconus is not possible. A cornea with keratoconus shows protrusion at the point of maximal thinning (typically in the inferior paracentral cornea), whereas one with pellucid marginal degeneration shows protrusion central to the area of maximum thinning, which is typically inferior but can be superior. No vascularization or lipid deposition occurs in pellucid marginal degeneration, but posterior stromal scarring has been noted within the thinned area. Decreased vision results from high regular and irregular astigmatism. Placido-based corneal topography classically demonstrates high against-the-rule astigmatism, with steepening nasally and temporally and circling inferiorly (see Fig 3-5). Corneal flattening is noted just inferior to the central cornea. Corneal refractive surgery should be avoided in this condition.

Post–penetrating keratoplasty

Corneal topography is very helpful in managing postoperative astigmatism following PKP. Complex peripheral patterns may result in a refractive axis of astigmatism that is not aligned with the topographic axis. It is important to remove all the sutures in the graft prior to performing refractive surgery, as the presence of sutures may affect the refractive error. It is also important to operate on the appropriate axis in this situation; otherwise, an unexpected result may occur. The appropriate axis depends on the type of surgery (incisional surgery is done on the steep axis; compression sutures and wedge resections are placed on the flat axis). In addition, after corneal transplantation, corneal topography may identify a component of irregular astigmatism. Wavefront- or topography-guided ablations may be considered in these eyes after all sutures have been removed and the refraction has stabilized, if a good wavefront map can be obtained.

Wavefront Analysis

The wave theory of light has one of its major applications in wavefront analysis. Currently, wavefront analysis can be performed clinically by 4 methods: Hartmann-Shack; Tscherning; thin-beam single ray tracing; and optical path difference, which combines retinoscopy with corneal topography. Each method results in a detailed report of lower- and higher-order aberrations (the latter are associated with irregular astigmatism). As discussed earlier, lower-order aberrations are sphere and cylinder, which can be corrected with glasses; higher-order aberrations cannot be corrected by sphere and cylinder. This information is useful in refractive surgery, both in aiding the calculation of custom ablations to enhance vision or correct optical problems and in explaining patients' visual symptoms.

Wavefront Analysis and Irregular Astigmatism

As discussed, irregular astigmatism is usually caused by irregularities of corneal shape resulting from such factors as keratoconus, refractive surgery, PKP, and scars following traumatic injury. Visually significant irregular astigmatism is a relatively uncommon problem typically associated with corneal grafts or scars and requiring a gas-permeable contact lens for visual rehabilitation. Spectacles do not correct irregular astigmatism. Conventional (non–wavefront-guided) refractive surgery treats lower-order aberrations (sphere and cylinder) but typically increases higher-order aberrations, depending on optical zone size. Wavefront-guided keratorefractive surgery also treats lower-order aberrations but tends to induce fewer higher-order aberrations and may, in principle, be able to treat preexisting optical aberrations. However, several obstacles need to be overcome before surgically induced optical aberration can be treated or prevented with high predictability.

Measurement of Wavefront Aberrations and Graphical Representations

Several techniques are available for measuring wavefront aberrations clinically, but the most popular is based on the Hartmann-Shack wavefront sensor. In this device, a low-power laser beam is focused on the retina. A point on the retina acts as a point source, and the reflected light is then propagated back through the optics of the eye. In a perfect eye, all the rays would emerge in parallel and the wavefront would be a flat plane. In reality, the wavefront is not flat. An array of lenses samples parts of the wavefront and focuses light on a detector (Fig 1-6). The wavefront shape can be determined from the position of the focus on each detector.

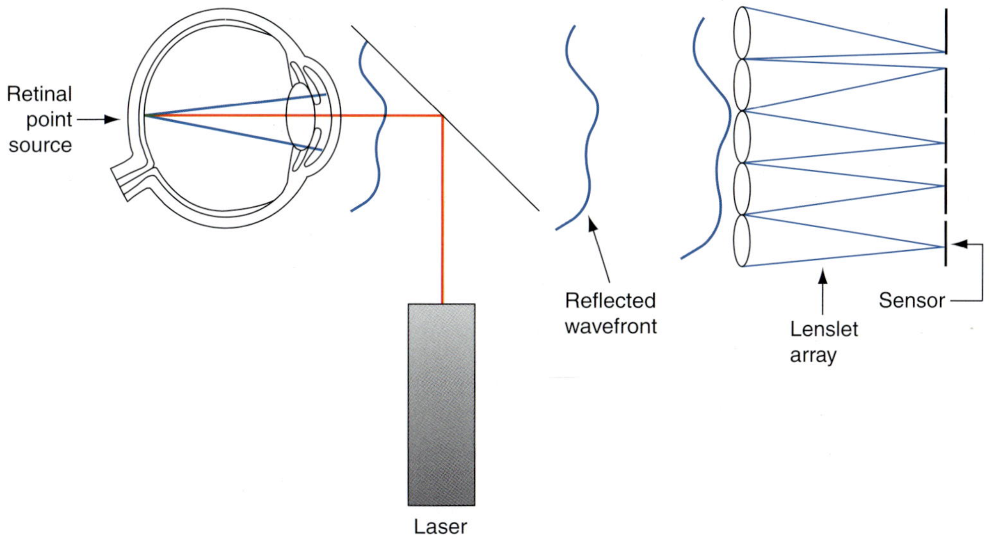

Figure 1-6 Schematic of a Hartmann-Shack wavefront sensor.

Wavefront aberrations can be represented in different ways. One approach is to represent the wavefront aberrations as 3-dimensional shapes. This is currently the approach most commonly adopted for refractive surgery. Two-dimensional contour plots may become more popular in the future. In both systems, optical aberrations can be resolved into a variety of basic shapes, the combination of which represents the total aberration of the system, just as conventional refractive error is a combination of sphere and cylinder.

Currently, wavefront aberrations are most commonly specified by Zernike polynomials, which are simply the mathematical formulas used to describe surfaces. The wavefront aberration surfaces are represented by 3-dimensional graphs generated using Zernike polynomials and mathematical graphing software. Each aberration, which may be positive or negative in value, can induce a predictable reduction in the quality of the image (such as that of a Snellen E chart). The magnitude of these aberrations is expressed as a root-mean-square (RMS) error, which is the deviation of the wavefront averaged over the entire wavefront. In a recent study that analyzed wavefront aberrometry data pooled from multiple studies looking at normal adult populations, mean total higher-order RMS was 0.33 μm for a 6.0-mm pupil. Most higher-order Zernike coefficients have mean values close to zero. The most prominent Zernike modes in this study were vertical coma, spherical aberration, and oblique trefoil, with mean absolute RMS values of 0.14, 0.13, and 0.11 μm (for a 6.0-mm pupil), respectively. At least 90% of normal eyes should have RMS values less than double these mean values.

Salmon TO, van de Pol C. Normal-eye Zernike coefficients and root-mean-square wavefront errors. *J Cataract Refract Surg.* 2006;32:2064–2074.

Fourier reconstruction is an alternative method of analyzing the output from an aberrometer. Fourier is a sine-wave-derived transformation of a complex shape. Compared with shapes derived from Zernike polynomial analysis, the shapes derived from Fourier analysis are more detailed, theoretically allowing for the measurement and treatment of more highly aberrated corneas.

Lower-Order Aberrations

Myopia, hyperopia, and regular astigmatism can be expressed as wavefront aberrations. Myopia produces an aberration that optical engineers call *positive defocus* (Fig 1-7); hyperopia, one called *negative defocus.* Regular (cylindrical) astigmatism produces a wavefront aberration that has orthogonal and oblique components (Fig 1-8). Defocus and astigmatism are second-order aberrations. Other lower-order aberrations are non–visually significant aberrations known as first-order aberrations, such as vertical and horizontal prisms (Fig 1-9), and zero-order aberrations (piston).

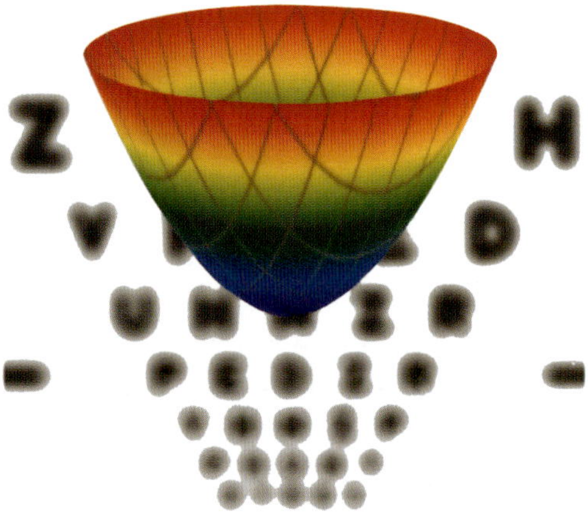

Figure 1-7 Zernike polynomial representation of defocus. *(Used with permission, Alcon Laboratories.)*

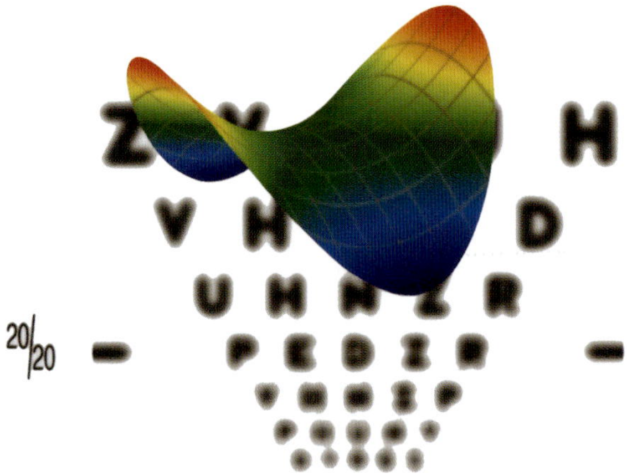

Figure 1-8 Representation of astigmatism using Zernike polynomials. *(Used with permission, Alcon Laboratories.)*

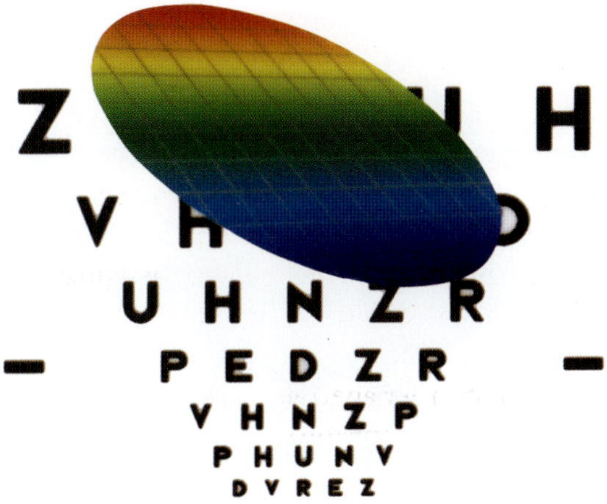

Figure 1-9 Representation of vertical prism using Zernike polynomials. *(Used with permission, Alcon Laboratories.)*

Higher-Order Aberrations

Wavefront aberration is a function of pupil size, with increased higher-order aberrations seen as the pupil dilates. Higher-order aberrations also increase with age, although the clinical effect is thought to be balanced by the increasing miosis of the pupil with age. Although lower-order aberrations decrease after laser vision correction, higher-order aberrations, particularly spherical aberration and coma, may increase after conventional PRK or LASIK for myopia. This increase is correlated with the degree of preoperative myopia. After standard hyperopic laser vision correction, higher-order aberrations increase even more than they do in myopic eyes but in the opposite (toward negative values) direction. Customized excimer laser treatments may decrease the number of induced higher-order aberrations compared with that induced by conventional treatments, thus providing a higher quality of vision, particularly in mesopic conditions.

Spherical aberrations

When peripheral light rays focus in front of more central rays, the effect is called *spherical aberration* (Fig 1-10). Clinically, this radially symmetric fourth-order aberration is the cause of night myopia and is commonly increased after myopic LASIK and PRK. It results in halos around point images. Spherical aberration is probably the most significant higher-order aberration. It may increase depth of field, but it is likely to decrease contrast sensitivity.

Coma and trefoil

A common aberration after refractive surgery is called *coma.* In this third-order aberration, rays at one edge of the pupil cross the finish line first, whereas rays at the opposite edge of the pupil cross the finish line last. The effect is that the image of each object point resembles a comet, having vertical and horizontal components (Fig 1-11). Coma is common in patients with decentered corneal grafts, keratoconus, and decentered laser ablations.

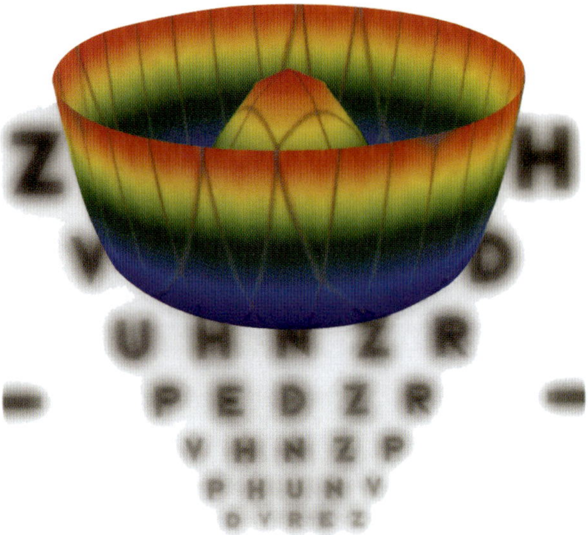

Figure 1-10 Zernike representation of spherical aberration. *(Used with permission, Alcon Laboratories.)*

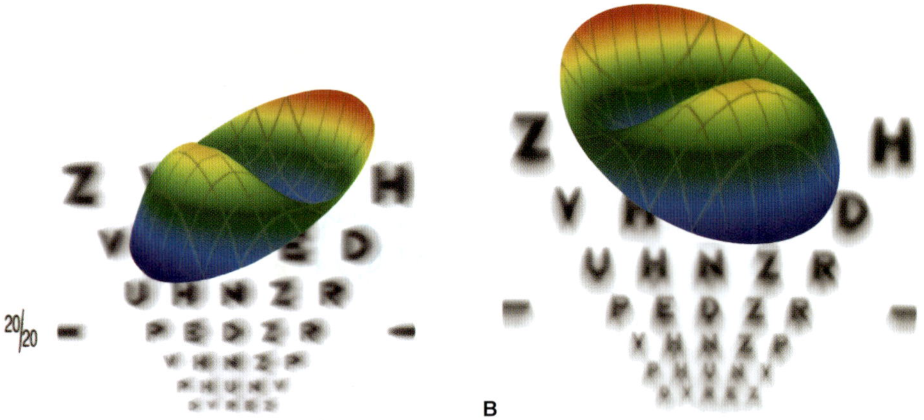

A B

Figure 1-11 Representation of horizontal coma **(A)** and vertical coma **(B)** using Zernike polynomials. *(Used with permission, Alcon Laboratories.)*

Trefoil is another third-order aberration seen after refractive surgery. It seems to be less detrimental to the quality of the image compared with coma of similar RMS magnitude (Fig 1-12).

Other higher-order aberrations

Optical engineers have found numerous basic types of aberrations, of which only a small number are of clinical interest. After refractive surgery, most patients have a combination of these aberrations. *Secondary astigmatism* (Fig 1-13) and *quadrafoil* (Fig 1-14) are forms of fourth-order aberration with dramatically different effects on vision. As knowledge of surgically induced aberration increases, more of the basic types of aberration may become clinically relevant.

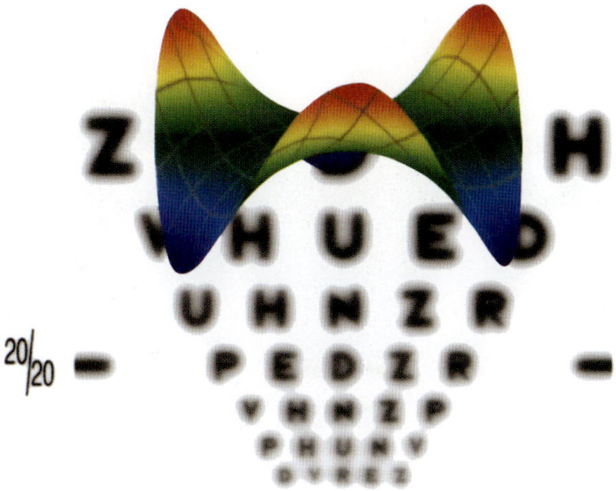

Figure 1-12 Zernike representation of trefoil. *(Used with permission, Alcon Laboratories.)*

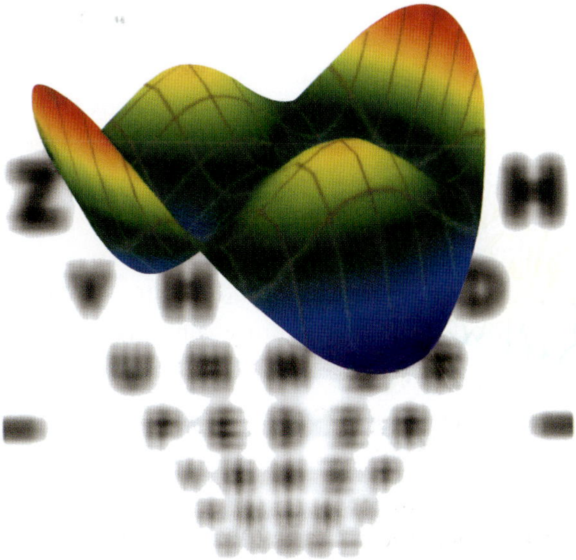

Figure 1-13 Zernike representation of secondary astigmatism. *(Used with permission, Alcon Laboratories.)*

Biomechanics of the Cornea

The cornea consists of collagen fibrils arranged in approximately 200 parallel lamellae that extend from limbus to limbus. The fibrils are oriented at angles to the fibrils in adjacent lamellae. This network of collagen is responsible for the mechanical strength of the cornea. The fibrils appear to be more closely packed in the axial, or prepupillary, cornea compared with the peripheral cornea.

When the cornea is in a dehydrated state, stress is distributed principally to the posterior layers or uniformly over the entire structure. When the cornea is healthy or edematous, the anterior lamellae take up the strain. There are differences in glycosaminoglycans

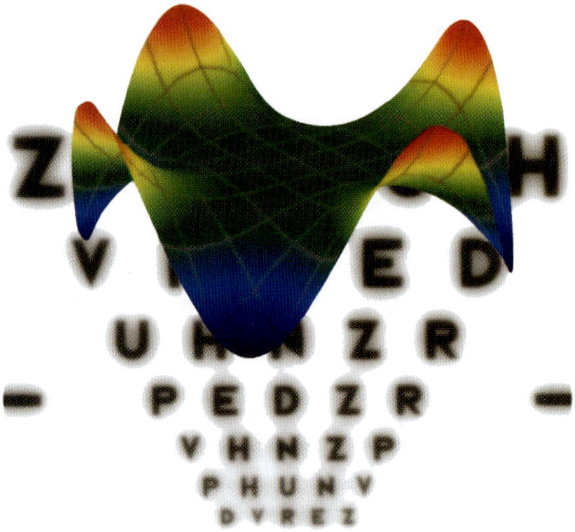

Figure 1-14 Zernike representation of quadrafoil. *(Used with permission, Alcon Laboratories.)*

between the anterior and posterior stroma, as well as more lamellar interweaving in the anterior corneal stroma, and thus the anterior cornea swells far less than the posterior cornea. Stress within the tissue is partly related to IOP but not in a linear manner under physiologic conditions (normal IOP range).

Effects of Keratorefractive Surgery

Corneal refractive procedures can be classified as lamellar, keratotomy, keratectomy, or collagen shrinkage (Table 1-1). These procedures can alter the corneal biomechanics in several ways:

- incisional effect
- tissue addition or subtraction
- alloplastic material addition
- laser effect
- collagen shrinkage

Incisional effect

Incisions perpendicular to the corneal surface predictably alter its shape, depending on direction, depth, location, and number (see Chapter 4). All incisions cause a local flattening of the cornea. Radial incisions lead to flattening in both the meridian of the incision and 90° away. Tangential (arcuate or linear) incisions (Fig 1-15) lead to flattening in the meridian of the incision and steepening in the meridian 90° away that may be equal to or less than the magnitude of the decrease in the primary meridian; this phenomenon is known as *coupling* (see Fig 4-5).

The closer that radial incisions approach the visual axis (ie, the smaller the optical zone), the greater their effect; similarly, the closer that tangential incisions are placed to the visual axis, the greater the effect. The longer a radial incision, the greater its effect until

Table 1-1 Classification of Corneal Refractive Surgery

Type of Refractive Surgery	Basic Surgical Technique	Variations of Surgical Technique or Material	Refractive Error Treated	Comment
Lamellar	Keratomileusis (cutting corneal disc with microkeratome)	*Microkeratome techniques:* • Manual or mechanical advance • Oscillating or femtosecond laser	Myopia, hyperopia, aphakia	
		Method of making refractive stromal cut: • Barraquer's cryolathe • Excimer laser (ArF, 193 nm)		Historical
		Source of tissue for disc: • Patient (autoplastic) • Donor (homoplastic)		
	Laser in situ keratomileusis	Excimer laser	Myopia, hyperopia, astigmatism, higher-order aberrations	FDA approved for −15.0 to +6.0 D; astigmatism to 6.0 D; most surgeons do not use for highest limits
	Epikeratoplasty	*Human donor lenticule:* • Cryolathe • Lyophilized Synthetic (eg, collagen and coated hydrogel)	Aphakia, hyperopia, astigmatism, myopia, keratoconus	Historical
	Intracorneal lens or ring	Microkeratome or femtosecond laser (lamellar bed) • Hydrogel lenticule	Myopia, hyperopia, presbyopia	Clinical trials for hyperopia and presbyopia
		Lamellar pocket • High index of refraction (eg, fenestration polysulfone)	Aphakia	
		Intracorneal ring segments	Myopia Keratoconus, ectasia	FDA approved for −1.0 to −3.0 D FDA approved for KC under HDE
Keratotomy	Radial	Nomogram-based Staged with repeated adjustments	Myopia	Rarely used
	Astigmatic (transverse keratotomy, arcuate keratotomy, limbal relaxing incisions)	Straight (T cuts)	Astigmatism: primary (naturally occurring); compound myopic astigmatism	Incision made in the steep corneal meridian (axis of plus refractive cylinder); rarely used

(Continued)

Table 1-1 *(continued)*

Type of Refractive Surgery	Basic Surgical Technique	Variations of Surgical Technique or Material	Refractive Error Treated	Comment
Keratotomy *(continued)*	Astigmatic *(continued)*	Modification of PKP (arcuate keratotomy)		Often staged under keratoscopic or keratometric control
		• Wound separation or incision in wound	Postoperative astigmatism	
		• Arcuate incision in donor		
	Astigmatic	Modification of cataract surgery • Intraoperative ☒ Limbal relaxing incision	Astigmatism	Limbal or corneal, cataract incision acts like arcuate keratotomy
Keratectomy	Laser	Photorefractive keratectomy, laser subepithelial keratomileusis, epi-LASIK • Excimer laser (ArF, 193 nm)	Myopia, astigmatism, hyperopia	FDA approved for −13.0 to +6.0 D; astigmatism to −4.0 D; most surgeons do not use for highest limits
		• Wavefront-guided	• Primary (naturally occurring)	
		• 5th harmonic Nd:YAG laser (213 nm)	• Secondary (eg, after radial keratotomy, epikeratoplasty, PKP)	
		Intrastromal photodisruption • Picosecond • Femtosecond	Myopia	In laboratory development
	Mechanical	Crescentic wedge • Wedge resection after PKP	Astigmatism	Limited use
Collagen shrinkage	Noncontact: holmium: YAG laser (2.06 μm)	Radial or circular pattern	Hyperopia, astigmatism	FDA approved for +0.75 to +2.5 D
		Treatment in flat meridian with or without concurrent treatment for hyperopia		Seldom used
	Contact	Peripheral, intrastromal, radial pattern	Hyperopia	Seldom used
	Conductive keratoplasty	Radiofrequency	Hyperopia, presbyopia	FDA approved for +0.75 to +3.25 D and for induction of myopia in presbyopic patients

For IOL implants, see BCSC Section 11, *Lens and Cataract*.

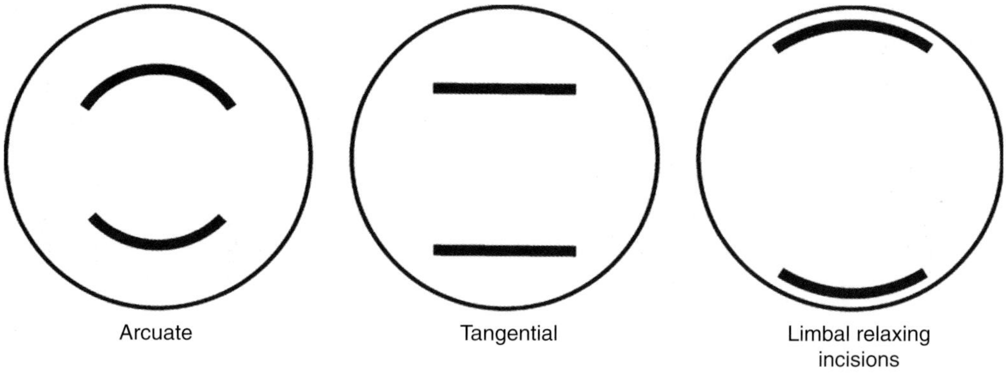

Figure 1-15 Astigmatic keratotomy. Flattening is induced in the axis of the incisions (at 90° in this case) and steepening is induced 90° away from the incisions (at 180° in this case). *(Illustration by C. H. Wooley.)*

approximately an 11-mm diameter is achieved, and then the effect reverses. The larger the angle severed by the tangential incision, the greater the effect.

For optimum effect, an incision should be 85%–90% deep to retain an intact posterior lamella and maximum anterior bowing of the other lamellae. Nomograms for numbers of incisions and optical zone size can be calculated based on finite element analysis, but they are typically generated empirically. The important variables for radial and astigmatic surgery include patient age and number, depth, and length of incisions. The same incision has greater effect in older patients than in younger patients. IOP and preoperative corneal curvature are not significant predictors of effect.

Tissue addition or subtraction

Lamellar surgery also alters the shape of the cornea. *Keratomileusis* was originated by Barraquer as "carving" of the anterior surface of the cornea. It is defined as a method of modifying the spherical or meridional surfaces of a healthy cornea by tissue subtraction. Tissue subtraction may be performed on the surface, by surface ablation (Fig 1-16), or intrastromally, by LASIK (Fig 1-17; see Chapter 6). The critical uncut depth of the cornea necessary to maintain normal integrity has not been determined, but most surgeons leave a minimum of 250 μm of residual stromal tissue (RST).

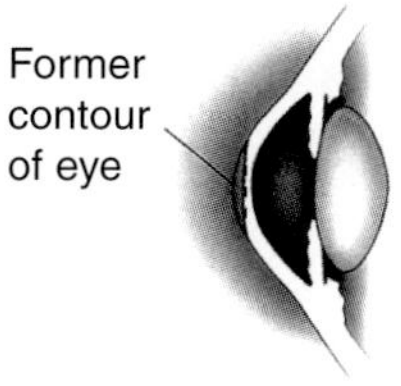

Figure 1-16 PRK for myopia.

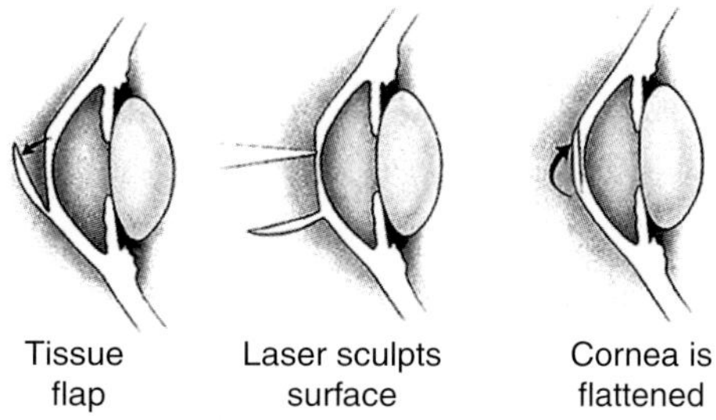

Figure 1-17 LASIK for myopia.

Epikeratoplasty (sometimes called *epikeratophakia*) adds carved donor tissue to the surface to cause hyperopic or myopic changes. *Keratophakia* requires the addition of a tissue lenticule or synthetic inlay intrastromally (see Chapter 5).

Alloplastic material addition

The shape of the cornea can be altered by adding alloplastic material such as hydrogel on the surface or into the corneal stroma to effect a change in the anterior shape or the refractive index of the cornea (Fig 1-18). For example, the 2 arc segments of an intrastromal corneal ring can be placed in 2 pockets of the stroma to directly alter the surface contour based on the profile of the individual rings (Fig 1-19).

Laser effect

In PRK, the depth of tissue that can be removed from the anterior surface is limited because of the possible complications of forward bowing and scarring. For low amounts of correction (<7 D), the amount of tissue to remove centrally is estimated by the Munnerlyn formula:

Ablation depth in micrometers (μm) ≈ diopters (D) of myopia multiplied by the square of the optical zone diameter (mm), divided by 3

Clinical experience has confirmed that the effective change is independent of the initial curvature of the cornea, although other proposed formulas take preoperative curvature into account. The Munnerlyn formula also highlights some of the problems and limitations

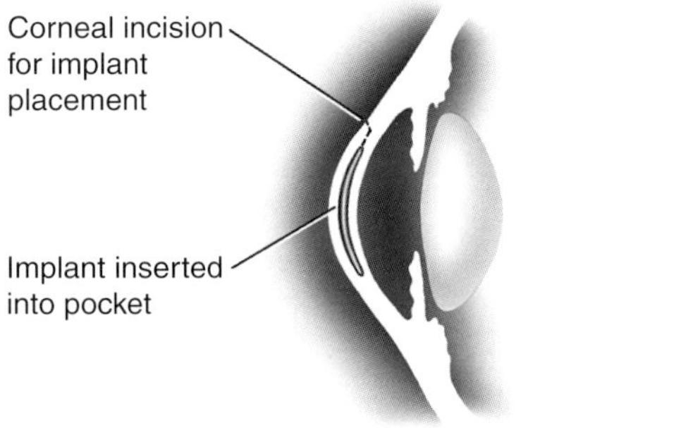

Figure 1-18 Intrastromal hydrogel implant. *(Illustration by Jeanne Koelling.)*

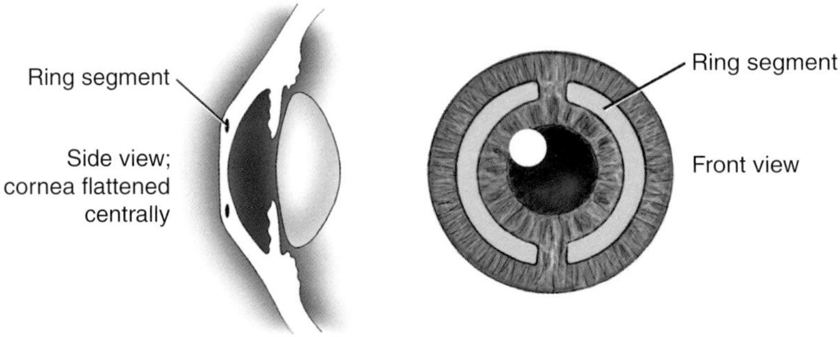

Figure 1-19 Intrastromal corneal ring segments. *(Illustration by Jeanne Koelling.)*

of laser vision correction. The amount of ablation increases by the square of the optical zone, but the complications of glare, halos, and regression increase when the optical zone decreases. To reduce these side effects, the optical zone should be 6 mm or larger.

Multizone keratectomies use several concentric optical zones to generate the total refraction required. This method can provide the full correction centrally, while the tapering peripheral zones reduce symptoms and allow higher degrees of myopia to be treated. For example, 12.00 D of myopia can be treated as follows: 6.00 D are corrected with a 4.5-mm optical zone, 3.00 D with a 5.5-mm optical zone, and 3.00 D with a 6.5-mm optical zone (Fig 1-20). Thus, the total 12.00 D correction is achieved in the center using a shallower ablation depth than would be necessary for a single pass (103 μm instead of 169 μm). Similarly, *bitoric ablations* (combining a myopic with a hyperopic ablation profile) can minimize ablation depth and provide a more physiologic postoperative topography.

LASIK combines a lamellar incision with ablation of the cornea, typically in the stromal bed (see Fig 1-16). The same theoretical limits for residual posterior cornea apply as with PRK, and the calculated effect is based on an empiric modification of the Munnerlyn formula. To reduce the complications of surface irregular astigmatism, the flap is typically cut 100–180 μm thick. The thickness and diameter of the LASIK flap depend on instrumentation, corneal diameter, corneal curvature, and corneal thickness.

Myopic treatments remove central corneal tissue, whereas hyperopic treatments steepen the cornea by removing a doughnut-shaped piece of midperipheral tissue. Hyperopic surface ablation and LASIK use a similar formula for determining the maximum ablation depth, but the ablation zone for hyperopia is much larger than the optical zone (Fig 1-21). The zone of maximal ablation coincides with the outer edge of the optical zone.

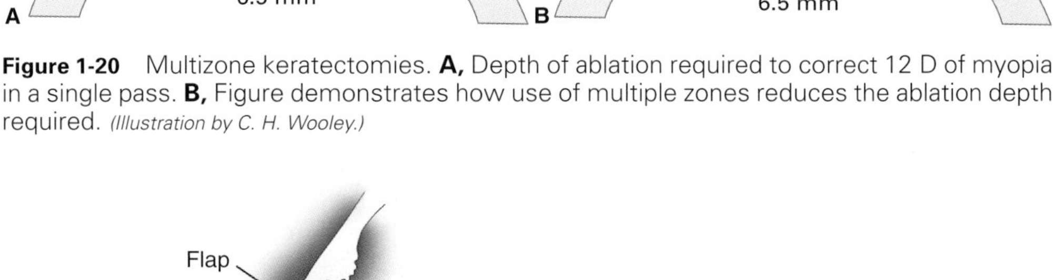

Figure 1-20 Multizone keratectomies. **A,** Depth of ablation required to correct 12 D of myopia in a single pass. **B,** Figure demonstrates how use of multiple zones reduces the ablation depth required. *(Illustration by C. H. Wooley.)*

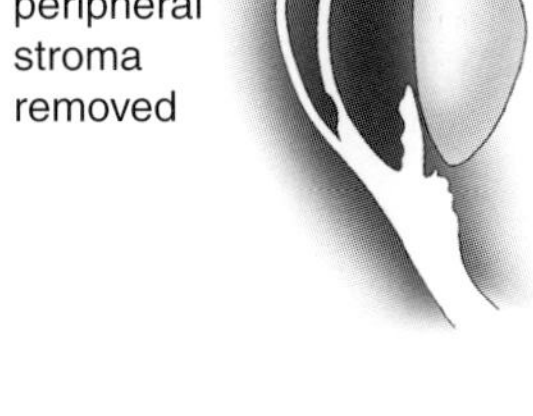

Figure 1-21 Hyperopic LASIK. *(Illustration by Jeanne Koelling.)*

A transition zone of ablated cornea is necessary to blend the edge of the optical zone to the peripheral cornea (Fig 1-22).

Care must be taken to ensure that adequate stromal tissue remains after ablation and creation of the LASIK flap. The historical standard has been to leave a minimum of 250 μm of tissue in the stromal bed. The exact amount of remaining tissue required to ensure biomechanical stability is not known and likely varies among individuals.

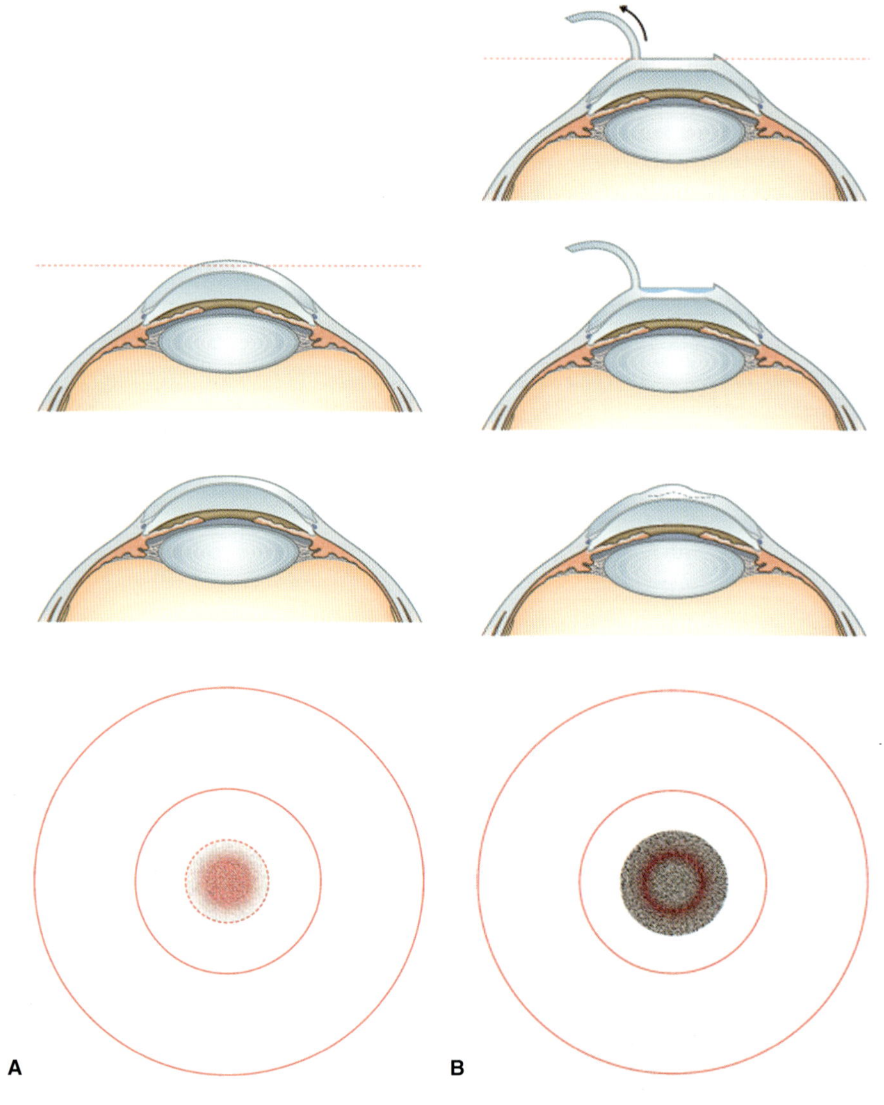

Figure 1-22 Ablation patterns. **A,** Myopic pattern (PRK). **B,** Hyperopic pattern (LASIK). *(Reproduced with permission from Azar DT, Damien G, Thanh Hoang-Xuan II, eds.* Refractive Surgery. *2nd ed. Philadelphia: Elsevier; 2007.)*

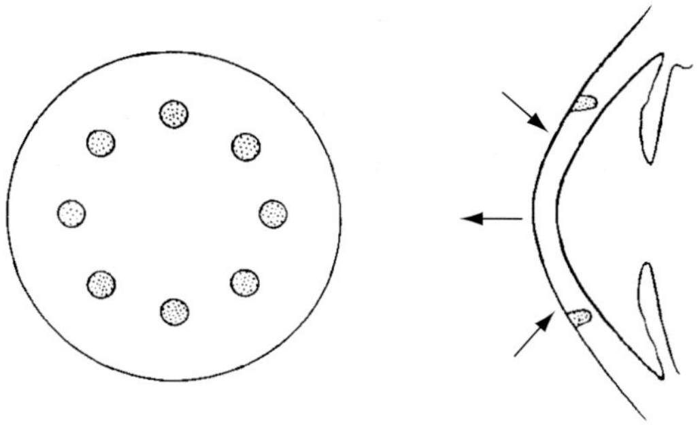

Figure 1-23 Thermokeratoplasty and CK: heat shrinks the peripheral cornea, causing central steepening.

Collagen shrinkage

Alteration in corneal biomechanics can also be achieved by collagen shrinkage. Heating collagen to a critical temperature of 55°–60°C causes it to shrink, inducing changes in the corneal curvature. *Thermokeratoplasty* and *conductive keratoplasty* are avoided in the central cornea because of scarring but can be used in the midperiphery (Fig 1-23; see Chapter 7). Corneal collagen can be heated with a holmium laser (noncontact) in thermokeratoplasty (although this technique is not commonly used) or with a radiofrequency diathermy probe inserted in the cornea (contact) in CK (Refractec, Bloomington, MN).

If the temperature is too high, local necrosis will occur, and if the source of heat is nonuniform or nonuniformly applied, irregular astigmatism will be induced.

Corneal Wound Healing

All forms of keratorefractive surgery are exquisitely dependent on the process of corneal wound healing. Satisfactory results after refractive surgery require either modifying or reducing wound healing or exploiting normal wound healing for the benefit of the patient. For example, astigmatic keratotomy requires initial weakening of the cornea followed by permanent corneal healing, with replacement of the epithelial plugs with collagen and remodeling of the collagen to ensure stability and avoid long-term hyperopic drift. PRK requires the epithelium to heal quickly, with minimal stimulation of the underlying keratocytes, to avoid corneal scarring and haze. Lamellar keratoplasty requires intact epithelium and healthy endothelium early in the postoperative period to seal the flap; later, the cornea must heal in the periphery to secure the flap in place and avoid late-term displacement while minimizing irregular astigmatism.

Our understanding of corneal wound healing has advanced tremendously with recognition of the multiple factors involved in the cascade of events initiated by corneal wounding. The cascade is somewhat dependent on the nature of the injury. Injury to the epithelium can lead to loss of underlying keratocytes from apoptosis. The remaining keratocytes respond by generating new glycosaminoglycans and collagen, to a degree dependent on the duration of the epithelial defect and the depth of the stromal injury. Corneal haze is localized in the subepithelial anterior stroma and may last for several years after surface ablation. Clinically significant haze, however, is present only in a small percentage of eyes. The tendency toward haze formation is greater with deeper ablations, surface irregularity, and prolonged absence of the epithelium. Despite loss of Bowman's layer, normal or even enhanced numbers of hemidesmosomes and anchoring fibrils form to secure the epithelium to the stroma.

Controversy persists over the value of different agents for modulating wound healing in surface ablation. Typically, clinicians in the United States use corticosteroids in a tapering manner following surgery to reduce inflammation. Other anti-inflammatory agents have also been tried, with no established effect. Mitomycin C has been applied to the stromal bed after excimer ablation to attempt to decrease haze formation (see Chapter 6). It has been proposed that vitamin C may play a role in protecting the cornea from ultraviolet light damage by the excimer laser, but a randomized, prospective clinical trial has not yet been performed. A number of growth factors that have been found to promote wound healing after PRK, including transforming growth factor β, may be useful in the future.

With the LASEK technique, the corneal epithelial basement membrane is cleaved between the lamina lucida and the lamina densa. Although several studies have shown faster visual rehabilitation, decreased pain, and decreased haze after LASEK compared with PRK, other studies have demonstrated the opposite effect. Theoretically, by maintaining initial epithelial integrity with LASEK, the activation of abnormal stromal wound healing should be reduced. In animal studies, there appear to be fewer apoptotic cells adjacent to the ablated stroma after LASEK, particularly in the setting of higher attempted corrections. Because alcohol exposure may cause necrosis of the epithelial cells, however, it is critical to limit alcohol exposure time to minimize toxicity.

Published information comparing epi-LASIK to PRK and LASEK is scarce. In epi-LASIK, the epithelium is lifted from the stroma with a mechanical blunt separator. The basement membrane is intact, with the plane of separation between the basement membrane and Bowman's layer. Because no alcohol is used and the epithelium is better preserved anatomically, the epithelial sheet consists of a greater percentage of cells that are viable in the short term. Although the epithelium regenerates in several days (similar to LASEK), it is thought to block some of the inflammatory pathways in the stroma that lead to apoptosis and myofibroblast transformation.

Haze formation does not seem to occur in the central flap interface following LASIK, which may be related either to lack of significant epithelial injury and consequent subcellular signaling or to maintenance of some intact surface neurons. LASIK shows very little long-term evidence of healing between the disrupted lamellae and only typical stromal healing at the peripheral wound. The lamellae are initially held in position by negative stromal pressure generated by the endothelial cells aided by an intact epithelial surface. Even after years, the lamellar interface can be broken and the flap lifted, indicating that only a minimal amount of healing occurs.

Aberrant healing can occur if the flap is placed with wrinkles (striae) or if epithelium grows into the interface (epithelial ingrowth). Epithelium in the interface acts as a barrier to nutrient flow and should be removed at any sign of thinning, inflammation, or obstruction of the visual axis. Interface debris can lead to inflammation or light scattering and should be minimized at the time of surgery.

Laser Biophysics

Laser–Tissue Interactions

Three laser–tissue interactions are exploited for keratorefractive surgery. *Photothermal* effects are achieved by focusing a holmium:YAG laser with a wavelength of 2.13 μm into the anterior stroma. The laser beam is absorbed by water, causing collagen shrinkage from heat. This technique is approved by the FDA for treating low hyperopia.

The femtosecond laser is approved by the FDA for creating corneal flaps for LASIK and may be used for lamellar or PKP. It uses a 1053-nm infrared beam that creates *photodisruption,* a process by which tissue is transformed into plasma, and high pressure and temperature create rapid tissue expansion, leading to microscopic cavities within the corneal stroma. Contiguous photodisruption allows for creation of the corneal flap or keratoplasty incision.

Photoablation, the most important laser–tissue interaction in refractive surgery, breaks chemical bonds using excimer (for "*exc*ited d*imer*") lasers or other lasers of the appropriate wavelength. Laser energy of more than 4 eV per photon is sufficient to break carbon–nitrogen or carbon–carbon tissue bonds. Argon-fluoride (ArF) lasers are excimer lasers that use electrical energy to stimulate argon to form dimers with the caustic fluorine gas. They generate a wavelength of 193 nm with 6.4 eV per photon. The 193-nm light is in the ultraviolet C (high ultraviolet) range, approaching the wavelength of x-rays. In addition to having high energy per photon, light at this end of the electromagnetic spectrum also has very low tissue penetrance and thus is suitable for operating on the surface of tissue. Not only is the laser energy capable of great precision, with little thermal spread in tissue, but its lack of penetrance or lethality to cells makes the 193-nm laser nonmutagenic, enhancing its safety. (DNA mutagenicity occurs in the range of 250 nm.) Solid-state lasers have been designed to generate wavelengths of light near 193 nm without the need for toxic gas, but the technical difficulties in manufacturing these lasers have limited their clinical use.

Types of Photoablating Lasers

Photoablating lasers can be divided into broad-beam lasers, scanning-slit lasers, and flying-spot lasers. *Broad-beam lasers* have larger-diameter beams and slower repetition rates and rely on optics or mirrors to create a smooth and homogeneous multimode laser beam of up to approximately 7 mm in diameter. These lasers have very high energy per pulse and require a small number of pulses to ablate the cornea. *Scanning-slit lasers* use excimer technology to generate a narrower slit beam that is scanned over the surface of the tissue to alter the photoablation profile, improving the smoothness of the ablated cornea and allowing for larger-diameter ablation zones. *Flying-spot lasers* use smaller-diameter beams (0.5–2.0 mm) that are scanned at a higher repetition rate, but to create the desired pattern of ablation, a tracking mechanism is required for precise placement. Broad-beam lasers and some scanning-slit lasers require a mechanical iris diaphragm or ablatable mask to create the desired shape in the cornea. The flying-spot lasers and some of the scanning-slit lasers use the pattern projected onto the surface to create the desired laser ablation profile without masking.

Wavefront-Optimized and Wavefront-Guided Laser Ablations

In the past, conventional treatments used laser profiles with smaller blend zones and created a more oblate corneal shape postoperatively, with induced higher-order aberrations, especially spherical aberration and coma. Wavefront-optimized laser ablations try to preserve the prolate shape of the cornea by increasing the number of peripheral pulses, which often results in better quality vision and fewer night vision complaints. This method also compensates for the decreased effect of the conventional laser in the periphery of the cornea due to the angle of the beam. As in conventional procedures, the refraction is used to program the wavefront-optimized laser ablation. This technology does not attempt to address preexisting higher-order aberrations but rather to minimize induction of spherical aberration caused by the laser ablation itself. It has the advantage of being quicker than wavefront-guided technology and avoids the additional expense of the aberrometer. There are currently few published studies comparing wavefront-optimized results with conventional or wavefront-guided laser results.

In wavefront-guided laser ablations, information obtained from a wavefront-sensing aberrometer (which quantifies the aberrations) is transferred electronically to the treatment laser to program the laser ablation. This is distinct from conventional excimer laser and wavefront-optimized laser treatments, where the subjective refraction is used to program the laser ablation. The wavefront-guided laser attempts to treat both lower-order (myopia or hyperopia and/or astigmatism) and higher-order aberrations.

Wavefront-guided lasers apply complex ablation patterns to the cornea to correct wavefront deviations from a desired final corneal shape. The correction of higher-order aberrations requires non–radially symmetric patterns of ablation (which are often much smaller in magnitude than ablations needed to correct defocus and astigmatism). Based on the difference between the desired and the actual wavefront, a 3-dimensional map of the ablation is generated. To match the intended ablation pattern with that which is ultimately delivered to the cornea, registration must be achieved using either marks at the limbus prior to obtaining the wavefront patterns or iris registration, which matches reference points in the natural iris pattern to compensate for cyclotorsion and pupil centroid shift. The wavefront-guided laser then uses a pupil-tracking system, which helps to maintain centration during treatment and allows the accurate delivery of the customized ablation profile.

The results of wavefront-guided ablations for low and moderate myopia are excellent, with well over 90% of eyes achieving 20/40 or better UCVA. Early results for wavefront-guided hyperopic and astigmatic corrections appear promising as well. Only a few published papers in the literature compare this technology to conventional treatments, however, and these do not show clear-cut superiority when the conventional procedures are performed with modern technology, including larger ablation zones, pupil-tracking systems, and anatomical registration. In general, fewer induced higher-order aberrations are found in eyes treated with wavefront technology compared with those treated with conventional treatments (although there is an increase postoperatively in both groups), but Snellen visual acuity parameters are similar. For enhancements, however, early results indicate that customized treatments appear to be better than conventional re-treatments. Investigations are ongoing in comparing wavefront-guided technology platforms and determining what constitutes the ideal optical correction.

Krueger RR, Applegate RA, MacRae SM, eds. *Wavefront Customized Visual Corrections: The Quest for Super Vision.* 2nd ed. Thorofare, NJ: Slack; 2004.

Netto MV, Dupps W, Wilson SE. Wavefront-guided ablation: evidence for efficacy compared to traditional ablation. *Am J Ophthalmol.* 2006;141:360–368.

CHAPTER 2

The Role of the FDA in Refractive Surgery

The field of refractive surgery is uniquely dependent on rapidly changing technology that dictates surgical technique. Many of the investigational devices discussed in the following chapters will receive Food and Drug Administration (FDA) approval by the time this book is published. Other "promising" devices or techniques may have already fallen out of favor.

Because of the continual introduction of new devices to the US market, the FDA approval process has particular influence in refractive surgery. Therefore, we have included this brief introduction to the FDA approval process. Table 2-1 gives a list of FDA-approved lasers for refractive surgery as of January 2007. The most current list can be found on the Web at www.fda.gov/cdrh/LASIK/lasers.htm.

The FDA

The scope of the FDA's work is established by legislation. The Food, Drug, and Cosmetic Act, passed by Congress in 1938, required for the first time that companies prove the safety of new drugs before placing them on the market and required regulation of cosmetics and therapeutic devices. The Medical Device Amendments of 1976 authorized the FDA to ensure that medical devices are safe and effective before they come to market in the United States. This amendment also provided for classification of medical devices into 3 categories, depending on potential risk of the device; established 3 pathways to market; and established advisory panels to assist the FDA in the review of devices. The Ophthalmic Devices Panel, for example, evaluates and advises on marketing and device applications for ophthalmic devices (see discussion later in the chapter).

Device Classification

All manufacturers of medical devices distributed in the United States must comply with basic regulations, or general controls. These include

- establishment (company) registration
- medical device listing
- quality systems regulation
- labeling requirements
- medical device reporting (of problems)

Table 2-1 FDA-Approved Lasers for Refractive Surgery

FDA-Approved Lasers for LASIK (from January 1, 2000, to January 25, 2007)		
Company and Model	**Approval Number and Date**	**Approved Indications (D = diopters)**
Alcon—LADARVision	P970043/S5; 5/9/00	Myopia ≤9.00 with or without astigmatism from –0.50 to –3.00 D
Alcon—LADARVision	P970043/S7; 9/22/00	Hyperopia <6.00 D with or without astigmatism ≤6.00 D
Alcon—LADARVision	P970043/S10; 10/18/02	Wavefront-guided LASIK: Myopia up to –7.00 D with or without astigmatism <0.50 D
Alcon—LADARVision	P970043/S15; 6/29/04	Wavefront-guided LASIK: Myopic astigmatism from –0.50 to –4.00 D
Bausch & Lomb Surgical—Technolas 217a	P990027; 2/23/00	Myopia from –1.00 to –7.00 D with or without astigmatism ≤3.00 D
Bausch & Lomb Surgical—Technolas 217a	P990027/S2; 5/15/02	Myopia ≤11.00 D with or without astigmatism ≤3.00 D
Bausch & Lomb Surgical—Technolas 217a	P990027/S4; 2/25/03	Hyperopia between 1.00 and 4.00 D with or without astigmatism up to 2.00 D
Bausch & Lomb Surgical—Technolas 217z	P990027/S6; 10/10/03	Wavefront-guided LASIK: Myopia up to –7.00 D with or without astigmatism up to –3.00 D
LaserSight—LaserScan LSX	P980008/S5; 9/28/01	Myopia from –0.50 to –6.00 D with or without astigmatism up to 4.50 D
Nidek—EC5000	P970053/S2; 4/14/00	Myopia from –1.00 to –14.00 D with or without astigmatism <4.00 D
Nidek—EC5000	P970053/S009; 10/11/06	Hyperopia from +0.50 to +5.00 D of sphere with or without astigmatic refractive errors from +0.50 to +2.00 D
VISX—Star S2 & S3	P930016/S12; 4/27/01	Hyperopia between 0.50 and 5.00 D with or without astigmatism up to 3.00 D
VISX—Star S2 & S3	P930016/S14; 11/16/01	Mixed astigmatism up to 6.00 D; cylinder is greater than sphere and of opposite sign
VISX—Star S3 (EyeTracker)	P990010/S1; 4/20/00	Same as S2, but w/eye tracker
VISX—Star S4 & WaveScan Wavefront System	P930016/S16; 5/23/03	Wavefront-guided LASIK: Myopia up to –6.00 D with or without astigmatism up to –3.00 D

(Continued)

Table 2-1 *(continued)*

Company and Model	Approval Number and Date	Approved Indications (D = diopters)
FDA-Approved Lasers for LASIK (from January 1, 2000, to January 25, 2007)		
VISX—Star S4 & WaveScan Wavefront System	P930016/S17; 12/14/04	Wavefront-guided LASIK: Hyperopia up to 3.00 D with or without astigmatism up to 2.00 D
VISX—Star S4 & WaveScan Wavefront System	P930016/S20; 3/17/05	Mixed astigmatism 1.00 to 5.00 D
VISX—Star S4 & WaveScan Wavefront System	P930016/S21; 8/30/05	Myopia 6.00 to 11.00 D with or without astigmatism up to –3.00 D
WaveLight—ALLEGRETTO WAVE	P020050; 10/07/03	Myopia up to –12.00 D with or without astigmatism up to –6.00 D
WaveLight—ALLEGRETTO WAVE	P030008; 10/10/03	Hyperopia up to 6.00 D with or without astigmatism up to 5.00 D
WaveLight—ALLEGRETTO WAVE	P020050/S004; 7/26/06	Myopia up to –7.00 D with or without astigmatism up to 3.00 D
Carl Zeiss—MEL 80	P060004; 8/11/06	Myopia up to –7.00 D, with or without astigmatism up to –3.00 D
FDA-Approved Lasers for PRK and Other Refractive Surgeries (from January 1, 2000, to January 25, 2007)		
Refractec—ViewPoint CK System	P010018; 4/11/02	Conductive keratoplasty; hyperopia from +0.75 to +3.25 D with or without astigmatism up to 0.75 D
Refractec—ViewPoint CK System	P010018/S5; 3/16/04	Conductive keratoplasty; monovision in patients with presbyopia with or without hyperopia
VISX—Star S2 & S3	P930016/S10; 10/18/00	PRK; hyperopia from 0.50 to 5.00 D with or without astigmatism 0.50 to 4.00 D
VISX—Star S2 & S3	P930016/S13; 3/19/01	Add myopia blend zone; increase overall ablation zone from 6.50 to 8.00 mm
VISX—Star S3	H000002; 12/19/01	Treatment of certain patients with symptomatic decentered ablations from previous laser surgery

In addition, devices are classified into 1 of 3 regulatory control groups (I, II, III). This classification of medical devices identifies any regulatory control specific to the class that is necessary to ensure the safety and effectiveness of a device.

Class I devices (eg, refractometers, perimeters, sunglasses, visual acuity charts) are usually considered minimal-risk devices. Although these devices are subject to general controls, most of them are exempt from premarket review by the FDA. With few exceptions, manufacturers can go directly to market with a class I device.

Class II devices (eg, phacoemulsification units, tonometers, vitrectomy machines, daily-wear contact lenses) are usually considered moderate-risk devices. Class II devices are those for which general controls alone are insufficient to ensure safety and effectiveness and for which methods exist to provide such assurances. These devices, in addition to general controls, are subject to special controls, which may include special labeling requirements, mandatory performance standards, and postmarket surveillance. With few exceptions, class II devices require premarket review by the FDA.

Class III devices (eg, excimer lasers, intraocular lenses, extended-wear contact lenses, intraocular fluids) are considered significant-risk devices that present a potential unreasonable risk of illness or injury. Class III devices are those for which insufficient information exists to ensure safety and effectiveness solely through general or special controls. Class III devices cannot be marketed in the United States until the FDA determines that there is a reasonable assurance of safety and effectiveness when used according to the approved indications for use. Most class III devices come to market through the *premarket approval (PMA)* process and require an extensive review by the FDA before approval is granted for marketing.

Collection of Clinical Data for an Unapproved Device

For all class III devices and many class II devices, clinical performance data are required to be included in the regulatory marketing submissions. An *investigational device exemption (IDE)* allows the investigational device to be shipped and used in a clinical trial to collect the safety and effectiveness data required to support an application to the FDA requesting clearance to market. The FDA has 30 days to review and grant approval of an IDE application. Applications containing deficiencies in such areas as bench testing, study design, or informed consent documents are denied or conditionally approved. The sponsor may begin enrollment and treatment of subjects for IDE applications that are conditionally approved, but the sponsor must respond to the deficiencies within 45 days of the date of the conditional approval letter. During the IDE process, the sponsor often meets with the FDA to discuss the details of the clinical trial in order to facilitate effective data collection for eventual review.

Pathways to Market

Premarket Notification 510(k)

Manufacturers of class I and class II devices that are not otherwise exempt from premarket review must submit a *premarket notification,* commonly referred to as a *510(k) application,* to the FDA before going to market. In the 510(k) application, a manufacturer must demonstrate that its device is substantially equivalent to a legally marketed device (commonly referred to as the "predicate device") of the same type and for the same intended use. The FDA must make its determination of substantial equivalence within 90 days. If a device is not found to be substantially equivalent, it is placed into class III, or alternatively, if the device is not of high risk, the sponsor may submit a de novo request stating that the device defines a new 510(k) device regulatory classification.

Humanitarian Device Exemption

Devices marketed under a *humanitarian device exemption (HDE)* are intended to treat or diagnose diseases or conditions that affect or are manifested in fewer than 4000 individuals per year in the United States. The sponsor is required to provide an HDE application to the FDA containing a reasonable assurance of safety. Efficacy information is limited to a demonstration of "probable benefits to health" rather than the higher standard of "reasonable assurance of effectiveness," as would be required for a PMA. These devices must be used in a facility with an institutional review board (IRB). The FDA has 75 days to review and make a decision on an HDE application.

Premarket Approval

The PMA process is the primary pathway to market for class III devices. Clinical data from the IDE study, along with manufacturing information, preclinical bench testing, animal data (if needed), and labeling, are submitted to the FDA as a PMA application. The FDA must decide within 180 days whether the information submitted in the application demonstrates the safety and effectiveness of the device in question. The time for making the decision is extended when the application lacks the required information or contains information that is incomplete or insufficient.

Ophthalmic Devices Panel

The Ophthalmic Devices Panel consists of 6 voting members, the Chair (who votes in case of a tie), 1 nonvoting consumer representative, and 1 nonvoting industry representative. The panel includes ophthalmologists as well as other experts, such as vision scientists, biostatisticians, and optometrists. Consultants are included on the panel as the need for their expertise dictates. All panel members are considered "special government employees" and are subject to the conflict-of-interest rules and ethics requirements for government employees.

The Ophthalmic Devices Panel meets in open public session to evaluate and advise on marketing applications for first-of-a-kind devices and for previously approved devices for which a firm is seeking a new indication for use, as well as on device applications that raise significant issues of safety and effectiveness. The panel also provides clinical input in the development of FDA and industry guidelines for the study of new devices.

During a panel meeting scheduled to review a specific device, panel deliberations focus on the clinical study data and the proposed physician and patient labeling (if applicable). After deliberation, the panel members must determine their recommendation regarding whether the information in the PMA application demonstrates a reasonable assurance of safety and effectiveness. At the conclusion of the meeting, the panel votes on its recommendation. However, because the committee is advisory in nature, the FDA is not bound to follow its recommendation.

Labeling

The sponsor defines the inclusion and exclusion criteria for the clinical trial. Prior to approval, the FDA reviews and makes recommendations for changes in the device labeling using the data from the population studied. For example, if dry eyes are an exclusion criteria for the PMA study, there will be no data on subjects with dry eyes. Consequently, the device is not approved in this subset of patients, and the labeling will indicate that dry eyes are an exclusion criteria. This does not mean that the device is contraindicated in dry-eye patients but that the safety and effectiveness of the device cannot be evaluated in this population because there are no data. Some exclusion criteria may be contraindications to treatment. For example, keratoconus could be an exclusion criterion as well as a contraindication to laser in situ keratomileusis (LASIK).

The clinical trial is performed for a limited range of refractive errors. Safety and effectiveness data guide the range of refractive error that is approved for use in the PMA labeling.

If a treating clinician does not follow the labeling recommendations for the device, he or she is using the device "off-label." Some off-label uses reflect the PMA's lack of data on safety and effectiveness—for example, use of the device in a patient listed within the exclusion criteria; other off-label uses reflect decreased or unknown safety or effectiveness—for example, use of the device beyond the refractive range of the labeling. Any modifications to the device to enable an off-label use, such as the addition of unapproved software, adulterates the device and causes it to be unapproved.

In the United States, ophthalmologists very commonly use devices off-label because the FDA does not control the practice of medicine. In some cases, off-label use has actually become the standard of care. For example, topical fluoroquinolones are FDA approved to treat bacterial conjunctivitis; however, these medications are commonly used to treat corneal ulcers as well, even though they are not FDA approved for this indication. Consequently, although use of fluoroquinolones for corneal ulcer treatment may be off-label, in some situations it may also be the community standard of care.

Conversely, use of an FDA-approved device in an off-label fashion that deviates from the community standard of care may place an ophthalmologist at increased risk of legal scrutiny, particularly if there is a poor result. In such a situation, the physician should seriously consider both informing the patient and having the patient sign an ancillary consent form.

Delays in FDA Approval

At times, deficiencies in the clinical trials of a PMA application may delay its presentation to the Ophthalmic Devices Panel. Sometimes a PMA application may be recommended for approval by the panel, but the manufacturer must wait for final FDA approval before marketing. Usually, a panel recommendation for approval is granted with conditions that must be met before final FDA approval is granted. For example, the panel may request that data obtained on study subjects with certain ophthalmic characteristics be submitted to the FDA to determine if visual results in this subset of patients demonstrate efficacy.

When delays occur, the public naturally wants to know why. The FDA and the Ophthalmic Devices Panel are legally bound to keep the result of the PMA application process confidential and are prohibited by law from revealing any information about the PMA, favorable or unfavorable. However, the company is not bound by these same rules and is not restricted in what it chooses to tell the public. The company's dissemination of information about the PMA often has financial motivation because such information may affect the company's stock price and the public's perception of the product. The FDA does not comment on statements made by the company; however, this does not indicate an FDA endorsement of any statement by the company. Even if a company releases incorrect or misleading information about the reasons for delay in FDA approval, the FDA is still prohibited from discussing details of the PMA application, which could include evidence contrary to statements made by the company. Only in the public sessions of the Ophthalmic Devices Panel is information about the PMA process legally allowed to be released to the public before a final decision on the application is made by the FDA. All other deliberations regarding the application, before and after the panel meeting, remain subject to FDA confidentiality rules. Consequently, before the FDA reaches its decision, the panel meeting is the best forum for the public to actually observe the true data from the PMA clinical trial. The executive summary minutes and a complete transcript of the panel meetings are placed on the FDA public website once the chair approves the minutes.

Reporting of Medical Device–Related Adverse Events

The FDA's involvement in medical devices is not limited to the premarket process. The FDA monitors postmarket reports of device-related adverse events (AEs), or product problems, through both voluntary and mandatory reporting. This monitoring is done to detect "signals" of potential public health safety issues.

Since 1984, device manufacturers and importers have been required to report device-related deaths, serious injuries, and malfunctions to the FDA. User facilities (hospitals, nursing homes, ambulatory surgical facilities, outpatient diagnostic and treatment facilities, ambulance services, and health care entities) are required to report deaths to the FDA and deaths and serious injuries to the manufacturer.

Voluntary reporting to the FDA of device-related problems is a critical professional and public health responsibility. Currently, voluntary reporting takes place under MedWatch, an FDA product-reporting program. MedWatch allows health care professionals and consumers to report serious problems that they suspect are associated with the medical devices they prescribe, dispense, or use. Reporting can be done online at www.fda.gov/medwatch/getforms.htm, by phone (1-800-FDA-1088), or by submitting the MedWatch 3500 form by mail or fax. Voluntary reporting to the FDA is an easy, minimally time-consuming task that has an enormous impact on public health.

The FDA relies on AE reports to maintain a safety surveillance of all FDA-regulated devices. Physician reports may be the critical action that prompts a modification in the use or design of a product, improves the safety profile of a device, and leads to increased patient safety.

Malvina Eydelman, Director of FDA Ophthalmic Devices Panel, personal communication, 2006.

CHAPTER 3

Patient Evaluation

A thorough preoperative patient evaluation is critically important in achieving a successful outcome following refractive surgery. It is during this encounter that the physician begins to develop an impression as to whether the patient is a good candidate for refractive surgery.

Patient History

The evaluation actually begins before the physician sees the patient. Receptionists or refractive surgical coordinators who speak with a patient prior to the visit may get a sense of the patient's goals and expectations regarding refractive surgery. If the patient is quarrelsome about the time or date of the appointment or argues about cost, the surgeon should be informed. Such a patient may be too demanding to be a good candidate for surgery.

Important parts of the preoperative evaluation include an assessment of the patient's expectations; his or her history; manifest and cycloplegic refractions; a complete ophthalmic evaluation, including slit-lamp and fundus examinations; and ancillary testing (Table 3-1). If the patient is a good candidate for surgery, the appropriate refractive surgery procedures, benefits, and risks need to be discussed, and informed consent must be obtained.

Because accurate testing results are critical to the success of refractive surgery, the refractive surgeon must closely supervise office staff who are performing the various tests (eg, corneal topography or pachymetry) in the preoperative evaluation. Likewise, the surgeon should make sure the instruments used in the evaluation are properly calibrated, as miscalibrated instruments can result in faulty data and poor surgical results.

Patient Expectations

One of the most crucial aspects of the entire evaluation is assessing the patient's expectations. Inappropriate patient expectations are probably the leading cause of patient dissatisfaction after refractive surgery. The results may be exactly what the surgeon expected, but if those expectations were not conveyed adequately to the patient before surgery, the patient may be quite disappointed.

The surgeon should explore expectations relating to both the refractive result (eg, uncorrected visual acuity [UCVA]) and the emotional result (eg, improved self-esteem). Patients need to understand that they should not expect refractive surgery

Table 3-1 Important Parts of the Preoperative Refractive Surgery Evaluation

PATIENT EXPECTATIONS AND MOTIVATIONS
Assessment of specific patient expectations
Discussion of uncorrected distance versus reading vision
HISTORY
Social history, including visual requirements of profession and hobbies
Medical history, including systemic medications and diseases such as diabetes and rheumatologic diseases
Ocular history, including history of contact lens wear
OCULAR EXAMINATION
Uncorrected near and distance vision
Manifest refraction (pushing plus)
Monovision demonstration, if indicated
External evaluation
Pupillary evaluation
Motility
Slit-lamp examination, including IOP measurement
Corneal topography
Wavefront analysis, if indicated
Pachymetry
Cycloplegic refraction (refining sphere, not cylinder)
Dilated fundus examination
INFORMED CONSENT
Discussion of findings
Discussion of medical and surgical alternatives and risks
Answering of patient questions
Having patient read informed consent document, undilated and unsedated, and ideally before the day of procedure, and sign prior to surgery

to improve their best-corrected visual acuity (BCVA). In addition, refractive surgery will not prevent possible future ocular problems such as cataract, glaucoma, or retinal detachment. If the patient has obviously unrealistic desires, such as a guarantee of 20/20 uncorrected visual acuity or perfect uncorrected reading *and* distance vision, even though he or she is presbyopic, the patient may need to be told that refractive surgery cannot currently fulfill his or her needs. The refractive surgeon should exclude patients with unrealistic expectations.

Social History

The social history and medical history can identify the visual requirements of the patient's profession. Certain jobs require that best vision be at a specific distance. For example, a preacher may desire that best uncorrected vision be at arm's length, so that reading can be done at the pulpit without glasses. Military personnel, firefighters, or police may have restrictions on minimal UCVA and BCVA and also on the type of refractive surgery they can have. The type of sports and recreational activities a patient prefers may help select the best refractive procedure or determine whether that patient is even a good candidate for refractive surgery. For example, a surface laser procedure may be preferable to a lamellar procedure for a patient who wrestles, boxes, or rides horses and is at high risk of ocular trauma. A highly myopic and presbyopic stamp collector or jeweler, who is used to examining objects without glasses a few inches from the eyes, may not be happy with postoperative emmetropia.

Medical History

The medical history should include systemic conditions, prior surgeries, and current and prior medications. Certain systemic conditions, such as connective tissue disorders, can lead to poor healing after refractive surgery. An immunocompromised state—for example from cancer or HIV/AIDS—may increase the risk of infection after refractive surgery (see Chapter 10). Medications that affect healing or the ability to fight infection, such as systemic corticosteroids or chemotherapeutic agents, should be specifically noted. The use of corticosteroids, and some diseases, such as diabetes, increase the risk of cataract development, which could compromise the long-term postoperative visual outcome. Certain medications—for example, isotretinoin (eg, Accutane) and amiodarone (eg, Cordarone)—have been traditionally thought to increase the risk of poor results with PRK and LASIK due to a potentially increased risk of poor corneal healing; however, there is no evidence for this in the peer-reviewed literature. Previous use of isotretinoin can damage the meibomian glands and predispose to dry-eye symptoms postoperatively. In addition, caution needs to be taken with patients using sumatriptan (eg, Imitrex) who are undergoing PRK and LASIK and with patients using hormone replacement therapy or antihistamines who are undergoing PRK due to a possible increased risk of delayed epithelial healing.

Although laser manufacturers do not recommend excimer laser surgery in patients with cardiac pacemakers and implanted defibrillators, many such patients have undergone the surgery without problems. It may be best to check with the pacemaker and defibrillator manufacturer prior to laser surgery. Refractive surgery is also generally contraindicated in pregnant and nursing women, due to possible changes in refraction and corneal hydration status. Many surgeons recommend waiting at least 3 months after delivery and cessation of nursing before performing the refractive surgery evaluation and procedure.

Pertinent Ocular History

The ocular history should focus on previous and current eye problems such as dry-eye symptoms, blepharitis, recurrent erosions, and retinal tears or detachments. Ocular medications should be noted. A history of previous methods of optical correction, such as glasses and contact lenses, should be taken. The stability of the current refraction is very important. Have the glasses or the contact lens prescription changed significantly in the past few years? A significant change is generally thought to be greater than 0.50 D in either sphere or cylinder over the past year. A contact lens history should be taken. Important information includes the type of lens (eg, soft, rigid gas-permeable [RGP], PMMA); the wearing schedule (eg, daily wear disposable, daily wear frequent replacement, overnight wear indicating number of nights worn in a row); the type of cleaning, disinfecting, and enzyming agents; and how old the lenses are. Occasionally, a patient may have been happy with contact lens wear and only need a change in lens material or wearing schedule to eliminate a recent onset of discomforting symptoms.

Because contact lens wear can change the shape of the cornea (corneal warpage), discontinuing contact lens wear is recommended prior to the refractive surgery evaluation and also prior to the surgery. The exact amount of time the patient should be out of contact lenses has not been established. Current clinical practice typically involves discontinuing soft contact lenses for at least 3 days to 2 weeks and rigid contact lenses for at least 2–3 weeks. Some surgeons keep patients out of rigid contact lenses for 1 month for every decade of contact lens wear. Patients with irregular or unstable corneas should discontinue their contact lenses for a longer period and then be rerefracted every few weeks until the refraction and corneal topography stabilize before being considered for refractive surgery. Some surgeons will have patients who wear RGP lenses and find glasses a significant hardship change to soft lenses for a period of time to aid stabilization and regularization of the corneal curvature.

Patient Age, Presbyopia, and Monovision

The age of a patient is very important in predicting postoperative patient satisfaction. The loss of near vision with aging should be discussed with all patients. Prior to age 40, emmetropic individuals generally do not require reading adds to see a near target. After this age, patients need to understand that if they are made emmetropic with refractive surgery, they will require reading glasses for near vision. This point cannot be overemphasized for myopic patients who are approaching age 40. These patients can read well with and without their glasses. Some may even read well with their contact lenses. If they are emmetropic after surgery, many will not read well without reading glasses. The patient needs to understand this phenomenon and must be willing to accept this result prior to undergoing any refractive surgery that aims for emmetropia. In patients wearing glasses, a trial with contact lenses will approximate the patient's reading ability after surgery.

A discussion of monovision (1 eye corrected for distance and the other eye for near) often fits well into the evaluation at this point. The alternative of monovision correction should be discussed with all patients in the prepresbyopic and presbyopic age groups. Many patients have successfully used monovision in contact lenses and want it after refractive surgery. Others have never tried it but would like to, and still others have no interest. If a patient has not used monovision before but is interested, the attempted surgical result should be demonstrated with glasses at near and distance. Generally, the dominant eye is corrected for distance and the nondominant eye is corrected to approximately –1.50 to –1.75 D. For most patients, such a refraction allows good uncorrected distance and near vision without intolerable anisometropia. Some surgeons prefer a "mini-monovision" procedure, where the near-vision eye is corrected to approximately –0.75 D, which allows some near vision with better distance vision and less anisometropia. The exact amount of monovision depends on the desires of the patient. Higher amounts of monovision (up to –2.50 D) can be used successfully in selected patients who want excellent postoperative near vision. However, in some patients with a higher degree of myopia, improving near vision may lead to the unwanted side effects of loss of depth perception and anisometropia. It is often advisable to have a patient try monovision with contact lenses prior to surgery to ensure that distance and near vision and stereovision are acceptable to them and also to ensure that no muscle imbalance is present, especially with higher degrees of monovision.

Although typically the nondominant eye is corrected for near, some patients prefer that the dominant eye be corrected for near. There are several methods for testing ocular dominance. One of the simplest is to have the patient point to a distant object, such as a small letter on an eye chart, and then close each eye to determine which eye he or she was using when pointing; this is the dominant eye. Another is to have a patient make an "okay sign" with one hand and look at the examiner through the opening.

Examination

Uncorrected Visual Acuity and Manifest and Cycloplegic Refraction Acuity

The refractive elements of the preoperative examination are critically important because they directly determine the amount of surgery that is performed. UCVA at distance and near should be measured. The current glasses prescription and vision with those glasses should also be measured, and a manifest refraction should be performed. The sharpest visual acuity with the least amount of minus ("pushing plus") should be the final endpoint. The Duochrome test should not be used as the final endpoint because it tends to overminus patients. Document the best visual acuity obtainable, even if it is better than 20/20. An automated refraction with an autorefractor or wavefront aberrometer may be helpful in refining the manifest refraction. A cycloplegic refraction is also necessary; sufficient waiting time must be allowed between the time the patient's eyes are dilated with appropriate cycloplegic drops—tropicamide 1% or cyclopentolate 1% is generally used—and the refraction. For full cycloplegia, waiting at least 30 minutes (with tropicamide 1%) or 60 minutes (with cyclopentolate 1%) is recommended. The cycloplegic refraction should refine the sphere and not the cylinder from the manifest refraction. For eyes with greater than 5.00 D of refractive error, a vertex distance measurement should be performed to obtain the most accurate refraction. When the difference between the manifest and cycloplegic refractions is large (eg, >0.50 D), a postcycloplegic manifest refraction should be performed to recheck the original. In myopic patients, such a large difference is often caused by an overminused manifest refraction. In hyperopic patients, significant latent hyperopia may be present, and in such cases the surgeon and patient need to decide exactly how much hyperopia to treat. If there is significant latent hyperopia, a pushed-plus spectacle or contact lens correction can be worn for several weeks preoperatively to reduce the postoperative adjustment from treating the true refraction.

Refractive surgeons have their own preferences on whether to program the laser using the manifest or cycloplegic refraction, based on their own individual nomogram and technique and on the patient's age. Many surgeons plan their laser input based on the manifest refraction, especially in younger patients, if that refraction has been performed with a careful pushed-plus technique.

Pupillary Examination

After the manifest refraction (but before dilating drops are administered), the external and anterior segment examinations are performed. Specific attention should be given to the pupillary examination; the pupil size should be evaluated in bright room light and dim illumination, and the surgeon should look for any afferent pupillary defect. A variety of techniques are available for measuring pupil size in dim illumination, including use of a near card with pupil sizes on the edge (with the patient fixating at distance), a light amplification pupillometer (eg, Colvard pupillometer), and an infrared pupillometer. The actual amount of light entering the eye during the dim-light measurement should closely approximate that entering the eye at night during normal nighttime activities, such as night driving; it should not necessarily be completely dark.

It is important to try to standardize pupil size measurements as much as possible. Large pupil size may be one of the risk factors for postoperative glare and halo symptoms after refractive surgery. Other risk factors for postoperative glare include higher degrees of myopia or astigmatism. As a general rule, pupil size greater than the effective optical zone (usually 6–8 mm) increases the risk of glare, but large pupil size is not the only determinant of glare. When asked, patients often note that they had glare under dim-light conditions even before refractive surgery. It is important that patients become aware of their glare and halo symptoms preoperatively, as this may minimize postoperative complaints.

Measuring the low-light pupil diameter preoperatively and using that measurement to direct surgery remains controversial. Conventional wisdom suggests that the optical zone should be larger than the pupil diameter to minimize visual disturbances such as glare and halos. However, it is not clear that pupil size can be used to predict which patients are more likely to have such symptoms. It is possible that the size of the effective optical zone, which is related to the ablation profile and the level of refractive error, is more important in minimizing visual side effects than the low-light pupil diameter.

Pop M, Payette Y. Risk factors for night vision complaints after LASIK for myopia. *Ophthalmology.* 2004;111:3–10.

Schallhorn SC, Kaupp SE, Tanzer DJ, Tidwell J, Laurent J, Bourque LB. Pupil size and quality of vision after LASIK. *Ophthalmology.* 2003;110:1606–1614.

Ocular Motility, Confrontation Fields, and Ocular Anatomy

Ocular motility should also be evaluated. Patients with an asymptomatic tropia or phoria may develop symptoms after refractive surgery if the change in refraction causes the motility status to break down. If there is a history of strabismus (see Chapter 10) or a concern regarding ocular alignment postoperatively, a trial with contact lenses before surgery should be considered. A sensory motor evaluation can be obtained preoperatively if strabismus is an issue.

Confrontation fields should be performed in all patients.

The general anatomy of the orbits should also be assessed. Patients with small palpebral fissures and/or large brows may not be ideal candidates for LASIK or epi-LASIK because there may be inadequate exposure and difficulty in achieving suction with the microkeratome.

Intraocular Pressure

The IOP should be checked after the manifest refraction is done and corneal topography measurements are taken. Patients with glaucoma (see Chapter 10) should be advised that during certain refractive surgery procedures the IOP is dramatically elevated, potentially aggravating optic nerve damage. Also, topical corticosteroids are used after most refractive surgery procedures and, after a surface ablation procedure, may be used for months. Long-term topical corticosteroids may cause a marked elevation of IOP in corticosteroid responders. Laser refractive surgery procedures such as surface ablation procedures and LASIK thin the cornea and typically cause a falsely low Goldmann applanation measurement of IOP postoperatively. Patients and surgeons need to be aware of this issue, especially if the patient has glaucoma or is a glaucoma suspect.

Slit-Lamp Examination

A complete slit-lamp examination of the eyelids and anterior segment should be performed. The eyelids should be checked for significant blepharitis and meibomitis, and the tear lake should be assessed for aqueous tear deficiency. The conjunctiva should be examined, specifically for conjunctival scarring, which may cause problems with microkeratome suction. The cornea should be evaluated for surface abnormalities such as decreased tear breakup time (Fig 3-1) and punctate epithelial erosions (Fig 3-2). Significant blepharitis (Fig 3-3), meibomitis, and dry-eye syndrome should be addressed prior to refractive surgery, as they are associated with increased postoperative discomfort and decreased vision. A careful examination for epithelial basement membrane dystrophy (Fig 3-4) is required, because its presence increases the risk of flap complications during LASIK. Patients with epithelial basement membrane dystrophy are not good candidates for LASIK, but they may be better candidates for a surface ablation procedure. Signs of keratoconus, such as corneal thinning and steepening, may also be found. Keratoconus is typically a contraindication to refractive surgery (see Chapter 5). The endothelium should be examined carefully for signs of cornea guttata and Fuchs and other dystrophies. Corneal edema is generally considered a contraindication to refractive surgery.

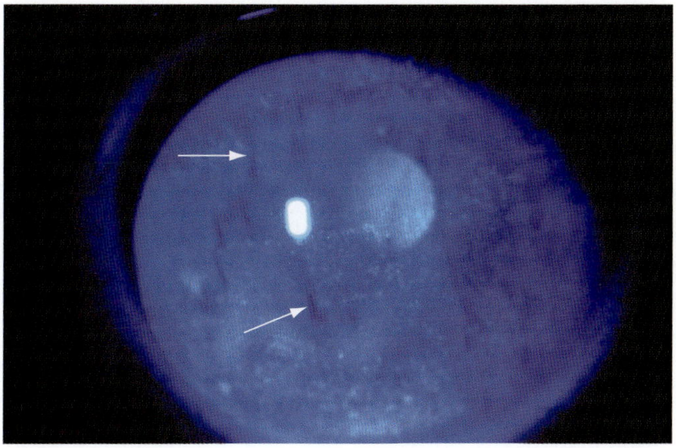

Figure 3-1 Decreased tear breakup time. After instillation of fluorescein dye, the patient keeps the eye open for 10 seconds and the tear film is examined with cobalt blue light. Breaks, or dry spots, in the tear film can be seen in this patient *(arrows)*. Punctate epithelial erosions are also present. *(Courtesy of Christopher J. Rapuano, MD.)*

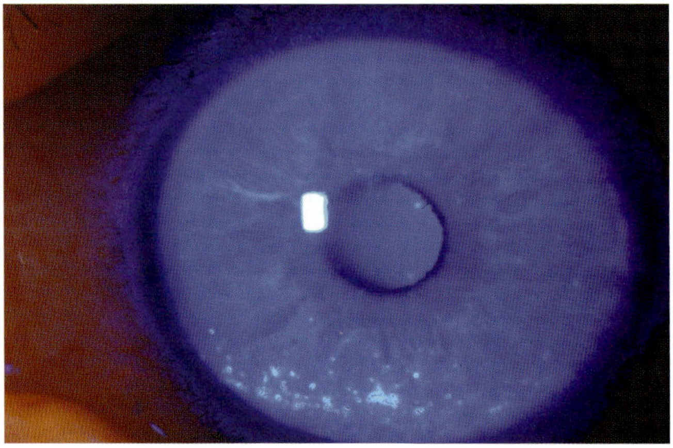

Figure 3-2 Punctate epithelial erosions. Inferior punctate fluorescein staining is noted in this patient with moderately dry eyes. *(Courtesy of Christopher J. Rapuano, MD.)*

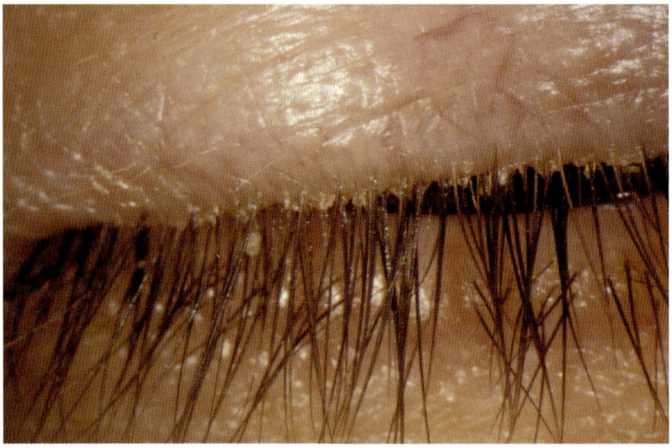

Figure 3-3 Blepharitis. Moderate crusting at the base of the lashes is found in this patient with seborrheic blepharitis. *(Courtesy of Christopher J. Rapuano, MD.)*

The anterior chamber, iris, and crystalline lens should also be examined. A shallow anterior chamber depth may be a contraindication for insertion of certain phakic IOLs (see Chapter 8). Careful undilated and dilated evaluation of the crystalline lens for clarity is essential, especially in patients over age 50. Patients with mild lens changes that are visually insignificant should be informed of these findings and advised that the changes may become more significant in the future, independent of refractive surgery. In patients with moderate lens opacities, cataract extraction may be the best form of refractive surgery. Patients with cataracts should be informed that if they do not undergo refractive surgery at this time, significant refractive error can be addressed at the time of future cataract surgery. Some surgeons give patients a record of their preoperative refractions and keratometry measurements along with the amount of laser ablation performed and the postoperative refraction. This information should help improve the accuracy of the IOL calculation should cataract surgery be required at a future date.

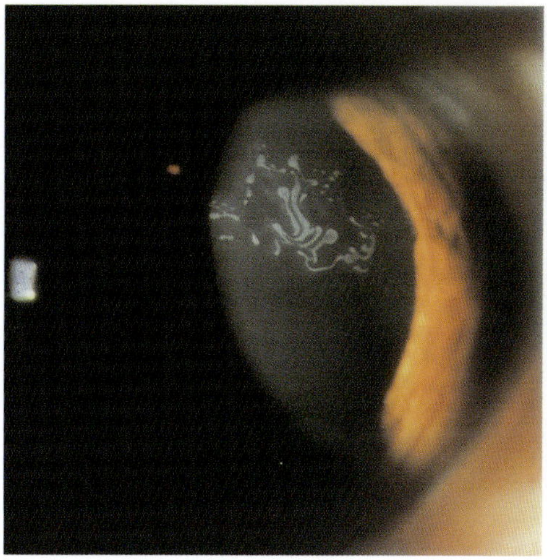

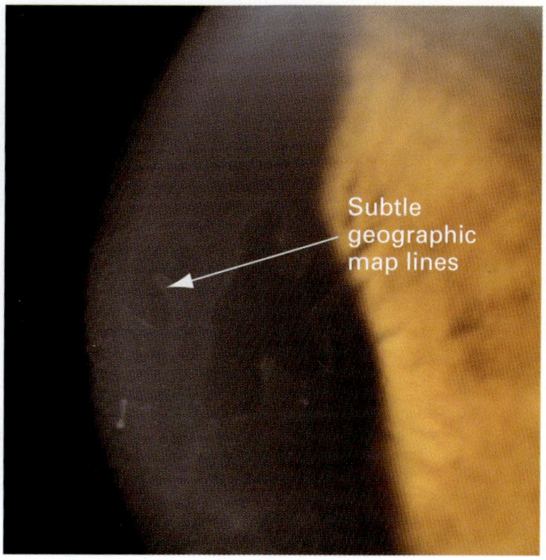

Figure 3-4 Epithelial basement membrane dystrophy. Epithelial map changes can be obvious **(A)** or subtle **(B)**. *Arrow* shows geographic map lines. *(Part A courtesy of Vincent P. deLuise, MD; part B courtesy of Christopher J. Rapuano, MD.)*

Dilated Fundus Examination

A dilated fundus examination is also important prior to refractive surgery to ensure that the posterior segment is normal. Special attention should be given to the optic nerve (glaucoma, optic nerve drusen) and peripheral retina (retinal breaks, detachment). Patients and surgeons should realize that highly myopic eyes (see Chapter 10) are at increased risk for retinal detachment, even after the refractive error has been corrected.

Ancillary Tests

Corneal Topography

The corneal curvature must be evaluated. Although manual keratometry readings can be quite informative, they have largely been replaced by computerized corneal topographic analyses. Several different methods are available to analyze the corneal curvature, including Placido disk, scanning-slit-beam, rotating Scheimpflug photography, high-frequency ultrasound, and ocular coherence tomography. (See also the extensive discussion of corneal topography in Chapter 1.) These techniques image the cornea and provide color maps showing corneal power and/or elevation. The analysis gives a "simulated keratometry" reading and an overall evaluation of the corneal curvature. Eyes with visually significant irregular astigmatism are generally not good candidates for corneal refractive surgery. Curvature analysis should reveal a spherical cornea or regular astigmatism. Early keratoconus, pellucid marginal degeneration (Fig 3-5), and contact lens warpage should be considered causes of visually significant irregular astigmatism. Irregular astigmatism secondary to contact lens warpage usually reverses over time, although it may take months. Serial corneal topography should be performed to document the disappearance of visually significant irregular astigmatism prior to any refractive surgery.

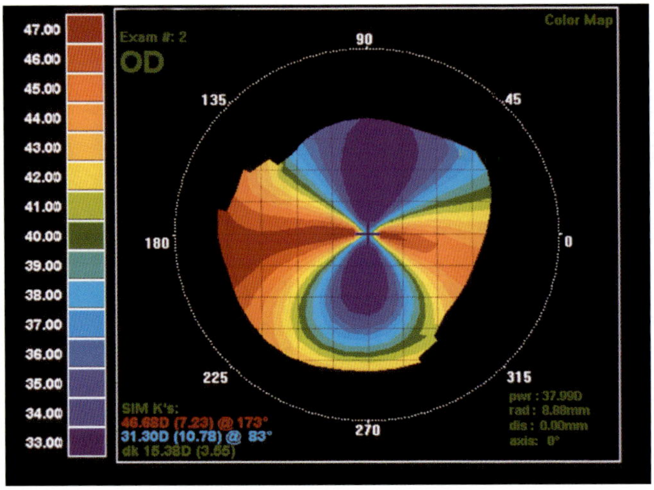

Figure 3-5 A corneal topographic map of the typical irregular against-the-rule astigmatism that is seen in eyes with pellucid marginal degeneration. Note that the steepening nasally and temporally connects inferiorly. *(Courtesy of Christopher J. Rapuano, MD.)*

Unusually steep or unusually flat corneas can increase the risk of poor flap creation with the microkeratome. Flat corneas (flatter than 40.00 D) increase the risk of small flaps and free caps, and steep corneas (steeper than 48.00 D) increase the risk of buttonhole flaps. Femtosecond laser flap creation theoretically may avoid these risks. Excessive corneal flattening (flatter than approximately 34.00 D) or excessive corneal steepening (steeper than approximately 50.00 D) after refractive surgery may increase the risk of poor quality vision. Postoperative keratometry for myopic patients is estimated by subtracting approximately 80% of the refractive correction from the average preoperative keratometry reading. For example, if the preoperative keratometry reading is 42.00 D, and 5.00 D of myopia is being corrected, an estimated postoperative keratometry reading would be $42.00 \text{ D} - (0.8 \times 5.00 \text{ D}) = 38.00 \text{ D}$. Postoperative keratometry for hyperopic patients is estimated by adding 100% of the refractive correction to the average preoperative keratometry reading. For example, if the preoperative keratometry reading is 42.00 D, and 3.00 D of hyperopia is being corrected, the estimated postoperative keratometry reading would be $42.00 \text{ D} + (1 \times 3.00 \text{ D}) = 45.00 \text{ D}$.

When keratometric or corneal topographic measurements reveal an amount or an axis of astigmatism significantly different from that seen at refraction, the refraction should be rechecked for accuracy. Lenticular astigmatism or posterior corneal curvature may account for the difference between refractive and keratometric/topographic astigmatism. Most surgeons will treat the amount and axis of the refractive astigmatism, as long as the patient understands that following future cataract surgery, some astigmatism may reappear (after the astigmatism contributed by the natural lens has been eliminated).

Pachymetry

Corneal thickness should be measured to determine if the cornea is of adequate thickness for keratorefractive surgery. This procedure is usually performed with ultrasound pachymetry; however, certain non–Placido disk corneal topography systems can also be used if properly calibrated. Most newer systems can provide a map showing the relative thickness of the cornea at various locations. The accuracy of the pachymetry measurements of scanning-slit systems decreases markedly after keratorefractive surgery is performed. Because the thinnest part of the cornea is typically located centrally, a central measurement should always be performed. Unusually thin corneas may reveal early keratoconus. Some surgeons also check the midperipheral corneal thickness for inferior thinning, which may also suggest early keratoconus. Unusually thick corneas may suggest mild Fuchs dystrophy. The thickness of the cornea is an important factor in determining whether the patient is a candidate for refractive surgery and which procedure may be best. In a study of 896 eyes undergoing LASIK, the mean central corneal thickness was 550 µm ± 33 µm, with a range of 472 µm to 651 µm. It is unclear whether an unusually thin cornea (beyond perhaps 2 standard deviations) suggests inherent instability that would not be ideal for any refractive surgery. Consequently, even if there is adequate stromal tissue for an excimer ablation, most refractive surgeons will not consider LASIK below a certain lower limit of corneal thickness. If LASIK is performed and results in a relatively thin residual stromal bed—for example around 250 µm—future enhancement surgery that further thins the stromal bed may not be possible. If there is a question of endothelial integrity causing an abnormally thick cornea, specular microscopy may be helpful in assessing the health of the endothelium.

Price FW Jr, Koller DL, Price MO. Central corneal pachymetry in patients undergoing laser in situ keratomileusis. *Ophthalmology.* 1999;106:2216–2220.

Wavefront Analysis

Wavefront analysis is a relatively new technique that can provide an objective refraction measurement (see also discussion of this topic in Chapters 1 and 6). Certain excimer lasers can use this wavefront analysis information directly to perform the ablation, a procedure called *wavefront-guided,* or *custom, ablation.* Some surgeons use wavefront analysis to document levels of preoperative higher-order aberrations. Refraction data from the wavefront analysis unit can also be used to refine the manifest refraction. If the manifest refraction and the wavefront analysis refraction are very dissimilar, the patient may not be a good candidate for wavefront treatment. Note that a custom wavefront ablation generally removes more tissue than a standard ablation in the same eye.

Calculation of Residual Stromal Bed Thickness After LASIK

A lamellar laser refractive procedure such as LASIK involves creation of a corneal flap, ablation of the stromal bed, and replacement of the flap. The strength and integrity of the cornea postoperatively depend on the thickness of the residual stromal bed (RST). Stromal bed thickness is calculated by taking the preoperative central corneal thickness and subtracting the flap thickness and the calculated laser ablation depth for the particular refraction. For example, if the central corneal thickness is 550 µm, the flap thickness is estimated to be 160 µm, and the ablation depth for the patient's refraction is 50 µm, the RST would be 550 µm – (160 µm + 50 µm) = 340 µm. When calculating RST, the amount of actual tissue removed should be based on the actual intended refractive correction, not on the nomogram-adjusted number entered into the laser computer. For example, if a −10.00 D myopic patient is being fully corrected, the amount of tissue removed is 128 µm for a 6.5-mm ablation zone for the VISX laser. Even if the surgeon usually takes off 15% of the refraction and enters that number into the laser computer, approximately 128 µm of tissue will be removed, not 85% of 128 µm.

Exactly how thick the residual stromal bed needs to be is unclear. However, most surgeons believe it should be at least 250 µm thick. Others want the RST to be greater than 50% of the original corneal thickness. If the calculation reveals an RST that is thinner than desired, LASIK may not be the best surgical option. In these cases, a surface ablation procedure may be a better option because no stromal flap is required.

Discussion of Findings and Informed Consent

Once the evaluation is complete, the surgeon must analyze all the information and discuss the findings with the patient. If the patient is a candidate for refractive surgery, the risks and benefits of the various medical and surgical alternatives must be discussed (Table 3-2). Important aspects of this discussion are the expected UCVA results for the amount of refractive error (including the need for distance and/or reading glasses, the chance of needing an enhancement, and whether maximal surgery is being performed during the initial procedure), the risk of decreased BCVA or severe visual loss, the side effects of glare and halos or dry eyes, the change in vision quality, and the need to revise a corneal flap (eg, for flap displacement, significant striae, or epithelial ingrowth). The patient should understand that the laser ablation might need to be aborted if there is an incomplete, decentered, or buttonholed flap. The pros and cons of surgery on 1 eye versus both eyes on the same day should also be discussed, and patients allowed to decide which is best for them. Although the risk of bilateral infection may be higher with bilateral surgery, serial unilateral surgery may result in temporary anisometropia and is more inconvenient. Nonsurgical alternatives, such as glasses and contact lenses, should also be discussed.

If a patient is considering refractive surgery, he or she should be given the informed consent document either prior to dilation or after dilation has worn off to take home and review. The patient should be given an opportunity to discuss any questions related to the surgery or the informed consent form with the surgeon preoperatively. The consent form should be signed prior to surgery and never when the patient is dilated and/or sedated. See Appendix 3-1 for a sample informed consent form.

Table 3-2 Summary of the Most Common Refractive Surgery Procedures

Procedure	Typical Spherical Range	Typical Cylinder Range	Limitations
LASIK	–10.00 to +4.00 D	Up to 4.00 D	Thin corneas (thin residual stromal bed); epithelial basement membrane dystrophy; small palpebral fissures; microkeratome flap complications, especially with flat and steep corneas; preoperative severe dry-eye syndrome; certain medications; wavefront-guided ablations may have more restricted FDA-approved treatment parameters
Surface ablation	–8.00 to +4.00 D	Up to 4.00 D	Postoperative haze at high end of treatment range but range may be extended with the use of mitomycin C; preoperative dry-eye syndrome; certain medications
Intrastromal corneal ring segments	–0.75 to –3.00 D	None	Not FDA approved to correct cylinder; glare symptoms; white opacities at edge of ring segments; not after radial keratotomy
Intrastromal corneal ring segments	FDA approved to treat myopia in keratoconus	NA	Approved for age greater than 21; contact lens intolerance; corneal thickness greater than 450 µm at incision site; no corneal scarring
Phakic intraocular lenses	–5.00 to –20.00 D	None	FDA approved for myopia; intraocular surgery; long-term complications such as glaucoma, iritis, cataract, pupil distortion, corneal edema
Refractive lens exchange	All ranges	Up to 3.00 D	Not FDA approved; same complications as with cataract extraction with a lens implant

APPENDIX 3-1: Example Informed Consent Form for LASIK

(Courtesy of Ophthalmic Mutual Insurance Company, www.OMIC.com)

NOTE: THIS FORM IS INTENDED AS A SAMPLE ONLY. PLEASE REVIEW IT AND MODIFY TO FIT YOUR ACTUAL PRACTICE. IT DOES NOT CONTAIN INFORMATION ABOUT LIMBAL RELAXING INCISIONS (LRIs), SO INCLUDE THAT IF YOU PERFORM LRIs DURING CATARACT SURGERY.

Version 071906

INFORMED CONSENT FOR LASER IN-SITU KERATOMILEUSIS (LASIK)

Introduction

This information is being provided to you so that you can make an informed decision about the use of a device known as a microkeratome, combined with the use of a device known as an excimer laser, to perform LASIK. LASIK is one of a number of alternatives for correcting nearsightedness, farsightedness, and astigmatism. In LASIK, the microkeratome is used to shave the cornea to create a flap. The flap then is opened like the page of a book to expose tissue just below the cornea's surface. Next, the excimer laser is used to remove ultra-thin layers from the cornea to reshape it to reduce nearsightedness. Finally, the flap is returned to its original position, without sutures.

LASIK is an elective procedure: There is no emergency condition or other reason that requires or demands that you have it performed. You could continue wearing contact lenses or glasses and have adequate visual acuity. This procedure, like all surgery, presents some risks, many of which are listed below. You should also understand that there may be other risks not known to your doctor, which may become known later. Despite the best of care, complications and side effects may occur; should this happen in your case, the result might be affected even to the extent of making your vision worse.

Alternatives to LASIK

If you decide not to have LASIK, there are other methods of correcting your nearsightedness, farsightedness, or astigmatism. These alternatives include, among others, eyeglasses, contact lenses, and other refractive surgical procedures.

Patient Consent

In giving my permission for LASIK, I understand the following: The long-term risks and effects of LASIK are unknown. I have received no guarantee as to the success of my particular case. I understand that the following risks are associated with the procedure:

Vision Threatening Complications

1. I understand that the microkeratome or the excimer laser could malfunction, requiring the procedure to be stopped before completion. Depending on the type of malfunction, this may or may not be accompanied by visual loss.

Patient Initials: _____

2. I understand that, in using the microkeratome, instead of making a flap, an entire portion of the central cornea could be cut off, and very rarely could be lost. If preserved, I understand that my doctor would put this tissue back on the eye after the laser treatment, using sutures, according to the ALK procedure method. It is also possible that the flap incision could result in an incomplete flap, or a flap that is too thin. If this happens, it is likely that the laser part of the procedure will have to be postponed until the cornea has a chance to heal sufficiently to try to create the flap again.
3. I understand that irregular healing of the flap could result in a distorted cornea. This would mean that glasses or contact lenses may not correct my vision to the level possible before undergoing LASIK. If this distortion in vision is severe, a partial or complete corneal transplant might be necessary to repair the cornea.
4. I understand that it is possible a perforation of the cornea could occur, causing devastating complications, including loss of some or all of my vision. This could also be caused by an internal or external eye infection that could not be controlled with antibiotics or other means.
5. I understand that mild or severe infection is possible. Mild infection can usually be treated with antibiotics and usually does not lead to permanent visual loss. Severe infection, even if successfully treated with antibiotics, could lead to permanent scarring and loss of vision that may require corrective laser surgery or, if very severe, corneal transplantation or even loss of the eye.
6. I understand that I could develop keratoconus. Keratoconus is a degenerative corneal disease affecting vision that occurs in approximately 1/2000 in the general population. While there are several tests that suggest which patients might be at risk, this condition can develop in patients who have normal preoperative topography (a map of the cornea obtained before surgery) and pachymetry (corneal thickness measurement). Since keratoconus may occur on its own, there is no absolute test that will ensure a patient will not develop keratoconus following laser vision correction. Severe keratoconus may need to be treated with a corneal transplant while mild keratoconus can be corrected by glasses or contact lenses.
7. I understand that other very rare complications threatening vision include, but are not limited to, corneal swelling, corneal thinning (ectasia), appearance of "floaters" and retinal detachment, hemorrhage, venous and arterial blockage, cataract formation, total blindness, and even loss of my eye.

Non–Vision Threatening Side Effects

1. I understand that there may be increased sensitivity to light, glare, and fluctuations in the sharpness of vision. I understand these conditions usually occur during the normal stabilization period of from one to three months, but they may also be permanent.
2. I understand that there is an increased risk of eye irritation related to drying of the corneal surface following the LASIK procedure. These symptoms may be

Patient Initials: _____

temporary or, on rare occasions, permanent, and may require frequent application of artificial tears and/or closure of the tear duct openings in the eyelid.

3. I understand that an overcorrection or undercorrection could occur, causing me to become farsighted or nearsighted or increase my astigmatism and that this could be either permanent or treatable. I understand an overcorrection or undercorrection is more likely in people over the age of 40 years and may require the use of glasses for reading or for distance vision some or all of the time.
4. After refractive surgery, a certain number of patients experience glare, a "starbursting" or halo effect around lights, or other low-light vision problems that may interfere with the ability to drive at night or see well in dim light. The exact cause of these visual problems is not currently known; some ophthalmologists theorize that the risk may be increased in patients with large pupils or high degrees of correction. For most patients, this is a temporary condition that diminishes with time or is correctable by wearing glasses at night or taking eye drops. For some patients, however, these visual problems are permanent. I understand that my vision may not seem as sharp at night as during the day and that I may need to wear glasses at night or take eye drops. I understand that it is not possible to predict whether I will experience these night vision or low-light problems, and that I may permanently lose the ability to drive at night or function in dim light because of them. I understand that I should not drive unless my vision is adequate.
5. I understand that I may not get a full correction from my LASIK procedure and this may require future enhancement procedures, such as more laser treatment or the use of glasses or contact lenses.
6. I understand that there may be a "balance" problem between my two eyes after LASIK has been performed on one eye, but not the other. This phenomenon is called anisometropia. I understand this would cause eyestrain and make judging distance or depth perception more difficult. I understand that my first eye may take longer to heal than is usual, prolonging the time I could experience anisometropia.
7. I understand that, after LASIK, the eye may be more fragile to trauma from impact. Evidence has shown that, as with any scar, the corneal incision will not be as strong as the cornea originally was at that site. I understand that the treated eye, therefore, is somewhat more vulnerable to all varieties of injuries, at least for the first year following LASIK. I understand it would be advisable for me to wear protective eyewear when engaging in sports or other activities in which the possibility of a ball, projectile, elbow, fist, or other traumatizing object contacting the eye may be high.
8. I understand that there is a natural tendency of the eyelids to droop with age and that eye surgery may hasten this process.
9. I understand that there may be pain or a foreign body sensation, particularly during the first 48 hours after surgery.
10. I understand that temporary glasses for either distance or reading may be necessary while healing occurs and that more than one pair of glasses may be needed.
11. I understand that the long-term effects of LASIK are unknown and that unforeseen complications or side effects could possibly occur.

Patient Initials: _____

12. I understand that visual acuity I initially gain from LASIK could regress, and that my vision may go partially back to a level that may require glasses or contact lens use to see clearly.
13. I understand that the correction that I can expect to gain from LASIK may not be perfect. I understand that it is not realistic to expect that this procedure will result in perfect vision, at all times, under all circumstances, for the rest of my life. I understand I may need glasses to refine my vision for some purposes requiring fine detailed vision after some point in my life, and that this might occur soon after surgery or years later.
14. I understand that I may be given medication in conjunction with the procedure and that my eye may be patched afterward. I therefore understand that I must not drive the day of surgery and not until I am certain that my vision is adequate for driving.
15. I understand that if I currently need reading glasses, I will still likely need reading glasses after this treatment. It is possible that dependence on reading glasses may increase or that reading glasses may be required at an earlier age if I have this surgery.
16. Even 90% clarity of vision is still slightly blurry. Enhancement surgeries can be performed when vision is stable UNLESS it is unwise or unsafe. If the enhancement is performed within the first six months following surgery, there generally is no need to make another cut with the microkeratome. The original flap can usually be lifted with specialized techniques. After 6 months of healing, a new LASIK incision **may be** required, incurring greater risk. In order to perform an enhancement surgery, there must be adequate tissue remaining. If there is inadequate tissue, it may not be possible to perform an enhancement. An assessment and consultation will be held with the surgeon at which time the benefits and risks of an enhancement surgery will be discussed.
17. I understand that, as with all types of surgery, there is a possibility of complications due to anesthesia, drug reactions, or other factors that may involve other parts of my body. I understand that, since it is impossible to state every complication that may occur as a result of any surgery, the list of complications in this form may not be complete.

For Presbyopic Patients (those requiring a separate prescription for reading)
The option of monovision has been discussed with my ophthalmologist.

Patient's Statement of Acceptance and Understanding

The details of the procedure known as LASIK have been presented to me in detail in this document and explained to me by my ophthalmologist. My ophthalmologist has answered all my questions to my satisfaction. I therefore consent to LASIK surgery on:

__________ Right eye ____________ Left eye __________ Both eyes

I give permission for my ophthalmologist to record on video or photographic equipment my procedure, for purposes of education, research, or training of other health care

Patient Initials: _____

professionals. I also give my permission for my ophthalmologist to use data about my procedure and subsequent treatment to further understand LASIK. I understand that my name will remain confidential, unless I give subsequent written permission for it to be disclosed outside my ophthalmologist's office or the center where my LASIK procedure will be performed.

______________________________________ ________________

Patient Name Date

______________________________________ ________________

Witness Name Date

I have been offered a copy of this consent form (please initial). _____

PART II

Specific Procedures in Refractive Surgery

CHAPTER 4

Incisional Corneal Surgery

Since its inception in the late 1890s, incisional corneal surgery has had periods of adoption, refinement, and abandonment. Incisional surgery for myopia and hyperopia has been replaced by excimer laser procedures and intraocular lens implantation, but astigmatic keratotomy still has a role in the treatment of primary and residual astigmatism after both cataract and keratorefractive surgery (limbal relaxing incisions) and following penetrating keratoplasty (PKP; arcuate keratotomy).

The first organized examination of incisional keratotomy has been attributed to a Dutch ophthalmologist, Lans, working in the 1890s. Lans examined astigmatic changes induced in rabbits after partial-thickness corneal incisions and thermal cautery. A Japanese ophthalmologist, Sato, made significant contributions to incisional refractive surgery in the 1930s and 1940s. He observed central corneal flattening and improvement in vision after the healing of spontaneous ruptures of Descemet's membrane (hydrops) in advanced keratoconus patients, which led him to develop a technique to induce artificial ruptures of Descemet's membrane. His long-term results in humans were poor, because incisions were made posteriorly through Descemet's layer, inducing late corneal edema in 75% of patients. In the 1960s and 1970s the Russian ophthalmologist Fyodorov, using radial incisions on the anterior cornea, established that the diameter of the central optical clear zone was inversely related to the amount of refractive correction: smaller central clear zones yield greater myopic corrections.

Incisional Correction of Myopia

Radial Keratotomy in the United States

Radial keratotomy (RK) is now largely considered an obsolete procedure, but it did play an important role in the history of refractive surgery. The excimer laser was originally applied to the cornea to produce more accurate RK incisions, not for surface ablation or laser in situ keratomileusis (LASIK), for which the excimer laser is now used. Following its introduction into the United States in 1978, the surgical technique was modified and advanced as researchers and clinicians sought to improve its safety and predictability. These advances included the use of better equipment (diamond blades, ultrasonic pachymetry, and so on) and more accurate nomograms (incorporating variables such as patient age and IOP), as well as technique modification (reduced number of incisions and mini-RK, with shorter incisions). Radial keratotomy differs from surface ablation and LASIK in that it does not involve removal of tissue from the central cornea.

To evaluate the safety and efficacy of RK, the Prospective Evaluation of Radial Keratotomy (PERK) study was undertaken in 1982 and 1983 for patients with myopia from −2.00 to −8.75 D (mean: −3.875 D). The sole surgical variable was the diameter of the central optical clear zone (3.00, 3.50, or 4.00 mm), based on the level of preoperative myopia. Eight radial incisions were used for all patients; repeat surgery, if necessary, involved an additional 8 incisions. Ten years after the procedure, 53% of the 435 study patients had 20/20 or better uncorrected visual acuity (UCVA) and 85% were 20/40 or better. Of the patients who had bilateral surgery, only 30% reported the use of spectacles or contact lenses for distance refractive correction at 10 years. Complications related to the procedure included loss of best-corrected visual acuity (BCVA; 3%), delayed bacterial keratitis, corneal scarring, irregular astigmatism, and epithelial erosions.

The most important finding in the 10-year PERK study was the continuing long-term instability of the procedure. A hyperopic shift of 1.00 D or greater was found in 43% of eyes between 6 months and 10 years postoperatively. There was an association between length of the incision and hyperopic shift, particularly if the incisions extended into the limbus. Two techniques were developed in response to the hyperopic shift after RK: intentional undercorrection and use of shorter incisions (mini-RK).

Waring GO III, Lynn MJ, McDonnell PJ; PERK Study Group. Results of the Prospective Evaluation of Radial Keratotomy (PERK) study 10 years after surgery. *Arch Ophthalmol.* 1994;112:1298–1308.

Patient Selection

Although it is no longer commonly used, RK was the primary procedure for treating patients with −1.00 to −4.00 D of myopia. Serious complications resulted from more aggressive treatment involving optical zones smaller than 3.0 mm or more than 8 incisions.

Surgical Technique

Radial corneal incisions sever collagen fibrils in the corneal stroma. This produced a wound gape that flattened it and decreased its refractive power, thereby decreasing myopia (Fig 4-1).

The design of the diamond-blade knife (angle and sharpness of cutting edge, width of blade, and footplate design) influenced both the depth and contour of incisions (Fig 4-2). The length of the knife blade was set based on the corneal thickness, which was usually measured with an ultrasonic pachymeter.

Outcomes

Variables affecting outcome

Variables in RK surgery included the following:

- *Centering.* Corneal surgical procedures preferably centered on the entrance pupil of the eye (although some surgeons centered on the visual axis).
- *Optical zone diameter.* Smaller optical clear zones produced more flattening and a greater reduction of myopia.

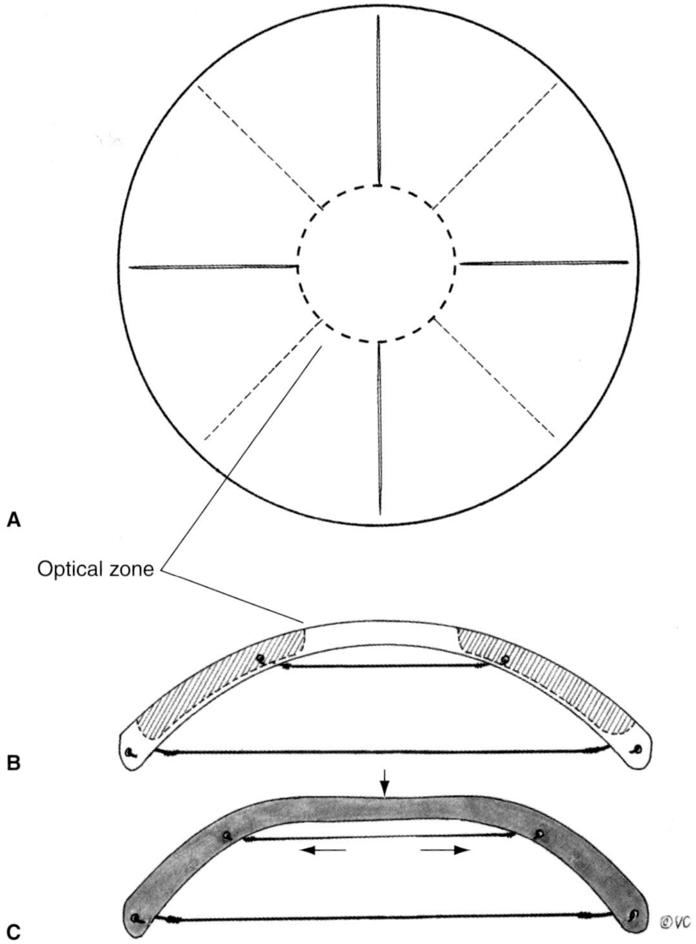

Figure 4-1 Effect of radial incisions. **A,** 8-incision RK with circular central optical zone *(dashed line),* which shows the limit of the inner incision length. **B,** Cross-sectional view of the cornea, showing RK incisions *(shaded areas).* **C,** Flattening is induced in the central cornea. *(Modified from Troutman RC, Buzard KA.* Corneal Astigmatism: Etiology, Prevention, and Management. *St. Louis: Mosby-Year Book; 1992.)*

- *Depth of incisions.* The ideal depth of radial incisions was 85%–90% of the corneal thickness. The deeper the incision, the greater the flattening; however, deeper incisions might have reduced the stability of the refractive outcome and increased the risk of perforation.
- *Age of the patient.* The older the patient, the greater the effect achieved with the same surgical technique. The increase was approximately 0.50 to 1.00 D per decade, which can be accounted for by nomograms.

Efficacy and predictability

The ideal result after surgery was mild residual myopia, on the order of –0.50 D because residual myopia delayed the onset of symptomatic presbyopia and to a degree offset the continued tendency toward hyperopia that occurred in some RK patients.

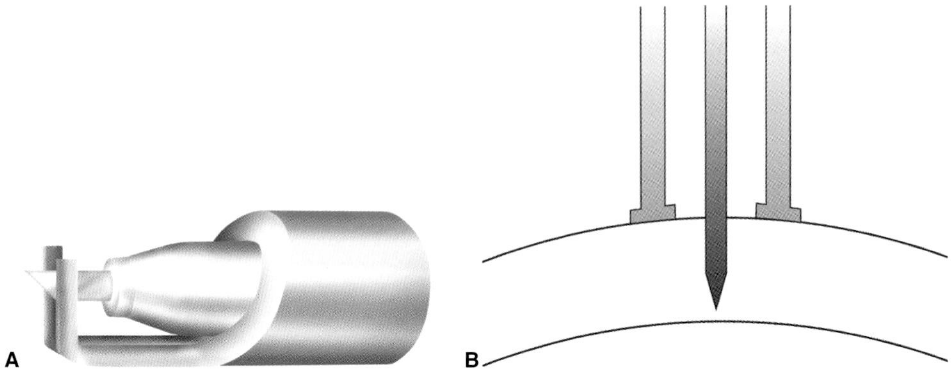

Figure 4-2 **A,** The guarded diamond knife used in RK surgery. Note the footplates and blade between them. The distance from the tip of the blade to the footplates is adjustable. **B,** Diagram of RK diamond blade with footplates that rest on the cornea, reducing the risk of penetration into the anterior chamber. *(Part A courtesy of KMI Surgical; redrawn by Cyndie Wooley.)*

The percentage of eyes with final spherical equivalent refractive error within ±1.00 D ranged from 54% to 96% in various studies. Series that included reoperations for undercorrection generally showed a higher percentage of emmetropic eyes. Among 310 patients with bilateral RK in the PERK study, 70% reported not wearing spectacles or contact lenses for distance vision at 10 years.

Postoperative refraction, visual acuity, and corneal topography

Radial keratotomy changed not only the curvature of the central cornea but also its overall topography, creating a multifocal cornea—flat in the center and steep in the periphery. The result was less correlation among refraction, central keratometry, and UCVA, presumably because the new corneal curvature created a more complex optical system. Thus, keratometric readings, which sample a limited number of points approximately 3.0 mm apart, might show amounts of astigmatism different from those detected by refraction. Similarly, UCVA might vary, particularly depending on pupil diameter: the smaller the pupil, the less the multifocal effect from postoperative corneal contour and the better the quality of vision.

Stability of refraction

Most eyes were generally stable by 3 months after RK surgery. However, 2 phenomena of postoperative refractive instability—diurnal fluctuation of vision and a progressive flattening effect of surgery—have been known to persist for several years.

Diurnal fluctuation of vision could occur because the cornea was flatter upon awakening and gradually steepened during the patient's waking hours. This was thought to be due to local edema of the incisions with the eyelids closed during sleep. In a subset of the PERK study at 10 years, the mean change in the spherical equivalent of refraction between the morning (waking) and evening examinations was an increase of 0.31 ± 0.58 D in minus power in first eyes.

The progressive flattening effect of surgery was one of the major unknowns with RK. The refractive error in 43% of eyes in the PERK study changed in the hyperopic direction by 1.00 D or more between 6 months and 10 years postoperatively. The hyperopic shift was statistically associated with decreasing diameter of the central optical clear zone.

Complications

Probably the best measure of the safety of ocular surgery is the incidence of loss of best spectacle-corrected visual acuity. After RK surgery, 1%–3% of eyes lost 2 or more Snellen lines. Mild to moderate irregular astigmatism has been known to cause visual distortion and glare, especially in patients who had more than 8 incisions, incisions extending inside a 3.0-mm central clear zone, or intersecting radial and transverse incisions (Fig 4-3A, B), and in patients with hypertrophic scarring.

Many patients reported seeing a starburst pattern around lights at night after RK. This presumably resulted from light scattering off the radial incisions and/or scars. Although most patients found the starburst effect comparable to looking through dirty spectacles or contact lenses, some patients could not drive at night because of this complication. Miotic agents such as brimonidine (eg, Alphagan) or pilocarpine could temporarily reduce symptoms by shrinking the pupil, which blocked light from the peripheral cornea. Side effects that did not reduce BCVA included postoperative pain, undercorrection and overcorrection, increased astigmatism, epithelial plugs (see Fig 4-3), vascularization of stromal scars, and nonprogressive endothelial disruption beneath the incisions.

Potentially blinding complications occurred only rarely after RK. These included

- perforation of the cornea, which can lead to endophthalmitis, epithelial downgrowth, and traumatic cataract
- traumatic rupture of the globe through a keratotomy incision (Fig 4-4); this complication has been reported as long as 13 years after RK

Ocular Surgery After Radial Keratotomy

Prior to the advent of excimer laser surgery, unacceptable residual myopia after RK was treated by opening the incisions with a blunt instrument and deepening or extending them to a smaller optical clear zone, or by making additional incisions between the initial ones.

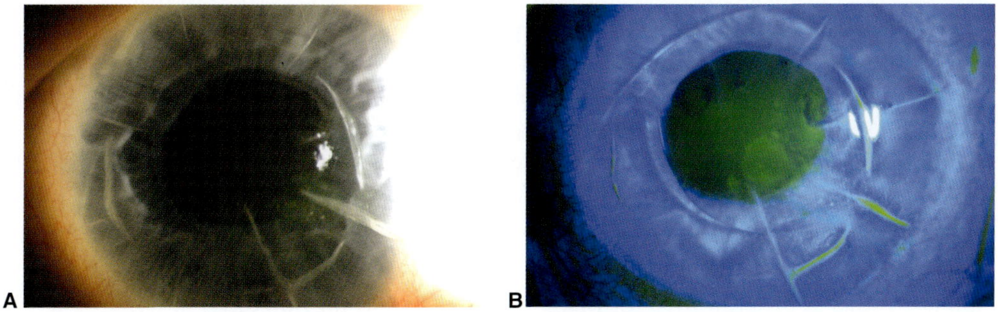

Figure 4-3 **A,** Crossed RK and arcuate keratotomy incisions with epithelial plugs in a patient who had intraoperative corneal perforation. **B,** Fluorescein staining demonstrates gaping of the incisions, causing persistent ocular irritation. *(Photographs courtesy of Jayne S. Weiss, MD.)*

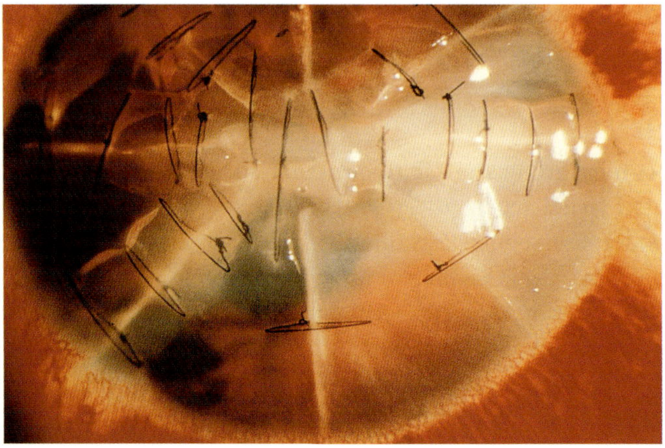

Figure 4-4 Traumatic rupture of an 8-incision RK, showing communication between 2 horizontal RK incisions. Interrupted 10-0 nylon sutures were used to close the incision. *(Reprinted with permission from* External Disease and Cornea: A Multimedia Collection. *San Francisco: American Academy of Ophthalmology; 2000.)*

It is not uncommon for RK patients to present years later with hyperopia, which may be related to the corneal incisions or to naturally occurring crystalline lens changes. LASIK and surface ablation have been shown to be effective in correcting residual hyperopia and myopia after RK. LASIK after RK engenders an increased risk of epithelial ingrowth, which can occur under the flap between the RK incisions and may prove challenging to treat. Performing a LASIK enhancement (flap lift re-treatment with a laser) after RK can cause the incision(s) to splay open, which can change corneal shape unpredictably, as well as increase the risk of epithelial ingrowth. Linebarger and colleagues have recommended modifications of the refractive correction for LASIK following RK. Surface ablation avoids the LASIK-related risks after RK but does increase the risk of postoperative cornea haze. The off-label use of mitomycin C 0.02% (0.2 mg/mL) applied to the cornea with a circular sponge for 12 seconds to 2 minutes has dramatically reduced surface ablation haze after RK and other prior cornea surgeries (eg, corneal transplant and LASIK). The drug should be copiously irrigated from the eye to reduce toxic effects. The refractive correction should be reduced 5%–15% when mitomycin C is used prophylactically.

Patients undergoing laser vision correction for refractive errors should understand that laser correction will not remove scars caused by RK incisions, so glare or fluctuation symptoms will remain after the laser surgery. In addition, obtaining wavefront analysis may not be possible due to complex optical irregularities associated with RK. Because of the progressive hyperopia that can occur with RK, it is prudent to aim for slight myopia with laser vision correction as some patients may still progress to hyperopia in the future. Finally, because of RK-related flattening, a nomogram adjustment must be made to reduce programmed laser correction in order to minimize the chance of significant overcorrection if the laser is programmed for myopia (risk of hyperopic outcome) or hyperopia (risk of myopic outcome).

In patients with endothelial dystrophy, corneal infection, irregular astigmatism, severe visual fluctuations, and starburst effects, PKP may be needed to restore visual functioning. PKP should be avoided if the patient's visual problems can be corrected with glasses or contact lenses. If PKP is deemed necessary, the RK incisions may need to be sutured before trephination to minimize the chance of their opening and to allow adequate suturing of the donor corneal graft to the recipient bed.

Joyal H, Gregoire J, Faucher A. Photorefractive keratectomy to correct hyperopic shift after radial keratotomy. *J Cataract Refract Surg.* 2003;29:1502–1506.

Linebarger EJ, Hardten DR, Lindstrom RL. Laser assisted in-situ keratomileusis for correction of secondary hyperopia after radial keratotomy. *Int Ophthalmol Clin.* 2000;40:125–132.

Salamon SA, Hjortdal JO, Ehlers N. Refractive results of radial keratotomy: a ten-year retrospective study. *Acta Ophthalmol Scand.* 2000;78:566–568.

Cataract extraction with IOL implantation may lead to unintentional hyperopia following RK. In the early postoperative period, corneal edema may be present that can flatten the central cornea and cause hyperopia temporarily. In addition, IOL power calculation may be problematic and may result in undercorrection and hyperopia. Calculation of implant power for cataract surgery after RK should be done using a third-generation formula (eg, Haigis, Hoffer Q, Holladay 2, or SRK/T) rather than a regression formula (eg, SRK I or SRK II) and then choosing the highest resulting IOL power. Keratometric power is determined in 1 of 3 ways: direct measurement using corneal topography; knowledge of pre-RK keratometry minus the refractive change; or adjustment of the base curve of a plano contact lens by the overrefraction (see Chapter 11).

Hill WE, Byrne SF. Complex axial length measurements and unusual IOL power calculations. *Focal Points: Clinical Modules for Ophthalmologists.* San Francisco: American Academy of Ophthalmology; 2004, module 9.

Seitz B, Langenbucher A. Intraocular lens calculations status after corneal refractive surgery. *Curr Opin Ophthalmol.* 2000;11:35–46.

Waring GO III. Radial keratotomy for myopia. *Focal Points: Clinical Modules for Ophthalmologists.* San Francisco: American Academy of Ophthalmology; 1992, module 5.

Incisional Correction of Astigmatism

Several techniques of incisional surgery have been used to correct astigmatism, including transverse (straight) keratotomy and arcuate (curved) keratotomy (AK), where incisions are typically placed in the cornea at the 7-mm optical zone; and limbal relaxing incisions (LRIs), which are curved at the limbus. Transverse keratotomy was frequently used in the past in combination with RK to correct myopic astigmatism, but it is seldom used today. Arcuate keratotomy was also used to correct naturally occurring astigmatism, but it is now used primarily to correct postkeratoplasty astigmatism. LRIs are used to help manage astigmatism during or after phacoemulsification and IOL implantation.

Coupling

When 1 meridian is flattened from an astigmatic incision, an amount of steepening occurs in the meridian 90° away (Fig 4-5). This phenomenon is known as *coupling.* When the coupling ratio (the amount of flattening in the meridian of the incision divided by

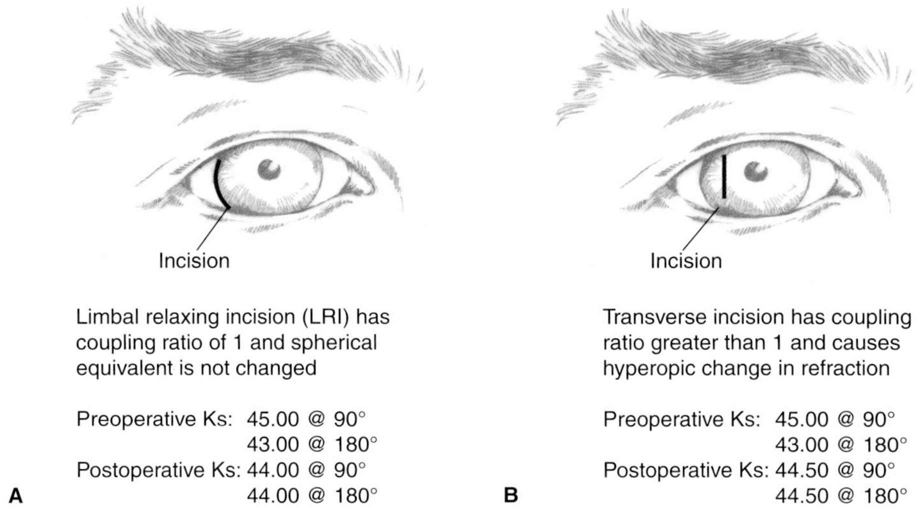

Figure 4-5 Coupling effect of astigmatic incisions. **A,** A limbal relaxing incision (LRI) has a coupling ratio of 1.0, and the spherical equivalent is not changed. **B,** A transverse incision has a coupling ratio greater than 1.0, which causes a hyperopic change in refraction. *(Illustration by Cyndie Wooley.)*

the induced steepening in the opposite meridian) is 1.0, the spherical equivalent remains unchanged. When there is a positive coupling ratio (greater than 1.0), a hyperopic shift occurs. The type of incision (arcuate vs tangential) and the length and number of parallel incisions can influence the coupling ratio. Long, straight, and tangential incisions tend to induce more positive coupling (greater than 1.0), and therefore more hyperopia, than do short, arcuate incisions. When a correction is less than 2.00 D of astigmatism, coupling is typically 1.0, whereas when a correction is greater than 2.00 D of astigmatism, coupling tends to be greater than 1.0. In general, LRIs do not change the spherical equivalent.

Rowsey JJ, Fouraker BD. Corneal coupling principles. *Int Ophthalmol Clin.* 1996;36:29–38.

Arcuate Keratotomy and Limbal Relaxing Incisions

Arcuate keratotomy is an incisional surgical procedure in which arcuate incisions of approximately 95% depth are made in the corneal midperipheral 7.0-mm zone placed in the steep meridian(s). LRIs are incisions set at approximately 600 μm depth, or 50 μm less than the thinnest pachymetry at the limbus, and placed just anterior to the limbus (Fig 4-6). Arcuate keratotomy differs from LRIs by its midperipheral location and its greater relative depth. Due to the concomitant steepening of the orthogonal meridian (coupling), AK and LRIs correct astigmatism without inducing a substantial hyperopic shift of the spherical equivalent of the preoperative refraction. Increased effect in LRIs is achieved primarily by increasing the length of the incision. For AK, cylindrical correction can be increased by increasing the length or depth of the incision, using multiple incisions, or reducing the distance between the AK incisions (Table 4-1).

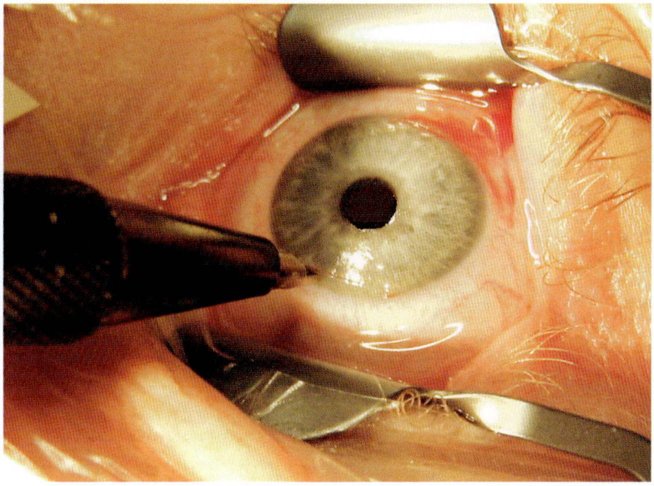

Figure 4-6 Limbal relaxing incision (LRI). A relaxing incision is made at the limbus using a diamond knife. The coupling ratio is typically 1.0. *(Courtesy of Eric Donnenfeld, MD, and Brian S. Boxer Wachler, MD.)*

Instrumentation

The instruments used in AK and LRIs are similar. Front-cutting diamond blades are more often used in AK, and back-cutting diamond blades are more often used in LRI surgery. A mechanized trephine, the Hanna arcuate trephine, has been shown to make smooth curvilinear AK incisions of specified optical zone and arc length. This has led to the development of other mechanized systems aimed at achieving smooth AK and LRI incisions, such as the Terry Astigmatome (Fig 4-7).

Table 4-1 Sample Nomogram for Limbal Relaxing Incisions to Correct Keratometric Astigmatism During Cataract Surgery

Preoperative Astigmatism (D)	Age (Years)	Number	Length (Degrees)
With-the-rule			
0.75–1.00	<65	2	45
	≥65	1	45
1.01–1.50	<65	2	60
	≥65	2	45 (or 1 × 60)
>1.50	<65	2	80
	≥65	2	60
Against-the-rule/oblique*			
1.00–1.25†	–	1	35
1.26–2.00	–	1	45
>2.00	–	2	45

*Combined with temporal corneal incision.

†Especially if cataract incision is not directly centered on the steep meridian.

From Wang L, Misra M, Koch DD. Peripheral corneal relaxing incisions combined with cataract surgery. *J Cataract Refract Surg.* 2003;29:712–722.

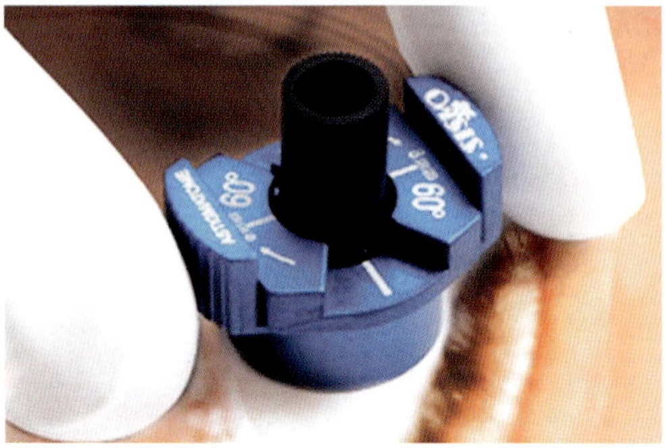

Figure 4-7 The Terry Astigmatome uses circular blades at preset depths for standardized astigmatic incisions of various arc lengths. The circular blades *(black)* are placed within the holder *(blue)* to maintain centration during the procedure. *(Courtesy of Oasis Medical, Inc.)*

Surgical Techniques

With any astigmatism correction system, accurate determination of the steep axis is essential. The plus cylinder axis of the manifest refraction is used, as this accounts for corneal and lenticular astigmatism, which are "manifest" in the refraction. If the crystalline lens is to be removed at the time of the astigmatic incisional surgery (ie, LRI), the correction should be based on the steep meridian and magnitude as measured with corneal topography or keratometry. The amount of treatment for a given degree of astigmatism can be determined from a nomogram, such as Table 4-1.

It is prudent to make horizontal reference marks using a surgical marking pen, with the patient sitting up, preferably at the slit lamp. Marking with the patient in this position avoids reference mark error due to cyclorotation of the eyes. Arcuate keratotomy incisions may be placed in pairs along the steep meridian and, because of induced glare and aberrations, no closer than 3.5 mm from the center of the pupil. LRIs are placed in the peripheral cornea. They result in lower amounts of astigmatic correction than do AK incisions. Arcuate keratotomy incisions used to correct post-PKP astigmatism are often made in the graft. When AK incisions are made in the graft–host junction or in the host, the effect of the incisions is reduced.

Outcomes

The outcome of AK and LRIs depends on several variables, including patient age; the distance separating the incision pairs; and the length, depth, and number of incisions. Few large prospective trials have been done. The ARC-T trial of AK, which used a 7.0-mm optical zone and varying arc lengths, showed a reduction in astigmatism of 1.6 ± 1.1 D in patients with preoperative naturally occurring astigmatism of 2.8 ± 1.2 D. Other studies have shown a final UCVA of 20/40 in 65%–80% of eyes. Overcorrections have been reported in 4%–20% of patients.

Studies of LRIs are limited, but these incisions are frequently used with seemingly good results in astigmatic patients undergoing cataract surgery. One study showed an absolute change in refractive astigmatism of 1.72 ± 0.81 D after LRIs in patients with mixed astigmatism. Astigmatism was decreased by 0.91 D, or 44%, in another series of LRIs in 22 eyes of 13 patients. Incisions in the horizontal meridian have been reported to cause approximately twice as much astigmatic correction as those in the vertical meridian (see Table 4-1).

Complications

Irregular astigmatism may occur following both AK and LRIs; however, it is more common with AK than with LRIs, probably because LRIs are farther from the cornea center, thus mitigating any effects of irregular incisions. Off-axis AK can lead to undercorrection or even worsening of preexisting astigmatism. To avoid creating an edge of cornea that swells and cannot be epithelialized, arcuate incisions and LRIs should not intersect other incisions (see Fig 4-3). Corneal infection and perforation have been reported.

Ocular Surgery After Arcuate Keratotomy and Limbal Relaxing Incisions

Arcuate keratotomy and LRIs can be combined with or done after cataract surgery, RK, surface ablation, or LASIK surgery. PKP can be done after extensive AK, but the wounds may have to be sutured before trephination, as discussed earlier for RK. A prerequisite for combining LRIs with cataract surgery is the use of astigmatically neutral, small-incision, phacoemulsification with self-sealing peripheral corneal incisions.

Bayramlar HH, Daglioglu MC, Borazan M. Limbal relaxing incisions for primary mixed astigmatism and mixed astigmatism after cataract surgery. *J Cataract Refract Surg.* 2003; 29:723–728.

Budak K, Yilmaz G, Aslan BS, Duman S. Limbal relaxing incisions in congenital astigmatism: 6 month follow-up. *J Cataract Refract Surg.* 2001;27:715–719.

Faktorovich EG, Maloney RK, Price FW Jr. Effect of astigmatic keratotomy on spherical equivalent: results of the Astigmatism Reduction Clinical Trial. *Am J Ophthalmol.* 1999;127:260–269.

Nichamin LD. Astigmatism control. *Ophthalmol Clin North Am.* 2006;19:485–493.

Price FW, Grene RB, Marks RG, Gonzales JS; ARC-T Study Group. Astigmatism Reduction Clinical Trial: a multicenter prospective evaluation of the predictability of arcuate keratotomy. Evolution of surgical nomogram predictability. *Arch Ophthalmol.* 1995;113:277–282.

CHAPTER 5

Onlays and Inlays

Refractive errors, including presbyopia, can be corrected by placing preformed tissue or synthetic material onto or into the cornea. This alters the optical power of the cornea by changing the shape of the anterior corneal surface or by creating a lens with a higher index of refraction than that of the corneal stroma. Tissue addition procedures, such as epikeratoplasty, have fallen out of favor because of the poor predictability of the refractive and visual results, loss of best-corrected visual acuity (BCVA), and difficulty in obtaining donor tissue. Synthetic material can be shaped to greater precision than donor tissue and can be mass produced. Because of problems with re-epithelialization of synthetic material placed on top of the cornea, synthetic material generally has to be placed within the corneal stroma. This requires a partial or complete lamellar dissection with specialized instruments. Early work using lenticules of glass and plastic resulted in necrosis of the overlying stroma because these substances are impermeable to water, oxygen, and nutrients. Current techniques use lenticule inlays made of more permeable substances such as hydrogel, with or without microperforations in the lenticule, to increase the transmission of nutrients. Another type of inlay indirectly alters the shape of the cornea using ring segments of polymethylmethacrylate (PMMA; Intacs [Addition Techology, Des Plaines, IL] and Ferrara rings [Ferrara Ophthalmics, Belo Horizonte, Brazil]). Because the ring segments are narrow, the overlying stroma can receive nutrients from surrounding tissue.

Keratophakia

In keratophakia, a plus-power lens is placed intrastromally to increase the curvature of the anterior cornea for the correction of hyperopia. After a central lamellar keratectomy with a microkeratome or femtosecond laser, the flap is lifted, the lenticule is placed onto the host bed, and the flap is replaced and adheres without sutures. The lenticule can be prepared either from donor cornea (homoplastic) or synthetic material (alloplastic). The homoplastic lenticule is created from a donor cornea by a lamellar keratectomy after removal of the epithelium and Bowman's layer. The lenticule (fresh or frozen) is then shaped into a lens with an automated lathe. The lens of tissue can be preserved fresh in refrigerated tissue culture medium, frozen at subzero temperatures, or freeze-dried.

Homoplastic Corneal Inlays

Keratophakia has been used to correct aphakia and hyperopia of up to 20 D, but few studies have been published on this procedure. Troutman and colleagues reported on 32 eyes treated with homoplastic keratophakia, 29 of which also underwent cataract extraction. Even when the surgeons were more experienced, in their second series, predictability was still low: 25% of patients were more than 3 D from the intended correction. Complications included irregular lamellar resection, wound dehiscence, and postoperative corneal edema. Although the procedure was originally intended to be used in conjunction with cataract extraction for the correction of aphakia, the complexity of the procedure and the unpredictable refractive results could not compete with aphakic contact lenses or the improved technology of intraocular lens (IOL) implantation in the early 1980s. Homoplastic keratophakia is largely obsolete.

Alloplastic Corneal Inlays

Synthetic inlays offer several potential advantages over homoplastic inlays, such as the ability to be mass produced in a wide range of sizes and powers that can be measured and verified. Also, synthetic material may have optical properties superior to those of tissue lenses, which are difficult to lathe accurately. Tissue lenticules, for example, can become distorted upon insertion and may undergo remodeling, which can prolong postoperative visual recovery and can lead to refractive instability—problems not found as much with synthetic material.

A variety of materials have been tried for inlays. Beginning in 1949, Barraquer experimented with flint glass and Plexiglas intracorneal lenses (6 mm diameter) in rabbits and cats, but he abandoned their use because of anterior corneal stromal necrosis and eventual implant extrusion. Polysulfone, another material tried, is impermeable, with excellent optical qualities and a high index of refraction (1.633). Because it can serve as an intrastromal lens, no change in anterior corneal curvature is required, as it is for hydrogel implants. For insertion of the inlay, a stromal pocket dissection can be performed; this is technically easier than a complete lamellar keratectomy. Experiments in the early 1980s had disappointing results because of corneal opacities, nonhealing epithelial erosions, and diurnal fluctuations in vision. These results led to the incorporation of microperforations into the inlay for the transfer of fluid and nutrients to the anterior cornea. Although fenestrated polysulfone (35-μm fenestrations) showed increased safety in cat corneas, it proved to be optically unsatisfactory. Smaller fenestrations (10 μm) may preserve the optical properties of implanted polysulfone and still provide adequate nourishment to the anterior cornea.

Knowles and many subsequent investigators demonstrated the importance of the implant's fluid and nutrient permeability to the nourishment of the overlying anterior stroma. Because of their work, most succeeding studies used water-permeable hydrogel implants. Hydrogel lenses have an index of refraction similar to that of the corneal stroma, so they have little intrinsic optical power when implanted. To be effective, they must change the curvature of the anterior cornea.

The AcuFocus corneal inlay (Bausch & Lomb/AcuFocus, Irvine, CA) is undergoing FDA clinical trials for the treatment of presbyopia. This device is composed of an ultrathin, biocompatible polymer that is microperforated to allow nutrient flow. The 3.8-mm-diameter inlay has a central aperture of 1.6 mm. In the nondominant eye, a thick corneal flap is created, and the inlay is placed on the stromal bed, centered on the pupil. Although the inlay has no refractive power, the goal of the device is to have the central aperture function as a pinhole to increase depth of focus and improve near vision without changing distance vision. (See also Chapter 9.)

Barraquer JI. Modification of refraction by means of intracorneal inclusions. *Int Ophthalmol Clin.* 1966;6:53–78.

Ismail MM. Correction of hyperopia with intracorneal implants. *J Cataract Refract Surg.* 2002;28:527–530.

Jankov M, Mrochen MC, Bueeler M, et al. Experimental results of preparing laser-shaped stromal implants for laser-assisted intrastromal keratophakia in extremely complicated laser in situ keratomileusis cases. *J Refract Surg.* 2002;18:S639–S643.

Epikeratoplasty

Background

To eliminate the complexity of the lamellar dissection and intraoperative lathing of early keratomileusis procedures, in which a corneal cap was dissected from the eye, shaped on a cryolathe, and then repositioned with sutures, Kaufman and Werblin developed *epikeratoplasty* (also called *epikeratophakia*) in the early 1980s. A largely obsolete procedure now, epikeratoplasty involves suturing a preformed lenticule of human donor corneal tissue directly onto Bowman's layer of the host cornea (Fig 5-1). Because no viable cells exist in the donor tissue, classic graft rejection does not occur. Epikeratoplasty was originally intended as a "living contact lens" for aphakic patients who were unable to wear contact lenses. Epikeratoplasty was later expanded to include the treatment of hyperopia, myopia, and keratoconus.

Werblin TP, Kaufman HE, Friedlander MH, Sehon KL, McDonald MB, Granet NS. A prospective study of the use of hyperopic epikeratophakia grafts for the correction of aphakia in adults. *Ophthalmology.* 1981;88:1137–1140.

Technique

To prepare the host cornea, the epithelium is removed and an annular keratectomy performed, with resection of a 0.5- to 1.0-mm wedge of Bowman's layer and anterior stroma

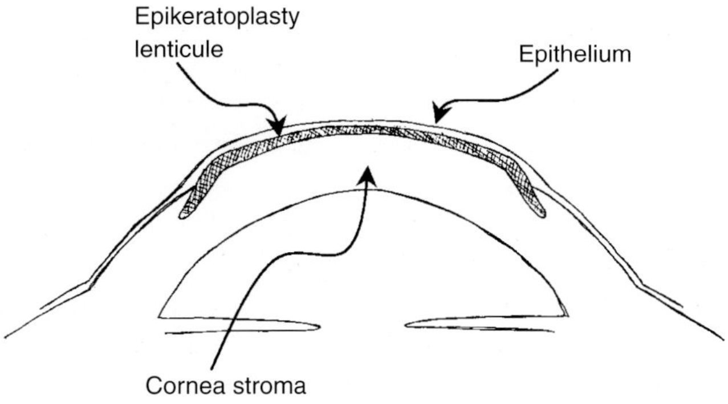

Figure 5-1 The lenticule in epikeratoplasty is sutured onto the cornea after removal of the epithelium. The edge of the lenticule is placed into a shallow lamellar dissection and tucked under the peripheral cornea.

from the inner aspect of a partial-thickness 7–8 mm trephine. A partial lamellar dissection peripheral to the trephine allows the edge of the lenticule to be tucked under the host tissue (Fig 5-2A, B). These lenticules can be removed at a later date by dissecting the periphery to find the interface and then bluntly separating the lenticule from Bowman's layer.

Outcomes

Studies were conducted initially on nonhuman primates and later expanded to include human adults. Four large nationwide studies (on adult and pediatric aphakia, keratoconus, and myopia), with a collective total of 1389 cases, were conducted after commercially prepared tissue became available in 1984. The refractive results of myopic epikeratoplasty, aphakic epikeratoplasty, and keratoconus epikeratoplasty were disappointing. Predictability of the refractive outcomes was poor.

Complications

Delayed re-epithelialization over the lenticule was a major complication in epikeratoplasty that was never fully overcome. Bandage contact lenses, patching, temporary tarsorrhaphies, and changes in lathing and preservation techniques of the lenticule were tried, but the incidence of nonhealing defects in the large nationwide series was 2.5%–3.5%. The consequences of failure to re-epithelialize were severe and included necrosis, infection, and melting of the graft. Other complications and causes for lenticule removal included graft haze and/or scar, infection, stromal infiltrates, melting, dehiscence, refractive error, irregular astigmatism, epithelial ingrowth, interface cysts, and severe glare symptoms. After lenticule removal, 14% of patients who had undergone epikeratoplasty for myopia had a reduction of BCVA.

Alloplastic Corneal Onlays

Laser-adjustable synthetic epikeratoplasty has been proposed as an adjustable and reversible refractive procedure. It is similar to standard epikeratoplasty, except that a synthetic lenticule is used. This procedure eliminates many of the disadvantages of human tissue, such as the difficulty of lathing, the production of consistent and measurable lenticules,

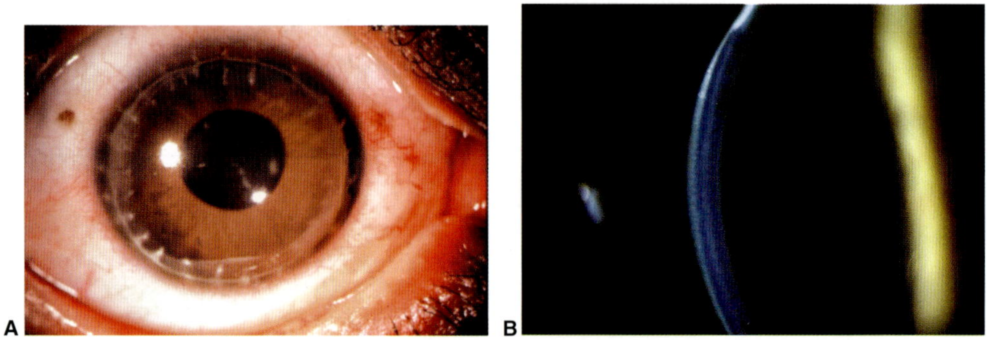

Figure 5-2 **A,** Epikeratoplasty after suture removal. **B,** A slit-lamp cross section shows the interface between the lenticule and the host cornea. *(Part A courtesy of Jayne S. Weiss, MD; part B courtesy of Steven C. Schallhorn, MD.)*

distortion upon suturing, and postoperative remodeling that causes changes in refraction. If further refractive correction is required after the synthetic lenticule is placed, a laser is used to remodel the anterior surface. The properties of the synthetic material are the key to the success of this technique. It must have satisfactory optical quality and biocompatibility without in vivo degradation, and it must be able to promote stable epithelial attachments. Because the ideal synthetic material has not yet been found, laser-adjustable synthetic epikeratoplasty has not progressed beyond the experimental stage.

Intrastromal Corneal Ring Segments

Background

Intrastromal corneal ring segments (ICRS; Intacs and Ferrara rings) can treat low amounts of myopia by displacing the lamellar bundles and shortening the corneal arc length. These circular rings of PMMA are placed in the midperipheral corneal stroma in a lamellar channel (Figs 5-3, 5-4). The thicker the segment, the greater the flattening of the cornea and the greater the reduction in myopia. Ferrara rings have a smaller optical zone and more of a flattening effect than Intacs. This section discusses Intacs, because Ferrara rings, although commonly used in South America, are not FDA approved in the United States.

Ring segments have several potential advantages over other forms of refractive surgery. The ring segments can be explanted, making the refractive result of the procedure potentially reversible, and the ring segments can be replaced with ring segments of a different thickness to titrate the refractive result. Unlike with surface ablation or LASIK, the central clear zone of the cornea is not directly treated. The normal cornea is generally prolate, or steeper centrally than peripherally: the central cornea profile after placement

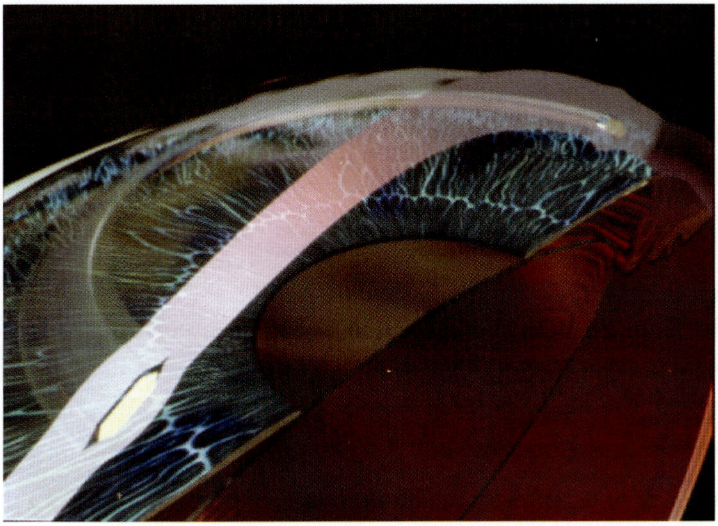

Figure 5-3 Cross section of the cornea with an intrastromal corneal ring segment. The ring segment displaces the lamellar bundles, which shortens the corneal arc length and reduces the myopia. *(Courtesy of Addition Technology.)*

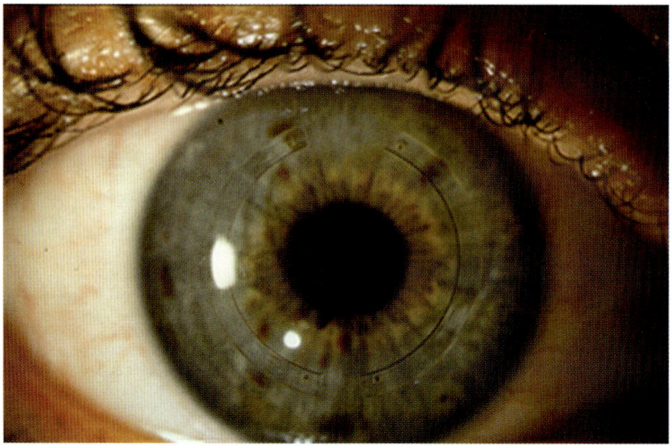

Figure 5-4 Ring segments implanted in an eye to treat low myopia. Note the vertical placement of the ring segments with a clear central zone. *(Courtesy of Steven C. Schallhorn, MD.)*

of ring segments has been shown to maintain an aspheric, prolate shape because the ring segments flatten the peripheral cornea more than the central cornea. It has been suggested that a prolate cornea may minimize visual disturbances, such as glare and halo symptoms. Conventional myopic excimer laser procedures flatten the central cornea more than the peripheral cornea, which typically produces an oblate (flattened) central corneal shape.

Intrastromal ring segments also have several disadvantages. Specialized equipment and training are required to create the lamellar channels and to insert the ring segments. The procedure generally takes longer to perform than LASIK. Patients can experience ocular discomfort after surgery, and some patients, especially those with large pupils, may complain of visual disturbances such as glare. Only low levels of myopia can be treated. Ring segments cannot currently correct hyperopia. Even in the low myopia range, ring segments have declined in popularity; excimer laser surgery remains much more popular for correcting myopia in the Intacs-approved range.

Patient Selection for Myopia

Intacs are approved by the FDA to treat low levels of myopia (−1.00 to −3.00 D spherical equivalent) and are not indicated for patients with astigmatism. Additional selection criteria are for patients

- 21 years or older
- with documented stability of refraction, as demonstrated by a change of ≤0.50 D for at least 12 months prior to the preoperative examination
- with 1.00 D of astigmatism or less

Intacs are typically contraindicated in

- patients with collagen vascular, autoimmune, or immunodeficiency diseases
- pregnant or nursing women
- the presence of ocular conditions (such as recurrent corneal erosion syndrome, or corneal dystrophy) that may predispose the patient to future complications

Intacs are generally not recommended in

- patients with a low-light pupil diameter of 7.0 mm or larger because of the predisposition to low-light visual symptoms (the inner segment diameter is 6.8 mm)
- patients with systemic diseases likely to affect wound healing, such as insulin-dependent diabetes or severe atopic disease
- patients with a history of ophthalmic herpes simplex or herpes zoster
- eyes with a central corneal thickness of less than 480 μm or a peripheral thickness of less than 570 μm
- eyes with a corneal keratometry steeper than 46.00 D or flatter than 40.00 D

Instrumentation

Initially, a 1-piece 330° Intacs segment was used in the procedure, but this was difficult to insert. The 1-piece segment was changed to 2 segments of 150° of arc. The segments have a fixed outer diameter of 8.10 mm and are available in 5 thicknesses: 0.250, 0.275, 0.300, 0.325, and 0.350 mm. Two additional segments, 0.400 and 0.450 mm, are available outside the United States. The amount of correction achieved is related to the thickness of the ring segments; the thicker ring segments are used for higher amounts of correction (Table 5-1).

A special set of surgical instruments has been developed for placing the ring segments. The set includes an incision and placement marker, glide tip, ring forceps, stromal spreader, vacuum centering guide with vacuum system, and clockwise and counterclockwise dissectors. Other necessary equipment includes an ultrasonic pachymeter and a guarded diamond knife. A femtosecond laser can also be used to create the channels.

Technique

The ring segment procedure involves creating a lamellar channel at approximately 68%–70% stromal depth and then inserting the ring segments. The procedure usually takes 10–15 minutes per eye to complete.

The eye is prepped with a topical anesthetic and an iodine solution, after which an eyelid speculum is inserted. The geometric center of the cornea or pupil is marked with a blunt

Table 5-1 Ring Segment Thickness and Predicted Correction for Intrastromal Corneal Ring Segments (Intacs)

Ring Segment Thickness	Predicted Correction	Recommended Prescribing Range
0.250 mm	−1.30 D	−1.00 to −1.63 D
0.275 mm	−1.65 D	−1.625 to −1.75 D
0.300 mm	−2.00 D	−1.75 to −2.25 D
0.325 mm	−2.35 D	−2.25 to −2.50 D
0.350 mm	−2.70 D	−2.375 to −3.00 D

Note: There is overlap in the prescribing ranges. For instance, the predicted correction for the 0.275-mm ring segments is −1.65 D and for the 0.300-mm ring segments is −2.00 D. To treat −1.75 D, the 0.275-mm ring segments would have a nominal postoperative refraction of −0.10 D, and the 0.300-mm ring segments would have a nominal postoperative refraction of +0.25 D. The choice of ring size, therefore, depends on whether the target is slightly myopic or slightly hyperopic.

hook using light pressure. The incision and placement device, using the center of the cornea as a reference, marks the radial entry incision at an optical zone of 7.5 mm and also indicates the ring segments' final positions. An ultrasound pachymeter is used to measure the thickness of the cornea over the radial incision mark. A diamond knife is set to 68%–70% of the stromal depth and then used to create a 1.0-mm radial incision. A lamellar channel is started using the stromal spreader tool. The vacuum centering guide is placed over the eye using the central corneal mark, and vacuum is applied and confirmed. The clockwise glide tip is placed in the lamellar channel, the clockwise dissector is engaged in the centering guide, and the tip is placed under the glide. While vacuum is maintained to stabilize the eye, the dissector is rotated clockwise to create the left-hand side of the intrastromal tunnel (Fig 5-5); then the counterclockwise dissection for the right-hand tunnel is performed, and the suction device is removed. A similar tunnel may be created using a spiral application of energy with a femtosecond laser. The tunnel is created as a ring at a desired inner and outer diameter. Once the tunnel is created, by either technique, an Intacs forceps is used to insert the first ring segment, rotating it into position, and then the second. One or two 10-0 nylon sutures may be used to close the radial incision at the corneal surface.

Outcomes

The FDA clinical trials provided the most complete outcome analysis of Intacs for myopia. A total of 452 patients enrolled in these trials. The patients received the 0.25-, 0.30-, or 0.35-mm ring segments to correct an average preoperative mean spherical equivalent of −2.240 D, with a range of −0.750 to −4.125 D. At 12 months postoperatively, 97% of eyes had 20/40 or better uncorrected vision and 74% had achieved 20/20 or better. In addition, 69% and 92% of eyes were within ±0.50 and 1.00 D of emmetropia, respectively. These clinical outcomes were similar to early PRK and LASIK results, although excimer laser studies generally had a broader range of preoperative myopia.

Patients who received the 0.35-mm ring segment were more likely to have a worse outcome, in terms of both refractive accuracy and postoperative uncorrected visual acuity. The larger ring segment was also associated with a higher rate of removal due to patient

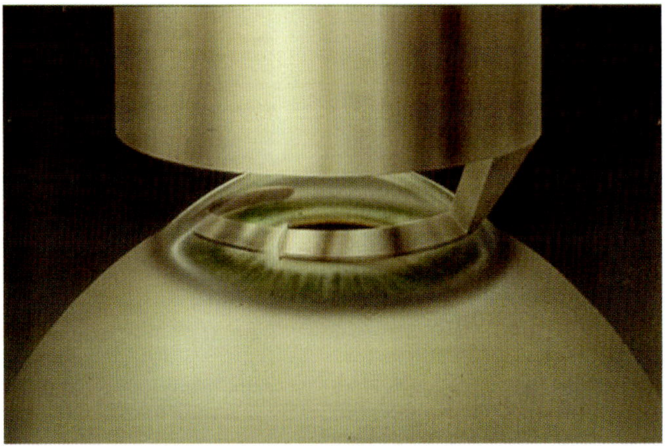

Figure 5-5 The Intacs dissector tool is being rotated to create the intrastromal tunnel. The suction ring and centering guide are not shown. *(Courtesy of Addition Technology.)*

dissatisfaction. In clinical trials, the 0.35-mm ring segments were removed at a rate of 13.3% versus a removal rate of 6.4% and 3.4% for the 0.30- and 0.25-mm ring segments, respectively.

The removal or exchange rate has been reported to vary between 3% and 15%. The most common reason for a ring segment exchange is residual myopia. Ring segment removal is most often performed for disabling visual symptoms such as glare, double vision, or photophobia. Few complications are associated with ring segment removal. In one series of 684 eyes that received Intacs, 46 underwent removal (6.7%). Most patients returned to their original preoperative myopia by 3 months postremoval (73% returned to within 0.50 D of preoperative mean spherical equivalent). No patient had a loss of BCVA of more than 2 lines. However, up to 15% of patients reported new or worsening symptoms after removal.

Intacs and Keratoconus

Other than penetrating and lamellar keratoplasty, very few surgical options are available for keratoconus. Excimer laser procedures, which correct ametropia by removing tissue, are generally not recommended in treating keratoconus due to the risk of exacerbating corneal structural weakening and ectasia.

Intacs received a Humanitarian Device Exemption (HDE; see Chapter 2) from the FDA in 2004 for use in reducing or eliminating myopia and astigmatism in certain patients with keratoconus, specifically those who are no longer able to achieve adequate vision with their contact lenses or spectacles. The intent is to restore functional vision and defer the need for a corneal transplant. Labeled selection criteria for patients include

- experience with a progressive deterioration in vision such that the patient can no longer achieve adequate functional vision on a daily basis with contact lenses or spectacles
- age 21 years or older
- clear central corneas
- a corneal thickness of 450 µm or greater at the proposed incision site
- corneal transplantation is the only remaining option for improving functional vision

Although these are FDA labeling parameters, many surgeons are performing Intacs insertion outside these criteria. In one study of 26 keratoconus patients, the ring segments were oriented horizontally, with a thick ring (0.45 mm, not currently available in the United States) in the inferior cornea and a thinner one (0.25 mm) in the superior cornea. In another study of 50 patients (74 eyes), the orientation of the ring segments was adjusted according to the refractive cylinder. Based on the level of myopia, either the 0.30-mm or the 0.35-mm ring (the largest currently available in the United States) was placed inferiorly, and the 0.25-mm ring was placed superiorly. Patients had mild to severe keratoconus with or without scarring. A superficial channel with Bowman's layer perforation in 1 eye was the only operative complication. A total of 6 rings were explanted for segment migration and externalization (1 ring) and foreign-body sensation (5 rings).

The visual improvement was significant. With an average follow-up of 9 months, the mean UCVA improved from approximately 20/200 (1.05 logMAR) to 20/80 (0.61 logMAR) ($P < .01$). The mean BCVA also improved, from approximately 20/50 (0.41 logMAR) to

20/32 (0.24 logMAR) ($P < .01$). Most patients still required optical correction to achieve their best-corrected vision. Eyes with corneal scarring had a similar improvement in UCVA and BCVA. Inferior steepening was reduced on topography. The dioptric power of the inferior cornea relative to the superior (I–S value) was reduced from a preoperative mean of 25.62 to 6.60 postoperatively.

One or two Intacs segments?

New data indicate that when the keratoconus is peripheral, not central, it may be preferable to place a single segment instead of 2 segments. The reason is that the keratoconic cornea has 2 optical areas of distortion within the pupil: a steep lower area and flat upper area. For peripheral keratoconus, instead of flattening the entire cornea, it is better to flatten the steep area and steepen the flat area. Single-segment placement can achieve that result (Fig 5-6). When a single segment is placed, it flattens the adjacent cornea but causes steepening of the cornea 180° away—the "bean bag effect" (when one sits on a bean bag, the bag flattens in one area and pops up in another area). This yields a more physiologic improvement than a global flattening effect from double segments. Intacs can also be combined with C3-R (corneal collagen cross-linking with riboflavin) to yield additional flattening and improved corneal strength. C3-R is not yet FDA approved.

Chan CC, Sharma M, Boxer Wachler BS. Effect of inferior-segment Intacs with and without C3-R on keratoconus. *J Cataract Refract Surg.* 2007;33:75–80.

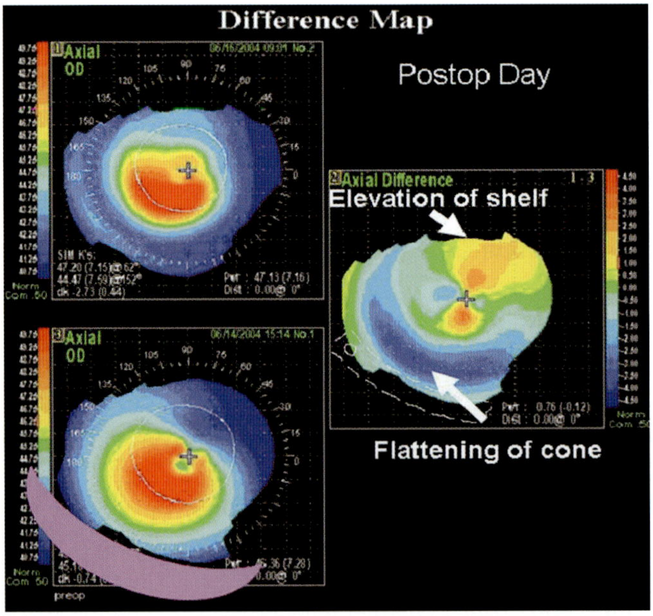

Figure 5-6 Corneal topography analysis before and after single-segment Intacs *(purple).* The preoperative topography *(lower left)* shows oblique steepening, and the postoperative topography *(upper left)* shows the result after a single-segment Intacs was placed outside the cone. The difference map (subtraction of pre- and postoperative topography) *(at right)* shows flattening over the cone *(blue)* and steepening *(red)* in the overly flat area. *(Courtesy of Brian S. Boxer Wachler, MD.)*

Sharma M, Boxer Wachler BS. Comparison of single-segment and double-segment Intacs for keratoconus and post-LASIK ectasia. *Am J Ophthalmol.* 2006;141:891–895.

Wollensak G, Spoerl E, Seiler T. Riboflavin/ultraviolet-a-induced collagen crosslinking for the treatment of keratoconus. *Am J Ophthalmol.* 2003;135:620–627.

Complications

The loss of BCVA (≥2 lines of vision) after Intacs insertion is approximately 1% at 1 year postoperatively. Adverse events (defined as events that, if left untreated, could be serious or result in permanent sequelae) occur in approximately 1% of patients. Reported adverse events include

- anterior chamber perforation
- microbial keratitis
- implant extrusion (Fig 5-7)
- shallow ring segment placement
- corneal thinning over Intacs (Fig 5-8)

Ocular complications (defined as clinically significant events that will not result in permanent sequelae) have been reported in 11% of patients at 12 months postoperatively. These include

- reduced corneal sensitivity (5.5%)
- induced astigmatism between 1 and 2 D (3.7%)
- deep neovascularization at the incision site (1.2%)

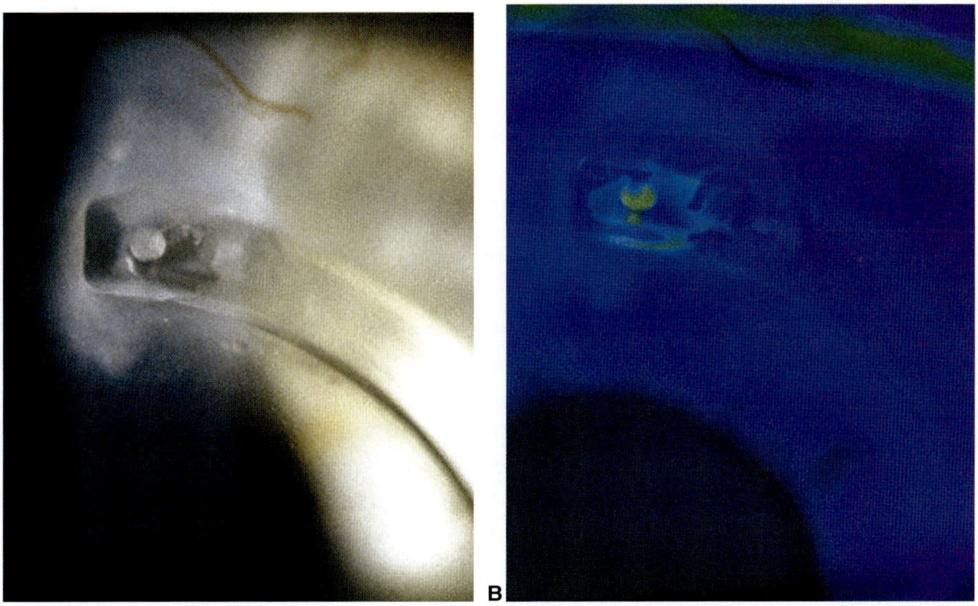

A B

Figure 5-7 Intacs extrusion. **A,** Tip extrusion. **B,** Tip extrusion easily seen with fluorescein. *(Courtesy of Brian S. Boxer Wachler, MD.)*

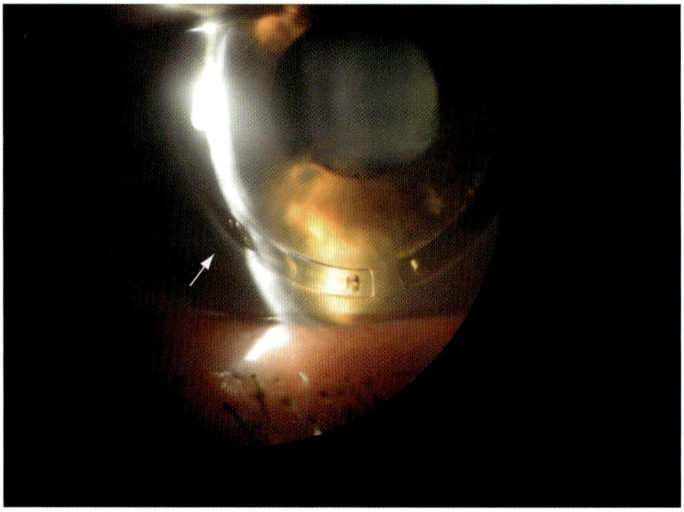

Figure 5-8 Complications of Intacs. Corneal thinning over Intacs segment from NSAID abuse. *(Courtesy of Brian S. Boxer Wachler, MD.)*

- persistent epithelial defect (0.2%)
- iritis/uveitis (0.2%)

Visual symptoms rated as always present and severe in nature have been reported in approximately 14% of patients and include

- difficulty with night vision (4.8%)
- blurred vision (2.9%)
- diplopia (1.6%)
- glare (1.3%)
- halos (1.3%)
- fluctuating distance vision (1.0%)
- fluctuating near vision (0.3%)
- photophobia (0.3%)

Fine white deposits occur frequently within the lamellar ring channels after Intacs placement (Fig 5-9). The incidence and density of the deposits increase with the ring segment thickness and the duration of implantation. Deposits do not seem to alter the optical performance of the ring segments or to result in corneal thinning or necrosis, although some patients are bothered by their appearance.

Intacs achieve the best results in eyes with mild to moderate keratoconus. The goals are generally to improve vision and reduce distortions and are based on degree of keratoconus. For example, a patient with mild keratoconus and best-corrected spectacle visual acuity (BCSVA) of 20/30 may have the goal of improved quality of vision in glasses or soft contact lenses. On the other hand, a contact lens–intolerant patient with more advanced keratoconus and BCSVA of 20/60 may have the goal of improved ability to wear a rigid gas-permeable contact lens. For some advanced cases of keratoconus, such as eyes with keratometry values over 60.00 D, the likelihood of functional vision improvement is less

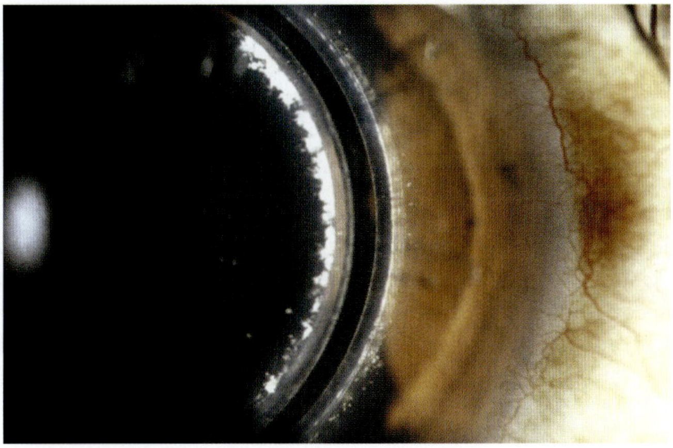

Figure 5-9 Grade 4 deposits around ring segments. The deposits can be graded on a 0 (none) to 4 (confluent) scale. These channel deposits are typically not seen until weeks or months after surgery. Although the corneal opacities may cause cosmetic complaints, they usually do not cause other ocular problems. *(Courtesy of Addition Technology.)*

compared to that for eyes with flatter keratometry values. In such cases, despite Intacs, a corneal transplant may not be avoided.

Ectasia after LASIK

Ring segments have also been used for the postoperative management of corneal ectasia after LASIK. As in the treatment of keratoconus, few surgical options are available to treat corneal ectasia. Use of the excimer laser to remove additional tissue is, in general, considered contraindicated. A lamellar graft or penetrating keratoplasty can have significant morbidity, such as irregular astigmatism, delayed visual recovery, and tissue rejection. In limited early trials using Intacs to treat post-LASIK ectasia, myopia was reduced and UCVA was improved. However, the long-term effect of such an approach for managing post-LASIK ectasia is still being evaluated. Use of Intacs for post-LASIK ectasia is off-label.

Kymionis GD, Tsiklis NS, Pallikaris AI, et al. Long-term follow-up of Intacs for post-LASIK corneal ectasia. *Ophthalmology.* 2006;113:1909–1917.

Uses for Intrastromal Corneal Ring Segments After LASIK

Corneal ring segments have been used to correct residual myopia following LASIK with good initial results. In such cases, a nomogram adjustment is necessary to reduce the risk of overcorrection. This procedure may be useful in patients whose stromal bed would not support repeat excimer laser ablation. Conversely, after ring segments have been removed from patients whose vision did not improve to a satisfactory level (eg, due to undercorrection or induced astigmatism), LASIK has been performed with good success. The flap is created in a plane superficial to the previous ring segment channel.

Boxer Wachler BS, Christie JP, Chandra NS, Chou B, Korn T, Nepomuceno R. Intacs for keratoconus. *Ophthalmology.* 2003;110:1031–1040.

Holmes-Higgin DK, Burris TE; Intacs Study Group. Corneal surface topography and associated visual performance with Intacs for myopia: phase III clinical trial results. *Ophthalmology.* 2000;107:2061–2071.

Kymionis GD, Siganos CS, Kounis G, Astyrakakis N, Kalyvianaki MI, Pallikaris IG. Management of post-LASIK corneal ectasia with Intacs inserts: one-year results. *Arch Ophthalmol.* 2003;121:322–326.

Rapuano CJ, Sugar A, Koch DD, et al. Intrastromal corneal ring segments for low myopia: a report by the American Academy of Ophthalmology. *Ophthalmology.* 2001;108:1922–1928.

Siganos CS, Kymionis GD, Kartakis N, Theodorakis MA, Astyrakakis N, Pallikaris IG. Management of keratoconus with Intacs. *Am J Ophthalmol.* 2003;135:64–70.

U.S. Food and Drug Administration. *KeraVision Intacs. Part 2. Summary of Safety and Effectiveness.* PMA P980031. April 30, 1999. http://www.fda.gov/cdrh/pdf/p980031.html.

Orthokeratology

Orthokeratology, or corneal refractive therapy, refers to the overnight use of rigid gas-permeable contact lenses to temporarily reduce myopia. The goal of this nonsurgical method of temporary myopia reduction is to achieve functional UCVA during the day. The contact lens is fitted at a base curve flatter than the corneal curvature. Temporary corneal flattening results from the flattening of corneal epithelium. A mean of 1.00 D temporary reduction of myopia was reported 20 years ago by Polse and colleagues in a National Eye Institute–sponsored orthokeratology clinical trial.

In 2002, the FDA approved a rigid contact lens (Paragon CRT, Paragon Vision Sciences, Mesa, AZ) for overnight orthokeratology for a temporary reduction of naturally occurring myopia of from –0.50 to –6.00 D of sphere, with up to 1.75 D of astigmatism. The contact lens used in this clinical trial had 3 zones. The center zone had an apical radius greater than the underlying corneal apical radius; the secondary midperipheral zone returned the contact lens to the proximity of the cornea; and the third zone was tangent to the cornea in the peripheral area. Special training was required for dispensing practitioners because of the unique challenges associated with fitting these contact lenses. The contact lenses were inserted every night before the patient went to sleep and were removed on awakening. Vision was optimal for 8 hours after removal. The refractive error increased to baseline after an undetermined period of time.

A total of 408 eyes were studied; 34.6% of patients discontinued orthokeratology contact lens use. The contact lenses did not affect the magnitude of pretreatment astigmatism. The mean reduction of myopia was 2.59 D. In the study, 89% of all eyes were within 1.00 D of emmetropia and 50% were within 0.50 D. At 9 months, UCVA of 20/20 was achieved in 58.4% of patients and UCVA of 20/40 was achieved in 89.8%. The study found that 90% of patients with 1.00–2.00 D of myopia achieved 20/40 UCVA, whereas 76% of patients with more than 4.00 D achieved 20/40 UCVA. At 9 months, 68% of patients had no change in BCVA, 13% had a 1-line increase in BCVA, 1.6% had more than a 2-line increase in BCVA, and 4% had a loss of 2 lines or more of BCVA. Safety and efficacy in patients under 18 years of age were not determined.

In this study, 75% of patients complained of some degree of discomfort, but this decreased to 20% by 9 months. There was 1 case of corneal abrasion and 18 cases of corneal edema. Corneal edema was reported more frequently in patients fitted at higher altitudes. No cases of corneal ulceration were reported in the FDA study, but after approval 2 cases of corneal ulcers in children were reported and aggressively treated with antibiotics without vision loss. Because the effect of the contact lens is temporary, a patient may notice blurring of vision during regression of effect at the end of the day. During this time, the gas-permeable contact lenses can be reinserted to achieve the BCVA. In addition, there is a significant increase in higher-order aberrations with orthokeratology, which may be associated with glare and halo.

Orthokeratology is most appropriate for highly motivated patients with low myopia who do not want refractive surgery but who want to be free of contact lenses and spectacles during the day. The contact lens does not treat astigmatism or hyperopia. Prospective patients should be informed that in clinical trials, approximately one third of patients discontinued contact lens use and most patients (75%) experienced discomfort at some point during contact lens wear.

Berntsen DA, Barr JT, Mitchell GL. The effect of overnight contact lens corneal reshaping on higher-order aberrations and best-corrected visual acuity. *Optom Vis Sci.* 2005;82:490–497.

Mascai MS. Corneal ulcers in two children wearing Paragon corneal refractive therapy lenses. *Eye Contact Lens.* 2005;31:9–11.

Saviola JF. The current FDA view on overnight orthokeratology: how we got here and where we are going. *Cornea.* 2005;24:770–771.

Schein OD. Microbial keratitis associated with overnight orthokeratology: what we need to know. *Cornea.* 2005;24:767–769.

U.S. Food and Drug Administration. Paragon CRT. PMA P870024/S043. June 13, 2002. http://www.fda.gov/cdrh/PDF/p870024s043b.pdf.

Watt K, Swarbrick HA. Microbial keratitis in overnight orthokeratology: review of the first 50 cases. *Eye Contact Lens.* 2005;31:201–208.

Conclusion

Corneal inlay and onlay procedures to correct ametropia have been performed for many years. Many procedures, such as epikeratoplasty, have been abandoned because of poor predictability or safety concerns. ICRS are unpopular for myopia but are becoming commonly used to treat keratoconus. Other uses are under investigation, including the treatment of residual myopia after LASIK and LASIK-induced ectasia. Alloplastic keratophakia inlays remain investigational but are promising. Although certain procedures have been relegated to history, their role in inspiring current and future techniques should be appreciated.

CHAPTER 6

Photoablation

The 193-nm argon-fluoride excimer laser decreases refractive error by ablating the anterior corneal stroma to create a new radius of curvature. Three major refractive surgical techniques use excimer laser ablation. In photorefractive keratectomy (PRK), the epithelium is debrided with a variety of techniques, including metal blades, brushes, and laser. In laser subepithelial keratomileusis (LASEK) and epi-LASIK, the epithelium may be preserved as an epithelial flap or excised with an epithelial microkeratome. All these forms are considered surface ablation. In laser in situ keratomileusis (LASIK), the excimer laser ablation is performed under a lamellar flap formed with a microkeratome or scanning pulsed laser.

Background

The excimer laser uses a high-voltage electrical charge to transiently combine molecules of argon and fluorine; when the molecule reverts back to its separate atoms, a charged photon is emitted. Srinivasan, an IBM engineer, was studying the far-UV (193-nm) argon-fluoride excimer laser for photoetching of computer chips. He and Trokel, an ophthalmologist, not only showed that the excimer laser could remove corneal tissue precisely, with minimal adjacent corneal damage—*photoablation*—but they also recognized the potential for refractive and therapeutic corneal surgery.

Photoablation occurs because the cornea has an extremely high absorption coefficient at 193 nm. A single 193-nm photon has sufficient energy to directly break carbon–carbon and carbon–nitrogen bonds that form the peptide backbone of the corneal collagen molecules. Excimer laser radiation ruptures the collagen polymer into small fragments, expelling a discrete volume of corneal tissue from the surface with each pulse of the laser (Fig 6-1). Because the laser removes tissue rather than incises it, the excimer laser is a poor replacement for a cutting scalpel.

PRK, the sculpting of the de-epithelialized corneal surface to alter refractive power, underwent extensive preclinical investigation before it was applied to sighted human eyes. Results of early animal studies provided evidence for relatively normal wound healing in laser-ablated corneas. McDonald and co-workers treated the first sighted human eye in 1988.

The popularity of PRK faded rapidly when LASIK began to be performed in the late 1990s because of LASIK's faster visual recovery and decreased postoperative discomfort. LASIK represents the combination of 2 refractive technologies: excimer laser stromal ablation and creation of a stromal flap by a microkeratome. The current microkeratomes

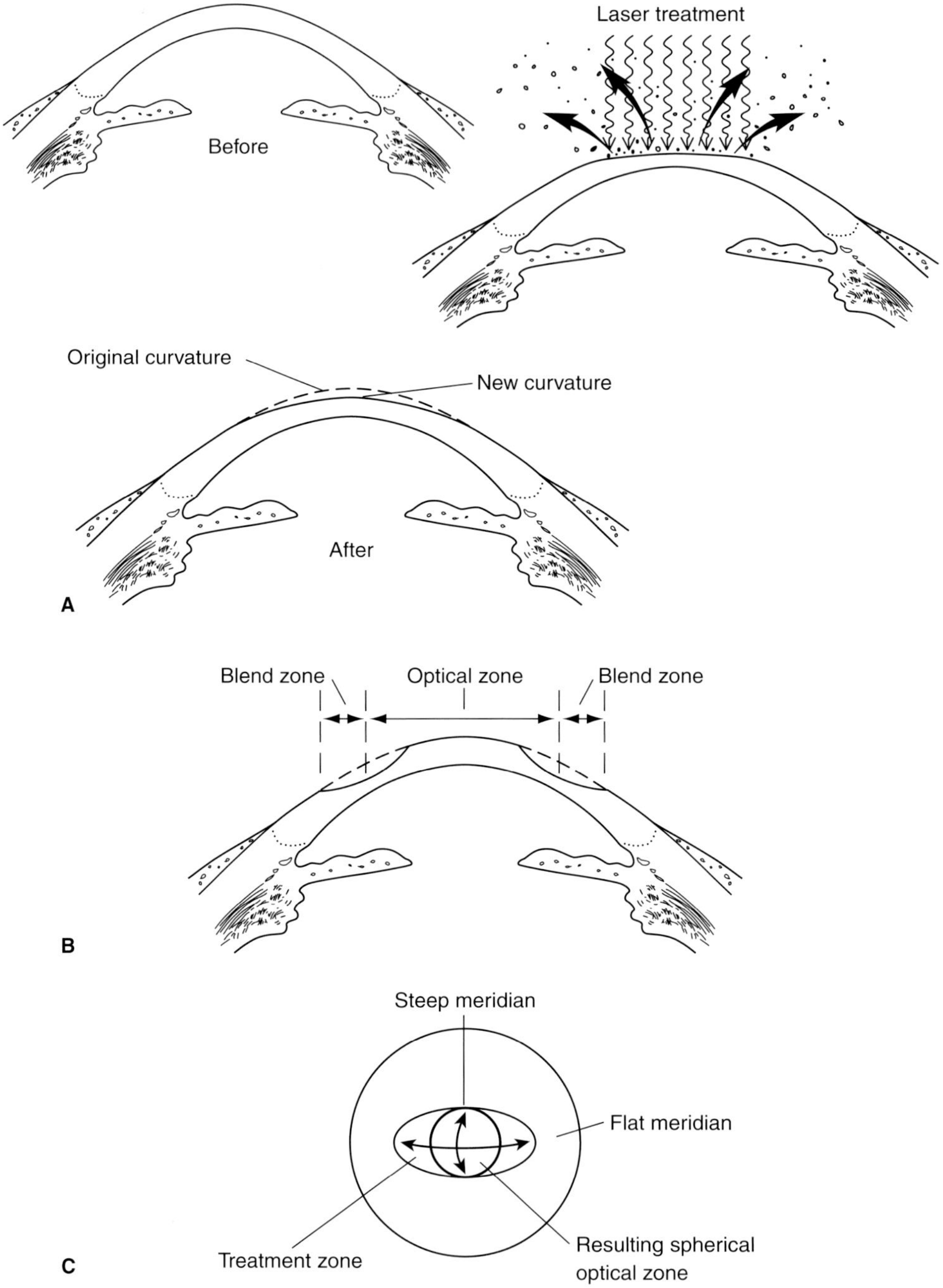

Figure 6-1 Schematic representation of corneal recontouring by the excimer laser. **A,** Correction of myopia by flattening the central cornea. **B,** Correction of hyperopia by relative steepening of the central corneal optical zone and blending the periphery. **C,** Correction of astigmatism by differential tissue removal 90° apart. Note that in correction of myopic astigmatism, the steeper meridian with more tissue removal corresponds to the smaller dimension of the ellipse. **D,** In LASIK, a flap is reflected back, the excimer laser ablation is performed on the exposed stromal bed, and then the flap is replaced. The altered corneal contour of the bed causes the same alteration in the anterior surface of the flap. *(Illustration by Jeanne Koelling.)* *(continued)*

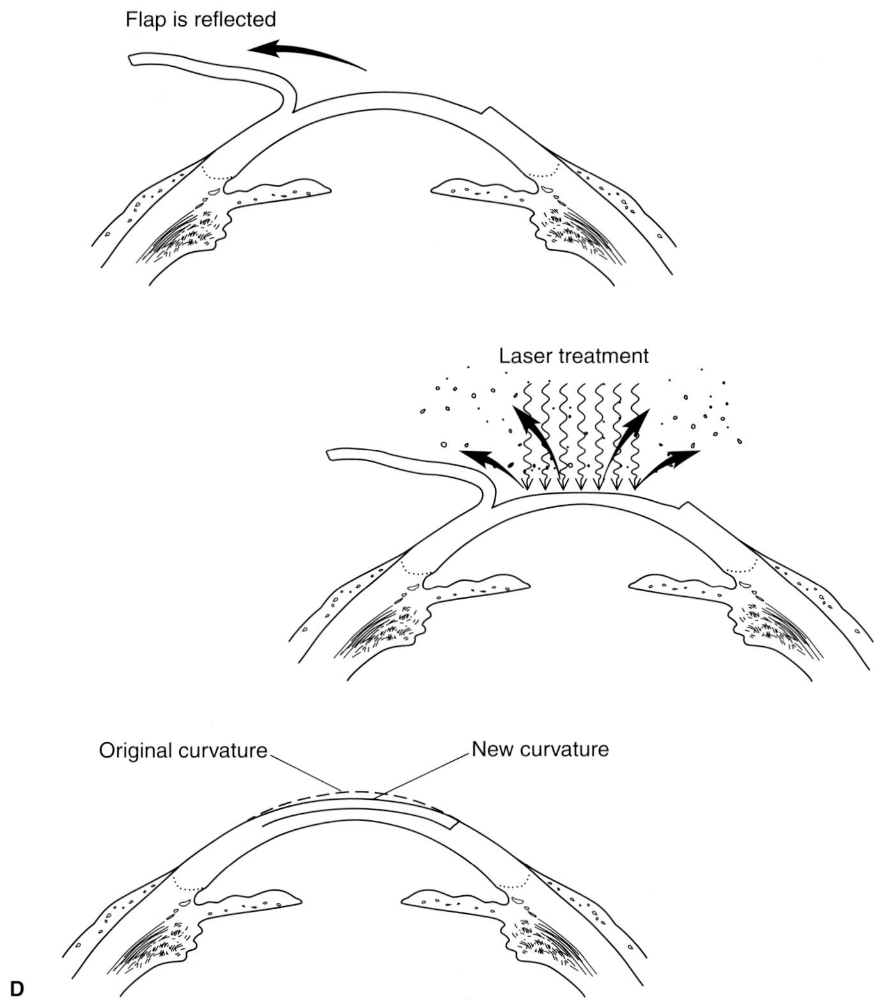

Figure 6-1 *(continued from previous page)*

evolved from the original version designed by Barraquer to perform his frozen-tissue keratomileusis procedures. Although more LASIK than surface ablation procedures continue to be performed, surface ablation is an attractive alternative in specific indications, such as irregular corneas, epithelial basement membrane disease (often called *map-dot-fingerprint dystrophy*), and thin corneas, and for treatment of some LASIK flap complications, such as incomplete or buttonholed flaps. Surface ablation eliminates the potential for stromal flap-related complications. With the advent of new epithelial removal techniques and wavefront-guided laser ablations, the popularity of surface ablation has been increasing. The LASIK flap itself is associated with a greater increase in postoperative higher-order optical aberrations than is surface ablation, so it is possible that the postoperative quality of vision may be higher with wavefront-guided surface ablation than with LASIK.

Srinivasan R. Ablation of polymers and biological tissue by ultraviolet lasers. *Science.* 1986;234:559–565.

Trokel SL, Srinivasan R, Braren B. Excimer laser surgery of the cornea. *Am J Ophthalmol.* 1983;96:710–715.

Surface Ablation: Photorefractive Keratectomy, Laser Subepithelial Keratomileusis, and Epithelial Laser in Situ Keratomileusis

Patient Selection

The preoperative evaluation of patients considering refractive surgery is presented in detail in Chapter 3. This section reviews only the aspects of the preoperative evaluation that are specific to surface ablation, which includes *photorefractive keratectomy (PRK), laser subepithelial keratomileusis (LASEK),* and *epithelial laser in situ keratomileusis (epi-LASIK).*

In general, any condition that delays epithelial healing is either a relative or absolute contraindication to surface ablation. A history of connective tissue diseases such as rheumatoid arthritis, systemic lupus erythematosus, or Sjögren syndrome is considered a relative contraindication to surface ablation because of less predictable corneal wound healing, with the potential for corneal melting; however, if the disease is well controlled, results may be very good. Patients with connective tissue disease seeking refractive surgery should have a thorough examination of the ocular surface, with attention to dry-eye disease. Although keloid scar formation was a contraindication to PRK in the FDA trials, one study found that African Americans with a history of keloid formation did well after PRK, and keloid formation is no longer considered a contraindication to surface ablation or LASIK. Prior herpes simplex keratitis is another commonly listed contraindication to PRK. Systemic antiviral prophylaxis preoperatively and for several months after surgery may reduce but not eliminate the risk of recurrence after PRK. Patients with a history of herpetic disease should have their corneal sensation evaluated and should be evaluated for stromal scarring. In patients with diabetes, blood sugar levels need to be well controlled preoperatively due to instability of the refractive error and potential poor wound healing with fluctuating blood sugar levels (see Chapter 10). Corneal sensation should be evaluated as well. Proliferative diabetic retinopathy remains a contraindication to surface ablation and LASIK. PRK is also contraindicated in patients actively taking isotretinoin (eg, Accutane) or amiodarone hydrochloride, both of which may affect corneal wound healing. PRK and LASIK are not approved by the FDA for use with patients younger than 18 and should not be performed except under special circumstances, such as treating anisometropic amblyopia in a child who cannot tolerate occlusion therapy or contact lenses.

The orbital anatomy must be carefully inspected. A narrow palpebral fissure and a prominent brow with deep-set globes both increase the difficulty of creating a successful corneal flap, and the presence of either may lead a surgeon to consider a surface ablation procedure over LASIK.

Measurement of the low-light scotopic pupil size is important in the preoperative assessment. High myopia and high astigmatism are the greatest risk factors for postoperative glare and halo. However, although the concept is controversial, pupil size may also play a role in postoperative visual complaints. Conventional wisdom previously suggested that, to minimize visual disturbances such as glare and halos, the ablation zone should be larger than the pupil diameter. More recent findings have demonstrated that this belief may be too simplistic; some patients with large pupils have no night vision complaints. Instead, it may be the interaction of pupil size with the increased higher-order optical aberrations that occur in the corneal periphery that explains complaints of poor night vision. In patients with larger pupils and thinner corneas, when an adequate stromal bed is not available for LASIK using a large ablation zone, surface ablation may be advisable.

Patients with epithelial basement membrane dystrophy are better candidates for PRK than for LASIK because PRK may be therapeutic, reducing epithelial irregularity and providing improved postoperative quality of vision while enhancing epithelial adhesion. In contrast, LASIK may cause a frank epithelial defect in eyes with basement membrane disease. If the surgeon is in doubt as to which procedure to use, he or she can perform a simple test for epithelial membrane dystrophy while the patient is under topical anesthesia by gently rubbing a cotton-tipped applicator over the corneal surface. If there is epithelial movement over the stroma, PRK is usually indicated.

Any patient undergoing excimer laser photoablation should have a pachymetric and topographic evaluation (Chapter 3). Patients with thin corneas or irregular topography may be at increased risk for the development of ectasia with LASIK. Patients with these topographic patterns who are stable could be offered surface ablation but with a clear acknowledgment, as well as a signed informed consent form, that they understand there may still be a risk of progression to corneal ectasia or keratoconus.

Binder PS, Lindstrom RL, Stulting RD, et al. Keratoconus and corneal ectasia after LASIK. *J Cataract Refract Surg.* 2005;31:2035–2038.

Cobo-Soriano R, Beltrán J, Baviera J. LASIK outcomes in patients with underlying systemic contraindications: a preliminary study. *Ophthalmology.* 2007;114:1032–1033.

Salib GM, McDonald MB, Smolek M. Safety and efficacy of cyclosporine 0.05% drops versus unpreserved artificial tears in dry-eye patients having laser in situ keratomileusis. *J Cataract Refract Surg.* 2006;32:772–778.

Schallhorn SC, Kaupp SE, Tanzer DJ, Tidwell J, Laurent J, Bourque LB. Pupil size and quality of vision after LASIK. *Ophthalmology*. 2003;110:1606–1614.

Smith RJ, Maloney RK. Laser in situ keratomileusis in patients with autoimmune diseases. *J Cataract Refract Surg.* 2006;32:1292–1295.

Surgical Technique

Calibration of the excimer laser

The laser should be checked daily and between patients by a technician for an adequate homogeneous beam profile, alignment, and power output, according to the instructions of the manufacturer.

Preoperative planning and laser programming

An important part of preoperative planning is programming the laser with the appropriate refraction. Often the manifest and cycloplegic refractions differ, or the amount and axis of astigmatism differ between the topographic evaluation and refractive examination. Thus, it may be unclear which refraction to enter into the laser. The surgeon's decision about whether to use the manifest or the cycloplegic refraction is based on his or her individual nomogram and technique. The manifest refraction is more accurate than the cycloplegic refraction in determining cylinder axis and amount. If the refractive cylinder is confirmed to differ from the topographic cylinder, lenticular astigmatism or posterior corneal curvature is assumed to be the cause. In this case, the laser is still programmed with the axis and amount of cylinder noted on refraction. The surgeon should take particular care to check the axis on the refraction and topography with the value programmed into the laser because entering an incorrect value is a common error, particularly when converting between plus and minus cylinder formats. Prior to all surgery, the surgeon and the technician should go over a checklist of information, confirming the patient's name, the refraction, and the eye on which surgery is to be performed.

In many laser models, the surgeon also must enter the size of the optical zone and indicate whether a blend of the ablation zone should be performed. If there is sufficient corneal tissue, an ablation zone larger than the scotopic pupil size is usually selected. A "blend zone" is an area of peripheral asphericity designed to reduce the possible undesirable effects of an abrupt transition from the optical zone to the untreated cornea (see Fig 6-1B). A common approach to the creation of a blend zone would be, for example, to have a –6.00 D correction consist of a –5.00 D correction at a 6-mm optical zone and to have a –1.00 D correction at an 8-mm optical zone. The larger the treatment area, the deeper will be the ablation. The surgeon must calculate whether an adequate stromal bed will remain, although this is rarely an issue for surface ablation. However, with thinner corneas and higher dioptric treatments, the amount of tissue may be inadequate for LASIK, which would be a reason to select surface ablation.

Preoperative preparation of the patient

Many surgeons use topical antibiotic prophylaxis preoperatively. The patient's skin is prepped with 5%–10% povidone-iodine (eg, Betadine) or alcohol wipes before or after entering the laser suite, and 5% povidone-iodine solution is sometimes applied as drops to the ocular surface and then irrigated out for further antisepsis. There is no consensus about the utility of these measures. In addition, prior to laser treatment, patients should be instructed regarding the sounds and smells they will encounter during the laser treatment. They may receive an oral antianxiety medication such as diazepam.

If a large amount of astigmatism is being treated, some surgeons elect to mark the cornea at the horizontal or vertical axis while the patient is sitting up to ensure accurate alignment under the laser. This is done to compensate for the cyclotorsion that commonly occurs when the patient goes from a sitting-up to a lying-down position. A 15° offset in the axis of treatment can decrease the effective cylinder change by 35% and can result in a significant axis shift.

After placing the patient under the laser, a sterile drape may be placed over the skin and eyelashes according to the surgeon's preference. Topical tetracaine and/or proparacaine anesthetic drops are placed in the eye. Anesthetic eyedrops should not be placed too early, as doing so may loosen the epithelium substantially. An eyelid speculum is placed in the operative eye and an opaque patch is placed over the fellow eye to avoid cross-fixation. A gauze pad may be taped over the temple between the operative eye and the ear to absorb any excess fluid. The patient is asked to fixate on the laser centration light (seen by the patient as a red light) while the surgeon focuses on the cornea and centers the laser. For most patients, voluntary fixation during laser vision ablation produces more accurate centration than does globe immobilization by the surgeon.

Epithelial debridement techniques for surface ablation

The epithelium can be removed by (Fig 6-2)

- a sharp blade
- a blunt spatula
- a rotating corneal brush
- application of 20% absolute alcohol for 20–45 seconds to the corneal surface to loosen the epithelium
- a mechanical microkeratome with an epi-LASIK blade
- transepithelial ablation from the excimer laser itself

With transepithelial ablation and epi-LASIK, the peripheral margin of the de-epithelialization is defined by the laser or keratome itself. For other epithelial debridement techniques, the surgeon defines the outer limit of de-epithelialization with an optical zone marker and then debrides from the periphery toward the center. An ophthalmic surgical cellulose sponge lightly moistened with an artificial tear lubricant such as carboxymethylcellulose 0.5% can be uniformly brushed over the surface of the cornea to remove any residual epithelium and to provide a smooth surface. The epithelium should be removed efficiently and consistently to prevent hydration changes in the stroma, because excessive corneal stromal dehydration may increase the rate of excimer laser ablation, resulting in an overcorrection. The optical zone must be free of epithelial cells, debris, and excess fluid before ablation.

Epithelial preservation techniques

LASEK In the LASEK variant of surface ablation, the goal is to preserve the patient's epithelium. Instead of debriding and discarding the epithelium or ablating the epithelium with the excimer laser, the surgeon folds back an intact sheet of epithelium (Fig 6-3). Placing a radial mark of gentian violet ink can help with later realignment of the epithelial flap. A solution of approximately 20% absolute alcohol is then applied for 20–30 seconds. An 8.0- to 9.0-mm-diameter optical zone marker pressed onto the corneal surface restricts the alcohol to the area to be de-epithelialized. After the desired exposure time, the alcohol is removed from the "well" of the optical zone marker by absorption into a microsurgical spear sponge. When the alcohol is fully absorbed and the optical zone marker is removed, the ocular surface is immediately irrigated with copious quantities of balanced salt solution to minimize toxicity to the limbal germinal epithelium. The surgeon then uses an instrument, often with a hoe or spatula configuration, to carefully separate a flap of full-thickness epithelium from the underlying Bowman's layer. The epithelium is delicately folded back on itself until all has been lifted except for a small "hinge," which is typically located superiorly.

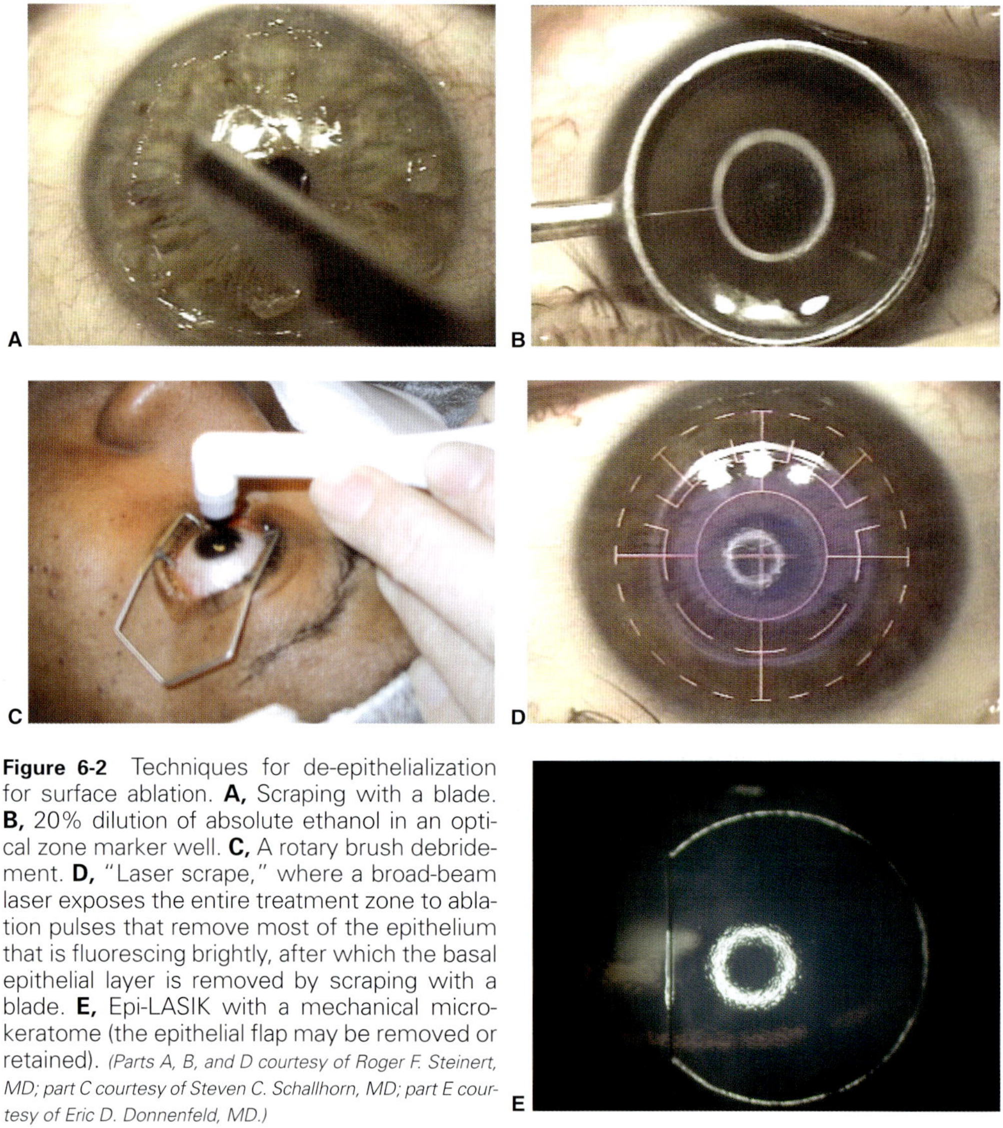

Figure 6-2 Techniques for de-epithelialization for surface ablation. **A,** Scraping with a blade. **B,** 20% dilution of absolute ethanol in an optical zone marker well. **C,** A rotary brush debridement. **D,** "Laser scrape," where a broad-beam laser exposes the entire treatment zone to ablation pulses that remove most of the epithelium that is fluorescing brightly, after which the basal epithelial layer is removed by scraping with a blade. **E,** Epi-LASIK with a mechanical microkeratome (the epithelial flap may be removed or retained). *(Parts A, B, and D courtesy of Roger F. Steinert, MD; part C courtesy of Steven C. Schallhorn, MD; part E courtesy of Eric D. Donnenfeld, MD.)*

Although the goal of LASEK is to reduce postoperative pain, speed the recovery of visual acuity, and decrease postoperative haze formation, controlled studies have had mixed results. With LASEK, vision may be slighter better on the first postoperative day compared with PRK, but some reports show more discomfort and a delay in recovery of vision with LASEK compared with PRK after the first day, which may be due to epithelial remodeling. In addition, the epithelial flap may not remain viable but may slough off, delaying healing and visual recovery.

Epi-LASIK Epi-LASIK, another technique for preserving the epithelium, has largely supplanted LASEK. In epi-LASIK, an epithelial flap is fashioned with a microkeratome fitted with a modified dull blade and a thin applanation plate that mechanically separates

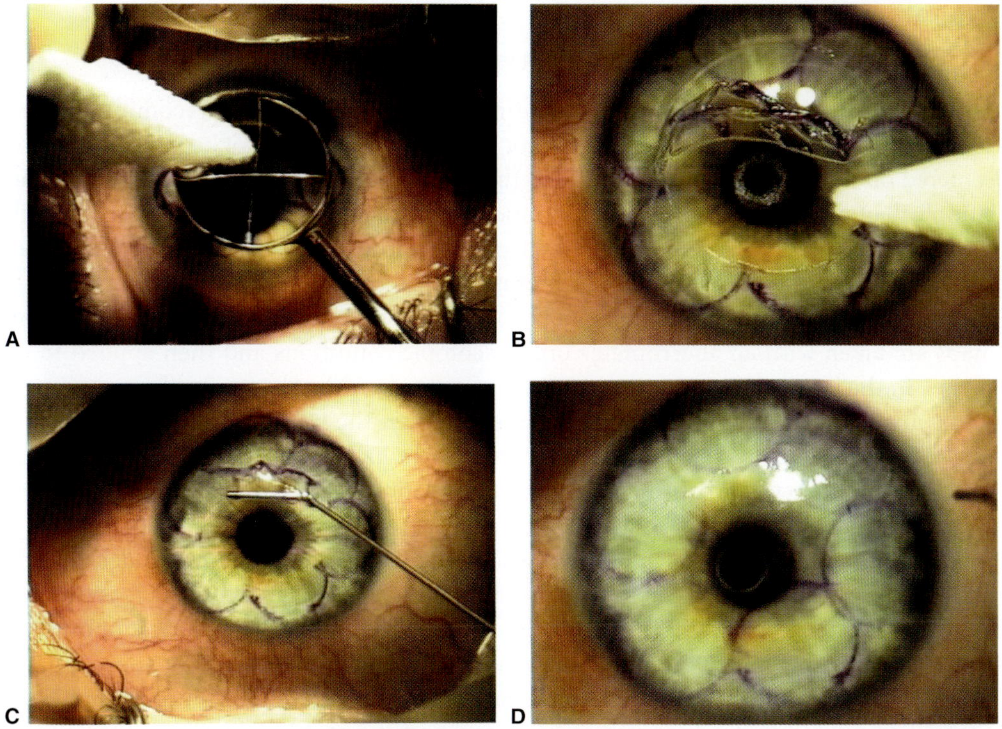

Figure 6-3 LASEK technique. **A,** 20% absolute alcohol (ethanol) is released into the marker well. Care is taken to avoid spillage by using a dry sponge to absorb any overflow. **B,** A dry, nonfragmenting sponge is used to peel the epithelial flap. **C,** After laser ablation is applied to the exposed Bowman's layer and stroma, a 30-gauge irrigating cannula is used to hydrate and reposition the epithelial flap. **D,** The flap edges are aligned, and no epithelial defects are noted after flap repositioning and during the 5-minute waiting period. A bandage soft contact lens is applied at the end of the procedure. *(Reprinted with permission from Azar DT, Ang RT. Laser subepithelial keratomileusis: evolution of alcohol-assisted flap surface ablation.* Int Ophthalmol Clin. *2002;42:89–97.)*

the epithelium without the use of epithelial toxic agents such as the alcohol used in LASEK. In this manner, epi-LASIK preserves more viable epithelial cells, may improve results compared with LASEK, and creates an epithelial flap that will successfully adhere postoperatively. Some surgeons use the epi-LASIK microkeratome to rapidly create a smooth corneal bed with regular epithelial borders and then discard the epithelial flap. To date, epi-LASIK and LASEK have not been proven advantageous over PRK for reducing corneal haze.

Ambrosio R Jr, Wilson S. LASIK vs LASEK vs PRK: advantages and indications. *Semin Ophthalmol.* 2003;18:2–10.

Gabler B, Winkler von Mohrenfels C, Dreiss AK, Marshall J, Lohmann CP. Vitality of epithelial cells after alcohol exposure during laser-assisted subepithelial keratectomy flap preparation. *J Cataract Refract Surg.* 2002;28:1841–1846.

Matsumoto JC, Chu YS. Epi-LASIK update: overview of techniques and patient management. *Int Ophthalmol Clin.* 2006;46:105–115.

Laser Treatment

Centration and ablation

The laser is centered and focused according to the manufacturer's recommendations. Tracking systems, although effective, do not lessen the importance of keeping the reticule centered on the patient's entrance pupil. If the patient begins to lose fixation, the laser ablation will often be automatically discontinued; if the ablation does not stop automatically, the surgeon should immediately stop the treatment until adequate refixation is achieved. It is still important for the surgeon to monitor for excessive eye roll, which can result in decentration despite the tracking device. For wavefront-guided ablations, the wavefront maps are taken with an aberrometer under scotopic conditions and then applied to the cornea in the laser suite under an operating microscope. The change in illumination can result in pupil centroid shift. For most patients, when the pupil is constricted, it moves nasally and superiorly. Registration is a technique in which a fixed landmark is used at the time of aberrometry and treatment to apply the ablation to the correct area of the cornea; it does not rely on the pupil for laser centration (Fig 6-4).

One of the major complications of surface ablation is corneal haze. To decrease the chance of post–surface ablation corneal haze after prior corneal surgery, such as previous PRK, LASIK, penetrating keratoplasty, or radial keratotomy, a soaked pledget of mitomycin C (usually 0.02% or 0.2 mg/mL) can be placed on the ablated surface for approximately 12 seconds to 2 minutes at the end of the laser exposure. The duration of mitomycin C application may vary by diagnosis and surgeon preference. Many surgeons also employ mitomycin C in primary surface ablation for moderate to high treatments or deeper ablation depths. Some surgeons reduce the amount of treatment when applying mitomycin C in surface ablation. The cornea is then copiously irrigated with balanced salt solution to

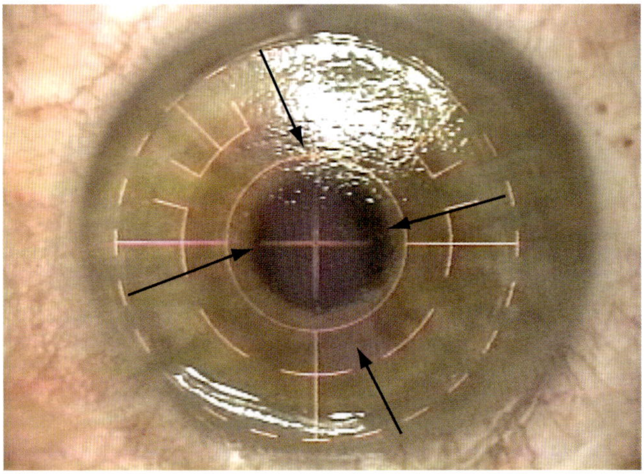

Figure 6-4 Excimer laser ablation of the stromal bed. Note the faint blue fluorescence of the stromal bed from the laser pulse *(arrows)*. The rectangular shape of the exposure by this broadbeam laser indicates that the laser is correcting the cylindrical portion of the treatment. (Photograph is enhanced to visualize fluorescence; the surgeon usually sees minimal or no fluorescence through the operating microscope.) *(Courtesy of Roger F. Steinert, MD.)*

remove excess mitomycin C. To avoid damage to limbal stem cells, care should be taken not to expose the limbus or conjunctiva to the mitomycin C. Human confocal microscopy studies have shown a reduced keratocyte population and less haze in eyes that had mitomycin C, but vision-threatening complications of mitomycin C have been reported in other settings, including glaucoma and pterygium surgery. In one study, there was a reduction in endothelial cell counts in patients receiving mitomycin C. The search continues for the ideal topical wound-healing modulator with high specificity for inhibiting collagen synthesis without toxic side effects.

Donnenfeld E. The pupil is a moving target: centration, repeatability, and registration. *J Refract Surg.* 2004;20:S593–S596.

Kapadia MS, Meisler DM, Wilson SE. Epithelial removal with the excimer laser (laser-scrape) in photorefractive keratectomy retreatment. *Ophthalmology.* 1999;106:29–34.

Lee DH, Chung HS, Jeon YC, Boo SD, Yoon YD, Kim JG. Photorefractive keratectomy with intraoperative mitomycin-C application. *J Cataract Refract Surg.* 2005;31:2293–2298.

Majmudar PA, Forstot SL, Dennis RF, et al. Topical mitomycin-C for subepithelial fibrosis after refractive corneal surgery. *Ophthalmology.* 2000;107:89–94.

Morales AJ, Zadok D, Mora-Retana R, Martinez-Gama E, Roblado NE, Chayet AS. Intraoperative mitomycin and corneal endothelium after photorefractive keratectomy. *Am J Ophthalmol.* 2006;142:400–404.

Immediate postablation measures

After the procedure is completed, drops of antibiotic, corticosteroid, and sometimes a nonsteroidal anti-inflammatory drug (NSAID) are placed on the eye, followed by a bandage soft contact lens. Some NSAIDs can be placed directly on the corneal bed and others should be placed on the surface of the contact lens. If the LASEK or epi-LASIK variant has been performed, the surgeon carefully floats and repositions the epithelial sheet back into position with balanced salt solution prior to applying the medications and the bandage soft contact lens. Some surgeons also apply sterile chilled balanced salt solution or a frozen cellulose sponge before and/or after the PRK procedure in the belief that cooling reduces pain and haze formation, although the advantage of this practice has not been substantiated in a controlled study. If the patient cannot tolerate a bandage soft contact lens, a pressure patch may be used.

Operative day postablation treatment

During the first 24–48 hours, patients experience a variable amount of pain, from minimal to severe, and some patients may need an oral narcotic pain medication. Studies have shown that topical NSAID drops reduce postoperative pain, although they may also slow the rate of re-epithelialization and promote sterile infiltrates (see Fig 6-8). Corneal melting and stromal scarring have been described after the use of some topical NSAIDs. For patients who are not healing normally following the surface ablation, any topical NSAID should be discontinued. Studies have also demonstrated a reduction in pain with the use of topical anesthetic drops. Patients must be carefully warned not to overuse topical anesthetic drops because, when used excessively over a prolonged period, the drops may cause severe corneal complications. Many patients benefit from oral NSAIDs preoperatively and postoperatively as well as from postoperative oral narcotics.

Subsequent postoperative care

Patients should be followed closely until the epithelium is completely healed, which usually occurs within 3–4 days. As long as the bandage soft contact lens is in place, patients are treated with topical broad-spectrum antibiotics and corticosteroids, usually 4 times daily. Once the epithelium is healed, the bandage soft contact lens, antibiotic drops, and NSAID drops (if used) may be discontinued. If topical anesthetic drops have been used, patients are strongly advised to stop their use.

The use of topical corticosteroids to modulate postoperative wound healing, reduce anterior stromal haze, and decrease regression of the refractive effect remains controversial. Although some studies have demonstrated that corticosteroids have no significant long-term effect on corneal haze or visual outcome after PRK, other studies have shown that corticosteroids are effective in limiting haze and myopic regression after PRK, particularly after higher myopic corrections. Some surgeons who advocate topical corticosteroids after the removal of the bandage soft contact lens restrict them to patients with higher levels of myopia (eg, myopia greater than –4.00 or –5.00 D). When used after bandage soft contact lens removal, corticosteroid drops are typically tapered over a 2- to 4-month period, depending on the patient's corneal haze and refractive outcome. For example, corticosteroids may be used 4 times daily for the first month, 3 times daily for the second month, 2 times daily for the third month, and once a day for the fourth month. For patients who receive mitomycin C, the duration of postoperative corticosteroid use may be shorter, due to the reduced risk of haze formation. Patients undergoing hyperopic PRK may experience prolonged epithelial healing time because of the larger ablation zone, as well as a temporary reduction in best-corrected distance visual acuity in the first week to month, which usually improves with time. Many hyperopic patients also experience a temporary myopic overcorrection, which regresses over several weeks to months.

Corbett MC, O'Brart DP, Marshall J. Do topical corticosteroids have a role following excimer laser photorefractive keratectomy? *J Refract Surg.* 1995;11:380–387.

Solomon KD, Donnenfeld ED, Raizman M, et al. Safety and efficacy of ketorolac tromethamine 0.4% ophthalmic solution in post-photorefractive keratectomy patients. *J Cataract Refract Surg.* 2004;30:1653–1660.

Outcomes

Evolving technology

As the early broad-beam excimer laser systems improved and as surgeon experience increased, surface ablation results improved markedly. The ablation zone diameter was enlarged because it was found that small ablation zones, originally selected to limit depth of tissue removal, produced more haze and regression as well as subjective glare and halos. The larger treatment diameters used today, including optical zones and gradual aspheric peripheral blend zones, improve optical quality and refractive stability in both myopic and hyperopic treatments. Central island elevations have become less common with improvements in beam quality and with the development of scanning and variable-spot-size excimer lasers.

Tracking devices

Today all excimer lasers employ tracking systems, which have improved outcomes. Two types of tracking technology are commonly used. With so-called closed-loop trackers, high-speed oscillating infrared beams scan across the edge of a fixed, dilated pupil. These beams detect the abrupt change in reflected light at the edge of the pupil. The signal then directs rapidly responding mirrors to create a space-stabilized image, and the laser treatment is located on the cornea based on that image. The second type of tracker, a so-called open-loop system, uses video technology to monitor the location of an infrared image of the pupil and to shift the laser beam accordingly.

Myopic spherical PRK

The first excimer lasers that were approved by the FDA for myopic PRK were manufactured by Summit and VISX. Clinical trials of conventional (non–wavefront-driven) excimer laser treatments limited to low myopia (generally less than –6.00 D) reveal that 56%–71% of eyes achieved uncorrected visual acuity (UCVA) of at least 20/20, 88%–97% achieved UCVA of at least 20/40, and 82%–94% were within 1.00 D of emmetropia. In the original Summit study, 6.8% had a loss of 2 or more lines of best-corrected visual acuity (BCVA). More recent clinical trials, however, have reported a 0% loss of BCVA postoperatively. FDA clinical trials of patients with moderate myopia (–6.00 to –10.00 D) report that 32%–49% of eyes achieved UCVA of at least 20/20, 67%–86% achieved at least 20/40 UCVA, 53%–77% were within 1.00 D of emmetropia, and up to 6.7% lost more than 2 lines of BCVA. In other published studies, of patients with high myopia (less than –10.00 D), 26%–42% achieved at least 20/40 UCVA, 28%–48% were within 1.00 D of emmetropia, and 7.7%–22% lost at least 2 lines of BCVA.

Greater amounts of attempted correction are associated with decreased predictability, increased severity of haze and loss of BCVA, increased regression, and decreased likelihood of obtaining 20/40 or better UCVA. Consequently, many surgeons limit their treatment to a maximum of approximately –10.00 D of myopia. However, pharmacologic mediators of wound healing, including but not limited to intraoperative topical mitomycin C and postoperative corticosteroid drops, may decrease the postoperative haze in patients with higher degrees of myopia who are undergoing excimer laser ablation. In one study of myopic PRK, refractive stability achieved at 1 year was maintained up to 12 years with no evidence of hyperopic shift, diurnal fluctuation, or late regression in the long term. Corneal haze decreased with time, with complete recovery of BCVA.

Toric PRK

Astigmatism is corrected with the excimer laser by performing an elliptical ablation to flatten the steeper meridian of the cornea to match the flatter meridian (see Fig 6-1C). Because the treatment zone becomes elliptical, the effective optical zone of the ablation is smaller than the treated area. The results of photoastigmatic keratectomy are difficult to interpret because the various studies use different techniques, nomograms, and variables to measure efficacy. In addition, a thorough evaluation of astigmatism requires vector analysis, which is not performed in many of the studies.

FDA clinical trials of photoastigmatic keratectomy revealed that 45%–64% of eyes achieved postoperative UCVA of 20/20 or better, 83%–93% achieved UCVA of 20/40, 80%–92% were within 1.00 D of emmetropia, and 1.6%–8.5% lost 2 or more lines of BCVA. Initial clinical trials of toric PRK showed that it was not as predictable as spherical PRK and that it tended to undercorrect the cylinder, probably because of conservative nomograms. By allowing more direct recontouring of the toric corneal surface into a sphere, in conjunction with simultaneous correction of hyperopia or myopia, the newer scanning lasers usually remove less tissue than the earlier broad-beam lasers.

Hyperopic PRK

In myopic PRK, the central cornea is flattened, whereas in hyperopic PRK, more tissue is removed from the midperiphery than from the central cornea, resulting in an effective steepening (see Fig 6-1B). However, a sharp transition between treated and untreated cornea in the periphery can cause significant haze and regression. For this reason, additional pulses are applied to blend the maximally ablated midperipheral area with the untreated peripheral cornea.

To ensure that the size of the central hyperopic treatment zone is adequate, a large ablation area is required for hyperopic PRK. Initial studies using hyperopic treatment zones of 4.0 mm combined with a total blended area out to 7.0 mm revealed an unacceptable regression of effect. In addition, a significant number of eyes lost BCVA, largely secondary to mild decentration combined with the small optical zones.

Later studies were performed using larger hyperopic treatment zones with transition zones out to 9.0–9.5 mm. FDA clinical trials of hyperopic PRK up to +6.00 D revealed postoperative UCVA of 20/20 or better in 46%–53% of eyes, postoperative UCVA of 20/40 or better in 92%–96%, 84%–91% within 1.00 D of emmetropia, and loss of greater than 2 lines of BCVA in 1%. The period from surgery to postoperative stabilization for the same quantity of correction is longer for hyperopic than for myopic corrections. Treatment of higher degrees of hyperopia results in poorer predictability and stability.

Hyperopic astigmatic PRK

The VISX FDA clinical trial of hyperopic astigmatic PRK up to +6.00 D sphere and +4.00 D cylinder reported an approximate postoperative UCVA of 20/20 or better in 50% of eyes, UCVA of 20/40 or better in 97%, and 87% within ±1.00 D of emmetropia, with loss of more than 2 lines of BCVA in 1.5%. Few other studies exist for hyperopic astigmatic PRK because hyperopic astigmatic LASIK has been approved with several other laser manufacturers.

Mixed astigmatic PRK

Mixed astigmatism occurs when the negative cylinder is greater than the positive sphere. According to vector analysis in one study, mean achieved vector magnitude was 80% of intended. Twenty eyes (50%) had a cylinder within ±0.50 D of emmetropia. Twenty-three eyes (57.5%) had a spherical component within ±0.50 D. Thirty-four eyes (85%) had postoperative UCVA of 20/40 or better. Four eyes (10%) lost 2 lines of Snellen BSCVA, whereas 14 eyes (35%) gained 1 or more lines.

Enhancements

After stabilization of the UCVA and refraction, typically around 3 to 6 months after the surface ablation, the patient and surgeon assess their satisfaction with the result of the surface ablation. If the patient is dissatisfied with the UCVA and the surgeon agrees it is prudent, reoperation or enhancement can be performed to treat the residual refractive error. The surgeon should avoid performing an enhancement for a patient with unrealistic expectations. The patient who wants enhancement to improve the UCVA of 20/20 in his "bad eye" to match the UCVA of "20/15" that his "good eye" has achieved should instead be re-educated about realistic results. However, patients with visual complaints and significant higher-order aberrations but good Snellen visual acuity may benefit from wavefront enhancements. When enhancement of myopic surface ablation is contemplated, the surgeon must be aware that the epithelium is often thickened (hyperplastic) centrally as a reaction to the flattened corneal profile created by the myopic ablation. Initial undercorrection of the laser ablation must be differentiated from regression of the initial ablation. Regression may be due to stromal collagen healing, epithelial hyperplasia, or a combination. A surface ablation enhancement may result in overcorrection if the regression due to epithelial hyperplasia is included in the enhancement and an equal amount of epithelial hyperplasia does not recur.

Hersh PS, Stulting RD, Steinert RF, et al. Results of phase III excimer laser photorefractive keratectomy for myopia. The Summit PRK Study Group. *Ophthalmology*. 1997;104:1535–1553.

Litwak S, Zadok D, Garcia-de Quevedo V, Robledo N, Chayet AS. Laser-assisted subepithelial keratectomy versus photorefractive keratectomy for the correction of myopia: a prospective comparative study. *J Cataract Refract Surg*. 2002;28:1330–1333.

McDonald MB, Deitz MR, Frantz JM, et al. Photorefractive keratectomy for low-to-moderate myopia and astigmatism with a small-beam, tracker-directed excimer laser. *Ophthalmology*. 1999;106:1481–1489.

Rajan MS, Jaycock P, O'Brart D, Nystrom HH, Marshall J. A long-term study of photorefractive keratectomy; 12-year follow-up. *Ophthalmology*. 2004;111:1813–1824.

Steinert RF, Hersh PS. Spherical and aspherical photorefractive keratectomy and laser in-situ keratomileusis for moderate to high myopia: two prospective, randomized clinical trials. Summit Technology PRK-LASIK Study Group. *Trans Am Ophthalmol Soc*. 1998;96:197–221.

Complications

Overcorrection

Overcorrection of more than +1.0 D at 1 year occurs in less than 5% of patients with myopia, and results have improved markedly with new technology. Myopic or hyperopic surface ablation typically undergoes regression for at least 3–6 months. In general, patients with higher degrees of myopia and hyperopia require more time to achieve refractive stability. Refractive stability must be achieved before a decision is made regarding whether the overcorrection requires re-treatment. For example, with myopic corrections, a 1-month low hyperopic response (expected overcorrection) is followed by regression of 0.50–1.00 D toward myopia over the next few months.

An overcorrection may occur if substantial stromal dehydration develops prior to beginning the laser treatment, because more stromal tissue will be ablated per pulse.

Overcorrection tends to occur more often in older individuals because they do not have as strong a wound-healing response and their corneas ablate at a more rapid rate due to their reduced hydration status. Studies reveal that older patients (ages 35–54) with moderate to high myopia have a greater response to the same amount of dioptric correction than younger patients do. Various modalities are available for treating small amounts of overcorrection. Myopic regression can be induced by the abrupt discontinuation of corticosteroids. The administration of topical NSAIDs (usually 4 times a day) in conjunction with a bandage soft contact lens over several months may decrease small amounts of overcorrection, although this is controversial (see Chapter 11). Patients with consecutive hyperopia, the hyperopia that occurs when an originally myopic patient is overcorrected, and patients who are myopic due to overcorrection of hyperopia require less treatment to return to emmetropia than previously untreated eyes. When re-treating these patients, care should be taken not to overcorrect a second time. With conventional ablation, most surgeons will reduce the ablation by 15%–50% for consecutive treatments.

Undercorrection

At higher degrees of myopia and hyperopia, undercorrection occurs much more frequently because of decreased predictability due to the greater frequency and severity of regression. Patients with regression after treatment of their first eye have an increased likelihood of regression in their second eye. Sometimes the regression may be reversed with aggressive topical corticosteroids. The patient may undergo a re-treatment after the refraction has remained stable for at least 3 months. A patient with significant corneal haze and regression is at higher risk after re-treatment for further regression and recurrence of visually significant corneal haze and loss of BCVA. Topical mitomycin C, administered at the time of re-treatment, can be used to modulate the response. It is recommended that the surgeon wait at least 6–12 months for the haze to improve naturally before repeating surface ablation. In patients with significant haze and regression, removal of haze with adjunctive use of mitomycin C should not be coupled with a refractive treatment as the resolution of the haze will commonly improve the refractive outcome.

Central islands

A central island is visualized by computerized corneal topography as an area of central corneal steepening surrounded by an area of flattening that corresponds to the myopic treatment zone in the paracentral region (Fig 6-5). A central island is defined as a steepening of at least 1.00 D with a diameter of more than 1 mm compared with the paracentral flattened area. Islands generally occur with the older broad-beam laser systems rather than with the newer scanning delivery systems. They have been reported to occur more frequently in ablations larger than 5.0 mm in diameter and with greater numbers of attempted corrections. Central islands may be associated with decreased visual acuity, monocular diplopia and multiplopia, ghost images, and decreased contrast sensitivity.

Central islands have been significantly reduced with the use of scanning and variable-spot-size lasers. Fortunately, after surface ablation, central islands typically resolve over time, although it may take 6–12 months. New treatment options such as wavefront technology and topography-based ablations may be helpful in treating persistent central islands.

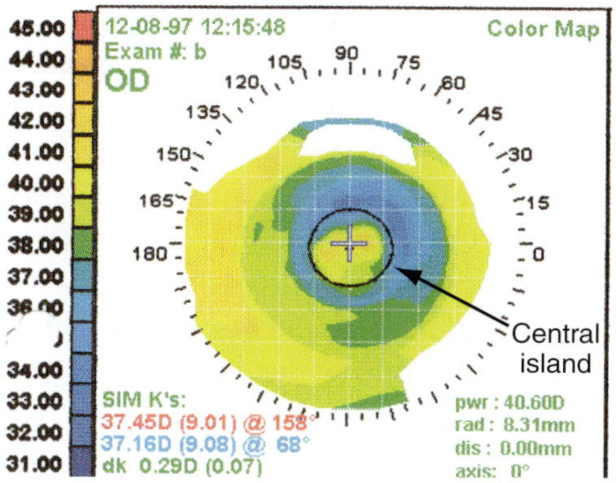

Figure 6-5 Corneal topography of a myopic ablation *(blue)* with a central island *(yellow)* in the visual axis. *(Courtesy of Roger F. Steinert, MD.)*

Optical aberrations

Some patients report optical aberrations after surface ablation, including glare, ghost images, and halos. These symptoms are most prevalent after treatment with smaller ablation zones and after attempted higher spherical and cylindrical correction. These complaints seem to be exacerbated at night. Wavefront mapping can reveal higher-order aberrations associated with these subjective complaints. In general, a larger, more uniform, and well-centered optical zone provides a better quality of vision, especially at night.

Night vision complaints are often caused by spherical aberration, although other higher-order aberrations also contribute to distortions. The cornea and lens have inherent spherical aberration. In addition, excimer laser ablation increases positive spherical aberration in the midperipheral cornea. Larger pupil size may correlate with frequency of complaints from aberrations because spherical aberration increases when the midperipheral corneal optics contribute to the light energy passing to the retina. Customized wavefront-guided corneal treatment patterns are designed to reduce existing aberrations and help prevent the creation of new aberrations, with the goal of achieving better quality of vision after laser ablation.

Decentered ablation

Accurate centration during the surface ablation procedure is important in optimizing the visual potential. Centration is even more critical for hyperopic than myopic treatments. A decentered stromal ablation may occur if the patient's eye slowly begins to drift and loses fixation or if the surgeon initially positions the patient's head improperly; if the patient's eye is not perpendicular to the laser treatment, it leads to parallax (Fig 6-6). In addition,

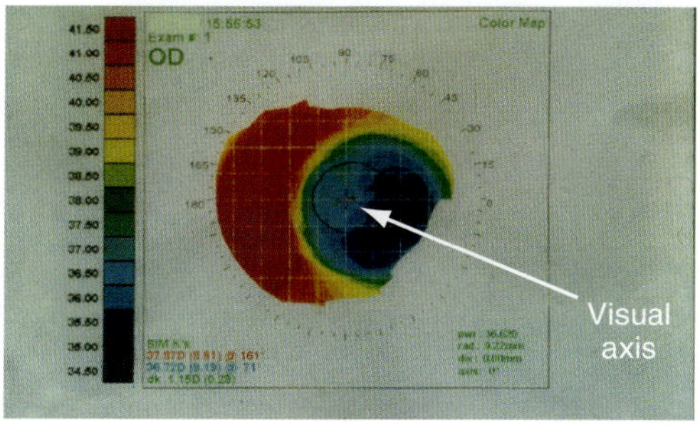

Figure 6-6 Corneal topography of a decentered ablation. *(Courtesy of Roger F. Steinert, MD.)*

centering the ablation on a pharmacologically miotic pupil may not be as accurate as centering it on a nonmiotic pupil. Miotics should not be used during photoablation because their use frequently leads to the pupil shifting nasally and sometimes superiorly. Decentration incidence increases with surgeon inexperience and with higher refractive correction, probably because the associated longer ablation time requires increased fixation time. Larger decentrations may lead to complaints of glare, halos, and decreased visual acuity. Patients with larger pupils may experience such symptoms with smaller amounts of decentration because the edge of the decentered ablation is perceived more easily within the patient's visual axis. Decentration may be reduced by ensuring that the patient's head is in the correct plane—that is, perpendicular to the laser—and that there is no head tilt. Treatment of decentration with wavefront and topographically guided technology has been effective.

Corneal haze

The type of wound healing after surface ablation is important in determining postoperative topical corticosteroid management. Patients who have haze and are undercorrected may benefit from increased corticosteroid use. Patients who have clear corneas following surface ablation and are overcorrected may benefit from a reduction in topical corticosteroid use, which may lead to regression of their refractive overcorrection.

Subepithelial corneal haze typically appears several weeks after surface ablation, peaks in intensity at 1–2 months, and gradually disappears over the following 6–12 months (Fig 6-7). Late-onset corneal haze has been described that occurs several months or even 1 year or more postoperatively after a prior period of a relatively clear cornea. Histologic studies in animals with corneal haze after PRK demonstrate abnormal glycosaminoglycans and/or nonlamellar collagen deposited in the anterior stroma as a consequence of epithelial-stromal wound healing. Most histologic studies from animals and humans show an increase in the number and activity of stromal keratocytes, which suggests that increased keratocyte activity may be the source of the extracellular deposits.

Persistent severe haze is usually associated with greater amounts of correction or smaller ablation diameters. Animal studies have demonstrated that UV-B exposure after

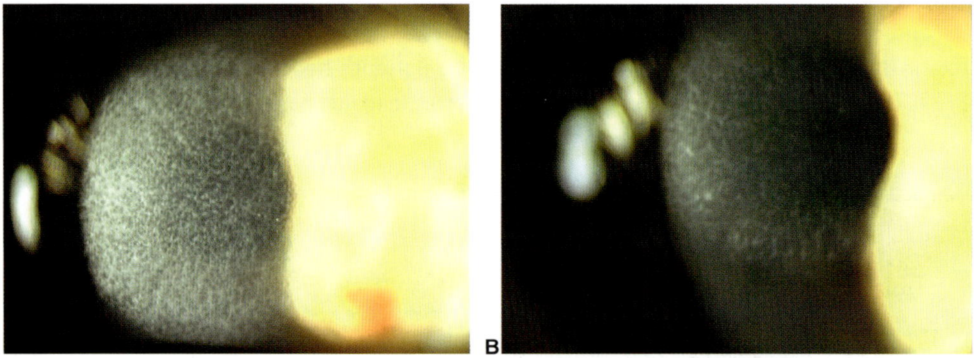

A B

Figure 6-7 PRK haze. **A,** Severe haze 5 months after PRK. The reticular pattern is characteristic of PRK-induced haze. **B,** Haze has improved to moderate level by 13 months postoperatively. *(Courtesy of Roger F. Steinert, MD.)*

PRK prolongs the stromal healing process with an increase in subepithelial haze. Clinical cases of haze after high UV exposure (such as at high altitude) corroborate these studies. Patients should be encouraged to wear UV-blocking sunglasses and brimmed hats for at least a year after surface ablation when they are in a sunny environment.

If clinically unacceptable haze persists, a superficial keratectomy or phototherapeutic keratectomy may be performed. In addition, topical mitomycin C (0.02%) may be used to prevent recurrence of subepithelial fibrosis after debridement or phototherapeutic keratectomy. Because haze is known to resolve spontaneously with normal wound remodeling, reablation should be delayed for at least 6–12 months. The clinician should be aware that in the presence of haze, refraction is often inaccurate, typically with an overestimation of the amount of myopia.

Epithelial defect

Usually, the epithelial defect created during PRK heals within 3–4 days with the aid of a bandage soft contact lens or pressure patching. A frequent cause of delayed re-epithelialization is keratoconjunctivitis sicca, which may be treated with increased lubrication, cyclosporine, and/or temporary punctal occlusion. Patients with undiagnosed autoimmune connective tissue disease or diabetes mellitus or patients who smoke may also have poor epithelial healing. Topical NSAIDs should be discontinued in any patient with delayed re-epithelialization. Oral tetracycline-family antibiotics may be beneficial in persistent epithelial defects. The importance of closely monitoring patients until re-epithelialization occurs cannot be overemphasized, as a persistent epithelial defect increases the risk of corneal haze, refractive instability, prolonged visual recovery, and infectious keratitis.

Infiltrates

The use of therapeutic contact lenses to aid in epithelial healing is associated with sterile infiltrates, especially in patients using topical NSAIDs for longer than 24 hours without concomitant topical corticosteroids. The infiltrates, which have been reported in approximately 1 in 300 cases, are secondary to an immune reaction (Fig 6-8). The incidence of

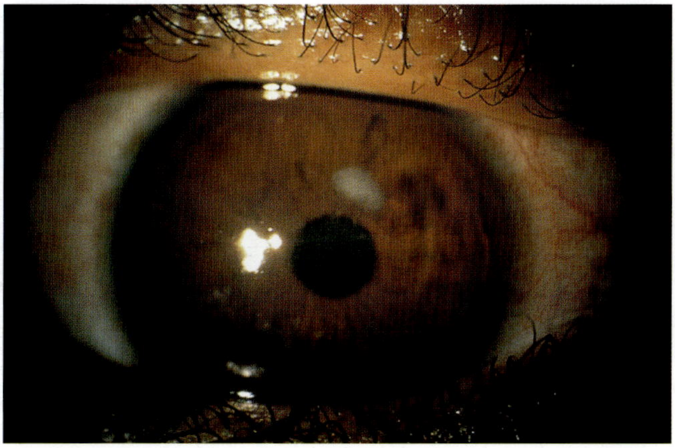

Figure 6-8 Stromal infiltrates seen with a bandage soft contact lens after PRK. *(Courtesy of Jayne S. Weiss, MD.)*

infectious keratitis has been reported as 0.2%. All infiltrates must be suspected of being infectious and managed appropriately. If infectious keratitis is suspected, the cornea should be scraped and cultured for suspected organisms.

Corticosteroid-induced complications

The incidence of increased intraocular pressure (IOP) after surface ablation has been reported to range from 11% to 25%. Occasionally, the IOP may be quite high. In one study, 2% of patients had IOP greater than 40 mm Hg. The majority of cases of elevated IOP are associated with prolonged topical corticosteroid therapy. Corticosteroid-induced elevated IOP occurs in 1.5%–3.0% of patients using fluorometholone but in up to 25% of patients using dexamethasone or stronger corticosteroids. The increase in IOP is usually controlled with topical IOP-lowering medications and typically normalizes after the corticosteroids are decreased or discontinued. Because of the changes in corneal curvature and/or corneal thickness, Goldmann tonometry readings after surface ablation are artifactually reduced (see Chapter 11). Measurement of IOP from the temporal rather than the central cornea may be more accurate, and pneumotonometry and Tono-Pen readings are also more reliable. Other corticosteroid-associated complications that have been reported after surface ablation are herpes simplex virus keratitis, ptosis, and cataracts.

Dry eye

Dry-eye conditions after surface ablation occur as a result of corneal denervation, as also happens after LASIK. Dry eye is generally less of a problem after surface ablation than after LASIK and generally resolves over 3–6 months (see Chapter 10).

Endothelial effects

In most studies, no significant change was found to have occurred in central endothelial cell density after PRK, unlike with radial keratotomy. In fact, the polymegethism associated with contact lens use typically improves after surface ablation, as demonstrated by the significant decrease in the peripheral coefficient of variation of cell size 2 years postoperatively.

Carones F, Vigo L, Scandola E, Vacchini L. Evaluation of the prophylactic use of mitomycin-C to inhibit haze formation after photorefractive keratectomy. *J Cataract Refract Surg.* 2002;28:2088–2095.

Corbett MC, Prydal JI, Verma S, Oliver KM, Pande M, Marshall J. An in vivo investigation of the structures responsible for corneal haze after photorefractive keratectomy and their effect on visual function. *Ophthalmology.* 1996;103:1366–1380.

Donnenfeld ED, O'Brien TP, Solomon R, Perry HD, Speaker MG, Wittpenn J. Infectious keratitis after photorefractive keratectomy. *Ophthalmology.* 2003;110:743–747.

Krueger RR, Saedy NF, McDonnell PJ. Clinical analysis of steep central islands after excimer laser photorefractive keratectomy. *Arch Ophthalmol.* 1996;114:377–381.

Matta CA, Piebenga LW, Deitz MR, Tauber J. Excimer retreatment for myopic photorefractive keratectomy failures. Six- to 18-month follow-up. *Ophthalmology.* 1996;103:444–451.

Conclusion

PRK, LASEK, and epi-LASIK are reasonably safe, effective, and predictable techniques for correcting myopia, astigmatism, and hyperopia. The primary disadvantages of surface ablation are the degree of postoperative discomfort, the length of time required for visual recovery, and the increase in corneal haze with treatment of higher refractive errors. There is also an increased risk of infectious keratitis with surface ablation as compared to LASIK due to the longer epithelial healing period. Wound-modulating agents such as mitomycin C are expanding the range of refractive errors that can be treated. Surface ablation may be preferable to LASIK in patients with epithelial basement membrane disease and in patients with thin corneas. PRK, LASEK, and epi-LASIK avoid the increase in higher-order aberrations associated with creation of a LASIK flap. In addition, surface ablation removes the risk of flap complications such as incomplete flaps, buttonholes, and striae. Surface ablation also reduces the risk of ectasia and dry eye compared with LASIK. For these reasons, the use of surface ablation has increased over the last several years.

Laser in Situ Keratomileusis

The term *keratomileusis* comes from the Greek words for "cornea" *(kerato)* and "to carve" *(mileusis). Laser in situ keratomileusis (LASIK),* which combines keratomileusis with excimer laser stromal ablation, has become the most popular refractive procedure performed today because of its safety, efficacy, quick visual recovery, and minimal patient discomfort.

Background

Barraquer first described corneal lamellar surgery for the correction of refractive error in 1949. The microkeratomes in use today employ many of the same general principles as Barraquer's original design of a manually advancing electric microkeratome for creating a corneal cap. Barraquer also invented a cryolathe, which froze the corneal cap and allowed for reasonably precise lenticular reshaping of the corneal tissue. The cryolathe did not gain popularity because it was technically difficult to use. In addition, the freezing process and subsequent suturing often resulted in irregular astigmatism and loss of BCVA.

Barraquer, Krumeich, and Swinger later developed a technique for removing corneal tissue without the complex cryolathe. After the corneal cap was cut by the microkeratome, it was stabilized with suction, and a refractive cut was made by a second pass of the microkeratome on the stromal side of the corneal cap. The reshaped free cap was sutured back onto the patient's corneal stromal bed. This procedure avoided the technical difficulties encountered with the cryolathe, but unpredictability and irregular astigmatism remained major obstacles.

In the late 1980s, Ruiz and Rowsey introduced the concept of removing tissue from the stromal bed rather than from the free corneal cap, a concept referred to as "in situ keratomileusis." In this technique, the microkeratome removed the corneal cap in a first pass. With a second pass of the microkeratome, a free lenticule of tissue was removed from the stromal bed. The diameter of the suction ring opening used in the second pass determined the thickness, and thus the dioptric power, of the lenticule removed. Although this technique involved less trauma to the corneal cap, the results remained suboptimal because of unpredictable refractive changes and irregular astigmatism. To improve the predictability of the microkeratome cut, Ruiz developed an automated microkeratome in the late 1980s. *Automated lamellar keratoplasty (ALK)* combined the advantages of an automated advancement of the microkeratome head with an adjustable suction ring for control of the second microkeratome cut. However, unacceptable optical aberrations often resulted from ALK because the amount of tissue removed in the second pass could not be predicted and the optical zone of the excised refractive lenticule was small.

In 1990, Pallikaris performed the first LASIK procedure when he used the excimer laser instead of the second microkeratome pass to remove tissue and induce refractive change. The excimer laser produced better optical results for 3 reasons:

1. The excimer laser ablates tissue with submicron accuracy.
2. The laser does not deform the tissue during the refractive reshaping.
3. Larger optical zones are achieved.

Modification in the microkeratome to stop the pass just short of creating a full free cap further improved results. With a narrow hinge of tissue, the outer cornea becomes a flap, which is reflected out of the way during the laser exposure. After the flap is returned to its original position, natural corneal dehydration causes it to adhere to the underlying stromal bed. The hinge allows for easier and more accurate repositioning of the flap, avoids the distortion induced by sutures, and reduces irregular astigmatism.

Instrumentation

Microkeratome

The basic principles of the microkeratome and the role of the suction ring and cutting head are illustrated in Figure 6-9. The suction ring has 2 functions:

1. to adhere to the globe, providing a stable platform for the microkeratome cutting head
2. to raise the IOP to a high level, which stiffens the cornea so it cannot move away from the cutting blade

The dimensions of the suction ring determine the diameter of the flap and the size of the stabilizing hinge. The thicker the vertical dimension of the suction ring and the smaller the diameter of the ring opening, the less the cornea will protrude, and hence a smaller-diameter flap will be produced. The suction ring is connected to a vacuum pump, which typically is controlled by an on–off foot pedal.

The microkeratome cutting head has several key components. The highly sharpened disposable cutting blade is discarded after each patient, either after a single eye or after bilateral treatment. The applanation head, or plate, flattens the cornea in advance of the cutting blade. The length of the blade that extends beyond the applanation plate and the clearance between the blade and the applanation surface are the principal determinants of flap thickness. The motor, either electrical or gas-driven turbine, oscillates the blade rapidly, typically between 6000 and 15,000 cycles per minute. The same motor or a second motor is often used to mechanically advance the cutting head, which is attached to the suction ring, across the cornea, although in several models the surgeon manually controls the advance of the cutting head.

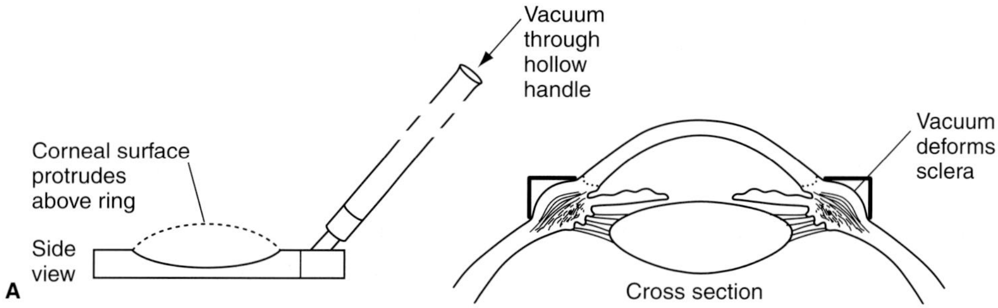

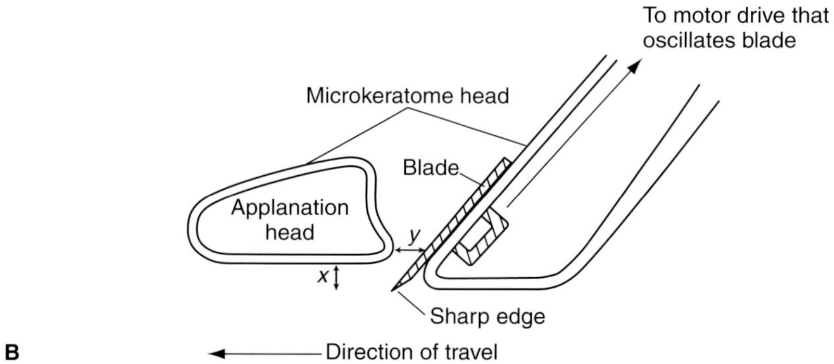

Figure 6-9 Schematic representation of the principles of a microkeratome. **A,** The suction ring serves as a platform for the microkeratome head, gripping the conjunctiva and sclera adjacent to the limbus. As the ring grips the globe, the vacuum deforms the scleral wall, increasing IOP by decreasing intraocular volume. Raising the IOP stiffens the cornea and prevents it from deforming away from the microkeratome blade when the flap is cut. The vertical dimension of the ring and the diameter of the opening are major factors in how much cornea protrudes and is exposed to the microkeratome blade, which determines the thickness and diameter of the flap. **B,** Simplified cross-section schematic of a typical microkeratome head. The protrusion of the cutting edge of the blade beyond the applanating head, or plate, of the microkeratome—that is, the distance *x* between the applanation head, which flattens the cornea, and the cutting edge of the blade—is the main determinant of flap thickness. The distance *y* allows the flap to curl up as it is cut. When *y* is larger than *x*, the flap tends to be thicker, as corneal tissue bunches up into this space. When *y* is the same as *x*, it tends to cause epithelial abrasions. **C,** Creation of the flap. When the microkeratome head passes across the cornea, the applanating surface of the head flattens the cornea in advance of the blade. The elevated IOP in the eye forces the cornea firmly against the cutting blade. **D,** Cross section of the flap after the cut. The flap has a beveled edge, which occurs when the blade cuts the edge of the flattened corneal dome, and a relatively flat lamellar separation from the underlying stromal bed. The flap and bed should be smooth. The blade advance is stopped short of full transection, leaving a hinge of tissue connecting the flap to the peripheral cornea. *(Illustration by Jeanne Koelling.)* *(continued)*

The Barraquer-designed sliding microkeratomes approached the cornea temporally for easy access, leaving a nasal hinge. Several microkeratomes developed later allowed the microkeratome head to pivot on a post, resulting in an arcing path with a superior hinge because the superior zone was the last to be cut. A superior hinge has the advantage that the up-down wiping motion of the eyelid helps prevent flap displacement. A nasal hinge does not have this advantage and also has the drawback that many pupils are located

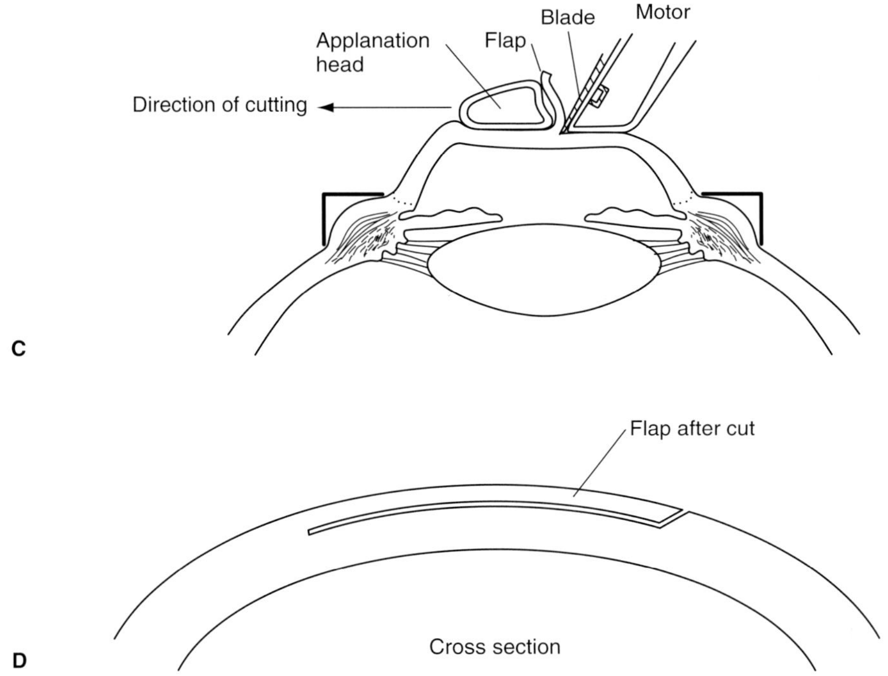

Figure 6-9 *(continued from previous page)*

somewhat nasal of the corneal center. As a result, the nasal hinge, even if shifted maximally to the nasal limbus, might impinge on a large treatment zone.

It is controversial which hinge position causes more prolonged corneal denervation and associated postoperative dry eye. Although nasal hinge location may spare some innervation of the flap because it does not transect the nasal long ciliary nerves as they enter the cornea, one study found that patients recover corneal sensation more rapidly with superior hinges. Smaller flap size and longer hinge cord length may be more important than hinge location in sparing the nerves and reducing the incidence and severity of dry eyes. Regardless of hinge type, patients generally recovered sensation to preoperative levels within 6–12 months after surgery.

Calvillo MP, McLaren JW, Hodge DO, Bourne WM. Corneal reinervation after LASIK: prospective 3-year longitudinal study. *Invest Ophthalmol Vis Sci.* 2004;45:3991–3996.

Kumano Y, Matsui H, Zushi I, et al. Recovery of corneal sensation after myopic correction by laser in situ keratomileusis with a nasal or superior hinge. *J Cataract Refract Surg.* 2003;29:757–761.

Lee KW, Joo CK. Clinical results of laser in situ keratomileusis with superior and nasal hinges. *J Cataract Refract Surg.* 2003;29:457–461.

Prior to surgery, the microkeratome and vacuum unit are assembled, carefully inspected, and tested to ensure proper function. The importance of meticulous maintenance of the microkeratome and of carefully following the manufacturer's recommendations cannot be overemphasized. Corneal perforation can result when certain microkeratome models are incorrectly assembled—for example, when the depth plate in the Automated Corneal Shaper (Chiron/B&L) is omitted.

Also, the surgeon should be aware that, regardless of the label describing the flap thickness of a specific device, the actual flap thickness varies with the type of microkeratome, patient age, preoperative corneal thickness, preoperative keratometry, preoperative astigmatism, corneal diameter, and translation speed of the microkeratome pass. It is important to maintain a steady translation speed to avoid creating bumps in the stromal bed.

Rosenfeld SI. Manual versus automated microkeratomes. In Feder RS, Rapuano CJ, eds. *The LASIK Handbook: A Case-based Approach.* Philadelphia: Lippincott Williams & Wilkins; 2007:33–43.

Femtosecond laser

The use of scanned intrastromal laser pulses to create the lamellar corneal flap for LASIK began around 1995 and has involved both picosecond and femtosecond lasers. The threshold energy for ablation is proportional to the square root of the pulse duration. The picosecond laser requires greater energy than does the femtosecond laser to photodisrupt corneal tissue and thus creates larger cavities of photodisruption and causes more tissue loss. Clinically, in picosecond-treated eyes, this leads to greater difficulty in separating the corneal lamellae and lifting the flap and to rougher stromal beds. For these reasons, the picosecond laser has generally been replaced by the femtosecond laser.

Kurtz RM, Horvath C, Liu HH, Krueger RR, Juhasz T. Lamellar refractive surgery with scanned intrastromal picosecond and femtosecond laser pulses in animal eyes. *J Refract Surg.* 1998;14:541–548.

A femtosecond Nd:YAG laser (eg, IntraLase) also creates flaps by performing a lamellar dissection within the stroma. Each laser pulse creates a discrete area of photodisruption of the collagen. The greater the number of laser spots and the more the spots overlap, the easier the tissue will separate when lifted. Although the goal is to try to minimize the total energy used in flap creation, a certain level of power is necessary to ensure complete photodisruption, and greater overlap of spots allows for easier flap lifting. With the computer programmed for flap diameter, depth, and hinge location and size, thousands of adjacent pulses are scanned across the cornea in a controlled pattern that results in a flap. It is unclear what, if any, effect removing tissue with photodisruption rather than cutting it with a traditional microkeratome has on the seating of the corneal flap. Advocates cite the potential for better depth control, lessening or avoiding such complications as buttonhole perforations, and precise control of flap dimension and location. One study of 208 eyes that underwent femtosecond laser flap creation showed that 1.9% had a loss of suction during femtosecond laser flap creation but that all had successful flap performance 5–45 minutes after reapplanation of the eye.

Holzer MP, Rabsilber TM, Auffarth GU. Femtosecond laser-assisted corneal flap cuts: morphology, accuracy, and histopathology. *Invest Ophthalmol Vis Sci.* 2006;47:2828–2831.

Preoperative inspection of the excimer laser

Prior to the LASIK procedure, the excimer laser beam should be tested for proper homogeneity, fluence, and centration, just as it is when preparing for surface ablation.

Patient Selection

The preoperative evaluation of patients prior to LASIK is similar to the evaluation prior to surface ablation. In this section, only the differences in evaluating a patient for LASIK surgery are discussed. The full preoperative evaluation of refractive surgery patients is discussed in Chapter 3.

As with surface ablation, careful attention must be given to preexisting systemic or ocular conditions that may interfere with healing. However, because LASIK violates the corneal surface less than surface ablation does, the healing response of the epithelium and superficial keratocytes is not as lengthy. Although in the past it was deemed otherwise, a history of keloid formation is not a contraindication to LASIK. In some systemic and ocular conditions, surface ablation may be more suitable than LASIK (see Chapter 10).

Many reports indicate that postoperative dry eye is more common with LASIK than with surface ablation. This is important to remember when considering refractive surgery in a patient with known dry-eye syndrome. Preoperative evaluation for dry eyes is performed by assessment of history, the tear meniscus, rose bengal or lissamine green staining, and/or Schirmer testing. Dry eyes should be treated preoperatively with artificial tear supplementation, topical anti-inflammatory medications (corticosteroids or cyclosporine), oral doxycycline, and/or punctal occlusion, to try and limit the postoperative keratopathy that can lead to flap irregularities and even regression or undercorrection.

When evaluating the cornea prior to LASIK, it is particularly important to look for signs of an epithelial basement membrane dystrophy that could predispose the patient to epithelial defects with the microkeratome pass, as well as to postoperative epithelial ingrowth. These patients are usually best served by having PRK, if their refractive error permits.

Corneal topography must be performed to assess corneal cylinder and rule out the presence of forme fruste keratoconus, pellucid marginal degeneration, or contact lens–induced corneal warpage. Corneas steeper than 48.00 D are more likely to have thin flaps or frank buttonholes (central perforation of the flap). Corneas flatter than 40.00 D are more likely to have smaller-diameter flaps and are at increased risk for creation of a free cap due to transection of the hinge. These problems may be reduced or eliminated by using a smaller or larger suction ring, which changes the flap diameter; modifying the hinge length; slowing passage of the microkeratome to create a thicker flap or using a microkeratome head designed to create thicker flaps; applying higher suction levels and creating a higher IOP; or selecting a femtosecond laser to create the lamellar flap. The surgeon must be aware that using the same blade to create the flap in a patient's second eye typically results in a flap that is 10–20 μm thinner than the flap in the first eye.

Solomon KD, Donnenfeld ED, Sandoval HP, et al. Flap thickness accuracy: comparison of 6 microkeratome models. *J Cataract Refract Surg.* 2004;30:964–977.

Preoperative pachymetric measurement of corneal thickness is mandatory because an adequate stromal bed must remain to decrease the possibility of postoperative corneal ectasia, although the definition of what constitutes an adequate residual stromal bed remains controversial. The following formula is used to calculate corneal thickness:

$$\text{Central corneal thickness} - \text{thickness of flap} - \text{depth of ablation} = \text{residual stromal bed thickness (RST)}$$

In calculating the likely RST, the surgeon must use the ablation depth based on the intended total correction, not the value of the nomogram-adjusted refractive error that is programmed into the laser. The true tissue ablation depth is closer to the value needed to achieve the refractive shift. A nomogram adjustment to a lower refractive error that is programmed into the laser does not mean that less tissue is removed.

Although most practitioners use as a guideline a minimum residual corneal bed thickness of 250 μm, this is a clinically derived figure and is not based on any definitive laboratory investigations or controlled prospective studies. Even 250 μm remaining in the stromal bed after ablation does not guarantee that postoperative corneal ectasia will not develop. In a retrospective study of 10 eyes from 7 patients who developed corneal ectasia after LASIK, 30% had a predicted RST of ≥250 μm. In this series, 88% of patients had previously undiagnosed forme fruste keratoconus. Also, the actual LASIK flap may be thicker than that noted on the label of the microkeratome head, making the stromal bed less than the calculated minimum of 250 μm. Consequently, an increasing number of surgeons are using intraoperative pachymetry, especially for high myopic corrections, enhancements, or thin corneas, to determine actual flap thickness.

A common approach to determining flap thickness and RST is to measure the central corneal thickness at the beginning of the procedure, create the LASIK flap with the surgeon's instrument of choice, lift the flap, measure the untreated stromal bed, and subtract the intended thickness of corneal ablation from the stromal bed to ascertain if the RST will be ≥250 μm or whatever safe threshold is desired. Flap thickness is then calculated by subtracting the untreated stromal bed measurement from the initial central corneal thickness.

Randleman JB, Russell B, Ward MA, Thompson KP, Stulting RD. Risk factors and prognosis for corneal ectasia after LASIK. *Ophthalmology.* 2003;110:267–275.

The surgeon should preoperatively inform patients with thinner corneas or higher corrections that future enhancement may not be possible because of inadequate RST.

Excessive corneal flattening or steepening after LASIK may reduce visual quality and increase aberrations. Although no controlled studies have established specific limits, many surgeons avoid creating a postoperative corneal power below about 34.00 D or above about 50.00 D because of the high amount of resulting spherical aberration. The surgeon should anticipate the postoperative keratometry by estimating a flattening of 0.80 D for every diopter of myopia treated and a steepening of 1.00 D for every diopter of hyperopia treated (see Chapter 3).

If wavefront-guided laser ablation is planned, wavefront error is measured preoperatively, as discussed in Chapter 1. Although wavefront data are used to program the laser, the surgeon must still compare these data to the manifest refraction prior to surgery to prevent data input errors. In general, one needs to be wary of significant differences between the manifest refraction and the wavefront refraction.

One company specifies that the safety and effectiveness of the wavefront-guided laser (VISX Star4 CustomVue) have not been established if the difference between the wavefront calculated power and the manifest power of sphere or cylinder is more minus than 0.50 D or more plus than 0.75 D or if the difference in manifest cylinder axis is greater than 15°. In such cases, the wavefront data and manifest refraction must be rechecked to detect and correct potential errors before the wavefront-guided ablation is performed. In addition, a minimum scotopic pupil size (eg, 5.0 mm for the VISX CustomVue) may be necessary to obtain adequate wavefront measurement data prior to the ablation.

Surgical Technique

Surgical suite conditions

The laser suite should have tightly controlled temperature and humidity to optimize results. The room needs to be clean but not sterile, and the lights should be adjustable. An observation window, if present, should have blinds to accommodate a patient's preference for privacy.

Preoperative preparation of the patient

A mild sedative, such as oral diazepam 5–10 mg, may be administered to the patient prior to the procedure. Topical anesthetic drops are instilled and the skin is usually prepped with povidone-iodine or another skin antiseptic. Preoperative topical antibiotics may be used.

Many surgeons drape the skin or eyelashes with a plastic drape or with Steri-Strips; others consider such measures unnecessary and a potential source of material to jam the microkeratome. An eyelid speculum is placed that has a configuration to accommodate the suction device and the path of the microkeratome. In patients with small interpalpebral fissures, various microkeratome suction rings may be applied without the need for an eyelid speculum. The cornea may be marked with an optical zone marker to assist in proper centration of the suction ring, and 1 or more lines may be placed across the intended flap edge to ensure proper realignment of the flap (Fig 6-10).

Programming the laser

The actual treatment value programmed into the laser is typically an adjustment of the final refractive goal, derived from each surgeon's individual nomogram, as developed by monitoring outcomes. The original LASIK FDA studies used nomograms based on PRK, and adjustments may be necessary in LASIK. In addition, each surgeon should analyze his or her first hundred cases and make personal adjustments as desired. Major variables that some but not all surgeons find to be important include specific laser, individual surgeon,

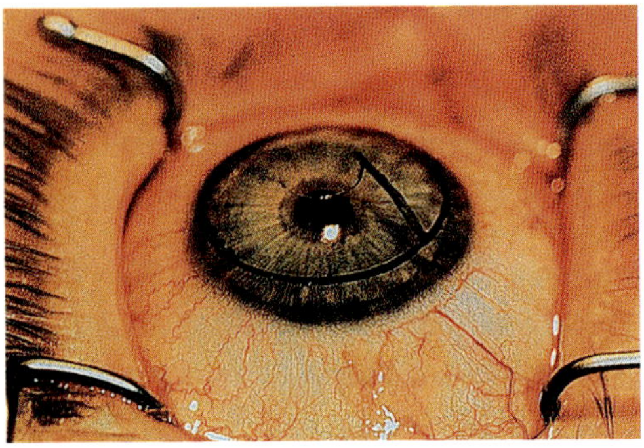

Figure 6-10 Proper corneal marking. *(Courtesy of Randy J. Epstein, MD.)*

amount of correction, age, temperature, and humidity. In addition, the size of the ablation zone and whether to include a blend are issues based on the patient's refractive error, the calculated residual stromal bed, and the pupillary diameter. In custom ablation, minor modifications can be made to the sphere and cylinder by the surgeon.

Creation of the flap by the microkeratome

The intended diameter of the flap is determined by the surgeon based on such variables as the type of refractive error to be treated (hyperopic corrections and wavefront-guided treatments require a larger flap because of the larger ablation diameter), the corneal curvature and microkeratome suction ring dimensions (flatter corneas result in a smaller flap for the same size ring), the patient's anatomy (presence of peripheral corneal blood vessels and size of the corneal diameter), and the surgeon's preference. Depending on the manufacturer, the suction ring is usually centered over the entrance pupil (Fig 6-11), but some surgeons prefer to displace the flap in the direction of the hinge to ensure that the hinge will not interfere with the laser ablation zone.

Thinner flaps leave greater stromal bed thickness for the ablation and possible enhancements but may be more prone to dislocation or striae. Thicker flaps have a lower risk of unexpected buttonholes and flap folds and may be more stable, but they leave a thinner residual stromal bed. Each type of microkeratome characteristically creates a flap with a range of thicknesses that the surgeon must know and include in the surgical plan to ensure an adequate residual stromal bed (ie, RST). The surgeon cannot accurately predict the flap thickness a microkeratome will create based only on the labeling of the microkeratome head.

Once the ring is properly positioned, suction is activated. The IOP should be assessed at this point because low IOP can result in a poor-quality, thin, or incomplete flap. It is essential to have both excellent exposure of the eye, allowing free movement of the microkeratome, and proper suction ring fixation. Inadequate suction may result from blockage of the suction ports from eyelashes under the suction ring or from redundant or scarred conjunctiva. To avoid the possibility of pseudosuction (occlusion of the suction port with

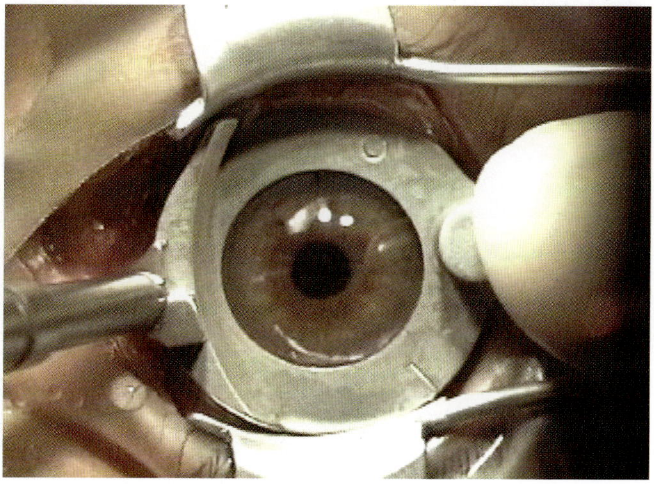

Figure 6-11 Placement of a suction ring. *(Courtesy of Roger F. Steinert, MD.)*

conjunctiva but not sclera), the surgeon can confirm that true suction is present by observing that the eye moves when the suction ring is gently moved, the pupil is mildly dilated, and the patient can no longer see the fixation light. Methods used to assess whether the IOP is adequately elevated include use of a Barraquer plastic applanator or a pneumotonometer or palpation of the eye by the surgeon. Beginning surgeons are advised to use an objective rather than only a subjective method.

Prior to the lamellar cut, the surface of the cornea is moistened with proparacaine with glycerin or with nonpreserved artificial tears. Balanced salt solution should be avoided at this point because mineral deposits may develop within the microkeratome and interfere with its proper function. The surgeon places the microkeratome on the suction ring and checks that its path is free of obstacles such as the eyelid speculum, drape, or overhanging eyelid. The microkeratome is then activated, passed over the cornea (Fig 6-12) until halted by the hinge-creating stopper, and then reversed off the cornea. With some models, epithelial defects may be reduced by lowering the vacuum or discontinuing the suction during the reversal; other models require the vacuum to remain at full pressure during reversal. Improvements in microkeratomes have decreased the incidence of epithelial defects. If a patient develops an epithelial defect in 1 eye during a microkeratome pass, an epithelial defect will usually develop in the second eye when it is treated, regardless of alterations in the microkeratome vacuum level. This implies that a subclinical epitheliopathy such as epithelial basement membrane disease may be present that is made manifest by the microkeratome pass.

Creation of the flap with the femtosecond laser

The femtosecond laser is gaining in popularity for creation of the LASIK flap. The femtosecond laser allows adjustments for several variables involved in making the flap, including flap thickness, flap diameter, hinge location, hinge angle, bed energy, and spot separation. A larger flap diameter is usually selected for hyperopic and wavefront-guided treatments.

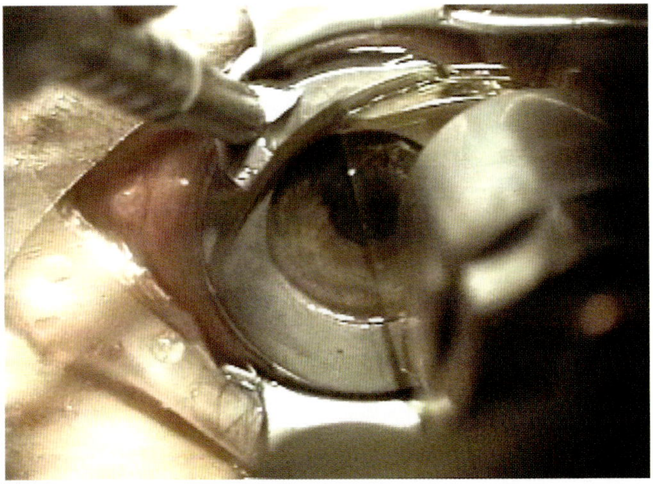

Figure 6-12 Movement of the microkeratome head across the cornea. *(Courtesy of Roger F. Steinert, MD.)*

The femtosecond laser creates a planar flap, whereas mechanical microkeratomes create a meniscus flap. With the femtosecond laser, the corneal morphology or curvature does not affect flap thickness.

The risk of certain flap-related complications, including epithelial defects, buttonholes, incomplete flaps, thin or thick flaps, postoperative striae, and dislocated flaps, seems to be reduced with the femtosecond laser. Certain other postoperative complications, however, may be more likely. One of these is diffuse lamellar keratitis (DLK), which has been reported to occur more commonly with inexperienced surgeons, who sometimes use higher laser energy levels than are needed. The surgeon must find a balance in the energy level: low enough to minimize DLK but high enough to allow easy tissue separation. Some surgeons also use more intensive and prolonged topical corticosteroid therapy when they use the femtosecond laser to reduce this risk of DLK. With both the mechanical microkeratome and the femtosecond laser, a suction ring must be applied, thus elevating IOP and increasing the potential for optic nerve damage, although for the latter, a more prolonged period of suction and elevated IOP is often needed.

The femtosecond laser may take longer to use than the mechanical microkeratome because it requires several extra steps. First, the suction ring is centered over the pupil and suction is applied. Proper centration of the suction ring is critical and is performed under a separate microscope, either the microscope from the adjacent excimer laser or an auxiliary microscope in the laser suite. The docking procedure is initiated under the femtosecond laser's microscope, while the patient's chin and forehead are kept level and the suction ring is kept parallel to the eye (Figs 6-13, 6-14). The applanation lens is then centered over the suction ring and lowered into place using the joystick, and the suction ring is unclipped to complete the attachment to the docking device (Fig 6-15). Complete applanation of the cornea must be achieved or an incomplete flap or incomplete side cut may occur.

Once the laser's computer has confirmed centration, the surgeon administers the femtosecond laser emission. The vacuum is then released, the suction ring is removed, and the patient is positioned under the excimer laser. A spatula with a semisharp edge identifies and scores the flap edge near the hinge (Fig 6-16). The instrument is then passed

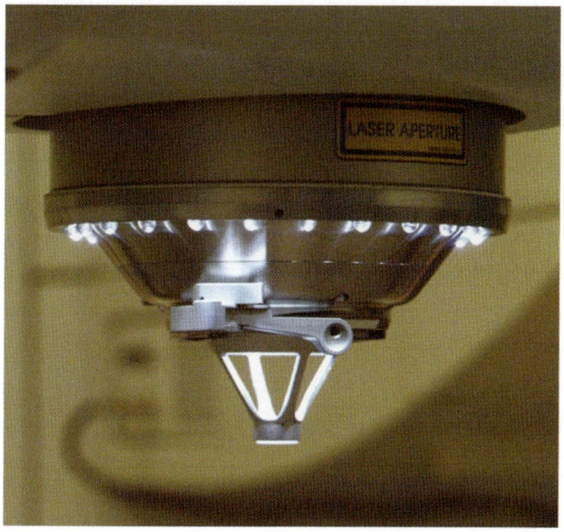

Figure 6-13 IntraLase with cone attached. *(Reproduced with permission from Feder RS, Rapuano CJ.* The LASIK Handbook: A Case-based Approach. *Philadelphia: Lippincott Williams & Wilkins; 2007:45, fig 2.7. Photograph courtesy of Robert Feder, MD.)*

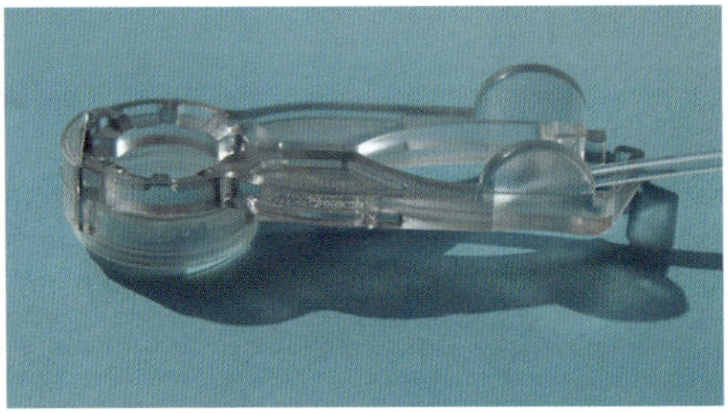

Figure 6-14 IntraLase suction ring. *(Reproduced with permission from Feder RS, Rapuano CJ.* The LASIK Handbook: A Case-based Approach. *Philadelphia: Lippincott Williams & Wilkins; 2007:45, fig 2.8. Photograph courtesy of Robert Feder, MD.)*

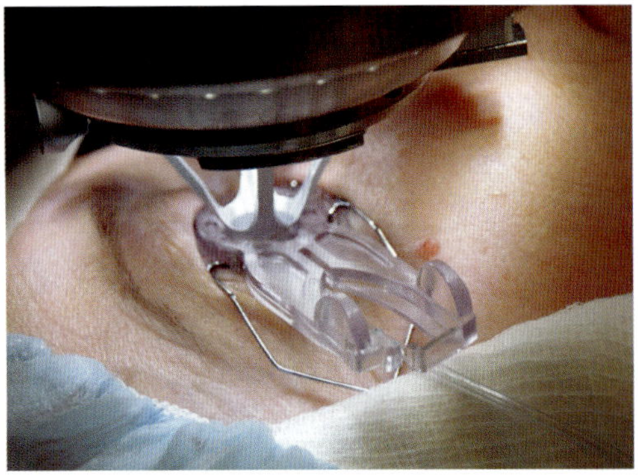

Figure 6-15 Docking of IntraLase cone with suction ring positioned on the eye. *(Reproduced with permission from Feder RS, Rapuano CJ.* The LASIK Handbook: A Case-based Approach. *Philadelphia: Lippincott Williams & Wilkins; 2007:46, fig 2.9. Photograph courtesy of Robert Feder, MD.)*

across the flap along the base of the hinge, and the flap is lifted by sweeping inferiorly and separating the flap interface, dissecting one third of the flap at a time and thus reducing the risk of tearing. If bilateral LASIK surgery is planned, a flap is usually created in both eyes before excimer ablation is performed.

Several recent studies have demonstrated the benefits of the femtosecond laser compared with those of the mechanical microkeratome in creating flaps, including more predictable flap thickness, thinner flaps, a reduction in the standard deviation for flap thickness, larger effective bed area for similar-sized flaps, less induction of astigmatism, fewer induced higher-order aberrations with flap formation, less reduction in contrast sensitivity, less epithelial injury, and better preservation of corneal sensitivity. Other studies have shown better UCVA and better manifest refractive outcomes with the femtosecond laser. See Table 6-1.

The disadvantages of the femtosecond laser compared with those of the mechanical microkeratome include significantly greater expense, increased time of operation, more prolonged suction and elevated IOP, more manipulation needed to lift the flap, greater difficulty lifting the flap beyond 6 months, the potential to create a dense *opaque bubble layer (OBL)* that may interfere with the laser ablation, and a greater risk of DLK. An OBL results from excessive cavitation bubbles that are produced by the interaction between the laser and the corneal tissue. When an OBL does occur, the surgeon may want to wait to allow the bubbles to resolve before proceeding with the ablation. Sometimes cavitation bubbles may appear in the anterior chamber, and in extreme cases, an OBL may interfere with the tracking and registration mechanisms. One rare complication unique to the femtosecond laser is the syndrome of delayed photosensitivity, or what some surgeons refer to as "good acuity plus photosensitivity (GAPP)." These cases of delayed photosensitivity generally occur weeks after an uneventful treatment; are associated with excellent vision; and usually respond to a short course of topical corticosteroids, although occasionally prolonged treatment is required.

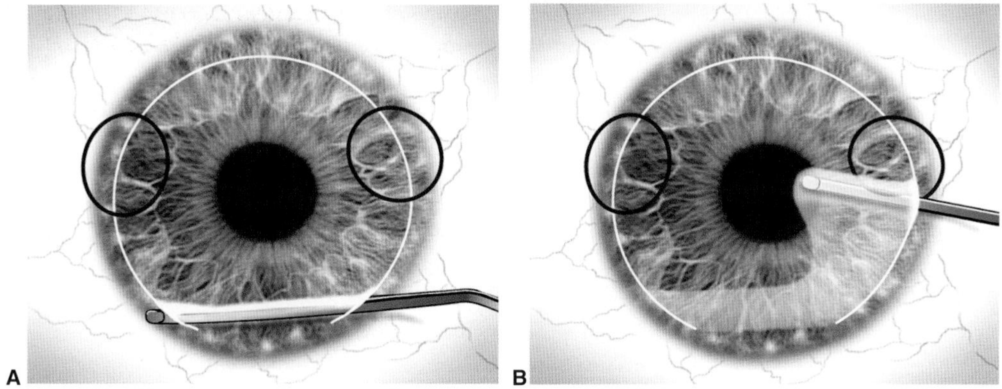

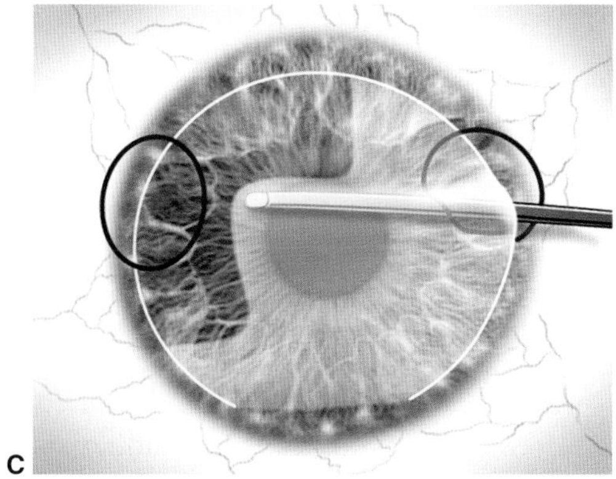

Figure 6-16 Flap lift technique following femtosecond laser application. **A,** After the flap edge is scored near the hinge on either side, a spatula is passed across the flap. **B,** The interface is separated by starting at the superior hinge and sweeping inferiorly. **C,** Dissecting one third of the flap at a time reduces the risk of tearing the hinge. *(Reproduced with permission from Feder RS, Rapuano CJ.* The LASIK Handbook: A Case-based Approach. *Philadelphia: Lippincott Williams & Wilkins; 2007:48, fig 2-12. Photograph courtesy of Robert Feder, MD.)*

Table 6-1 Advantages and Disadvantages of the Femtosecond Laser

Advantages	Disadvantages
Less increase in IOP required	Longer suction time
More control over flap diameter	More flap manipulation
Size and thickness of flap less dependent on corneal contour	Opaque bubble layer (OBL) may interfere with excimer ablation
Centration easier to control	Bubbles in the anterior chamber may interfere with tracking and registration
Epithelial defects on flap are rare	
Less risk of free cap and buttonhole	Increased overall treatment time
More reliable flap thickness	Difficulty lifting flap > 6 months
Hemorrhage from limbal vessels less likely	Increased risk of DLK
	Increased cost
Ability to re-treat immediately if incomplete femtosecond laser ablation	Need to acquire new skills
	Delayed photosensitivity or good acuity plus photosensitivity (GAPP), which may require prolonged topical corticosteroid therapy

Modified with permission from Feder RS, Rapuano CJ. *The LASIK Handbook: A Case-based Approach.* Philadelphia: Lippincott Williams & Wilkins; 2007.

Durrie DS, Kezirian GM. Femtosecond laser versus mechanical keratome flaps in wavefront-guided laser in situ keratomileusis: prospective contralateral eye study. *J Cataract Refract Surg.* 2005;31:120–126.

Kezirian GM, Stonecipher KG. Comparison of the IntraLase femtosecond laser and mechanical microkeratomes for laser in situ keratomileusis. *J Cataract Refract Surg.* 2004;30:804–811.

Lim T, Yang S, Kim M, Tchah H. Comparison of the IntraLase femtosecond laser and mechanical microkeratome for laser in situ keratomileusis. *Am J Ophthalmol.* 2006;141:833–839.

Nordan LT, Slade SG, Baker RN, Suarez C, Juhasz T, Kurtz R. Femtosecond laser flap creation for laser in situ keratomileusis: 6-month follow-up of initial U.S. clinical series. *J Refract Surg.* 2003;19:8–14.

Patel SV, Maguire LJ, McLaren JW, Hodge DO, Bourne WM. Femtosecond laser versus mechanical microkeratome for LASIK: a randomized controlled study. *Ophthalmology.* 2007; 114:1482–1490.

Tran DB, Sarayba MA, Bor Z, et al. Randomized prospective clinical study comparing induced aberrations with IntraLase and Hansatome flap creation in fellow eyes: potential impact on wavefront-guided laser in situ keratomileusis. *J Cataract Refract Surg.* 2005;31:97–105.

The excimer laser ablation

Once the flap has been created and reflected, the excimer laser system is focused and centered over the pupil, and the patient is asked to look at the fixation light (Fig 6-17). The lights in the room and laser may need to be adjusted so the patient can continue to see the fixation light through the irregular stromal surface after the flap has been lifted. The lights under the laser's microscope may need to be adjusted as well, as some tracking systems depend on pupil size and iris configuration. If excess moisture is noted, the stromal bed is dried with a microsurgical debris-free sponge. The laser is then refocused on the stromal bed and centered, most commonly on the pupil. A tracking system, if present, is activated (see the discussion of laser tracking systems earlier in this chapter in Laser Treatment). It is important to keep the patient's head parallel to the laser in order to prevent eye rolling or parallax. Once the patient confirms that the fixation light of the excimer laser is still

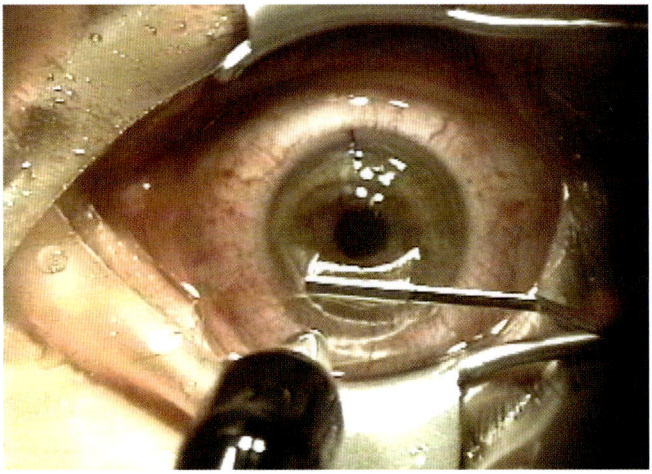

Figure 6-17 Reflecting the LASIK flap. *(Courtesy of Roger F. Steinert, MD.)*

visible and that he or she is looking directly at it, ablation begins (see Fig 6-4). With or without a tracking device, the surgeon must monitor the patient to ensure that fixation is maintained throughout the treatment. Neither tracking nor iris registration is a substitute for accurate patient fixation. It is important to initiate stromal ablation promptly, before excessive stromal dehydration takes place. If centration is lost, however, the ablation should be halted immediately and fixation regained prior to finishing the treatment. During larger-diameter ablations, a flap protector may be needed to shield the underside of the flap near the hinge from the laser pulses.

Replacing the flap

After the ablation is completed, the flap is replaced onto the stromal bed. The interface is irrigated until all interface debris is eliminated (which is better seen with oblique rather than coaxial illumination). The surface of the flap is gently stroked with a smooth instrument, such as an irrigation cannula or a moistened microsurgical spear sponge, from the hinge, or center, to the periphery to ensure that wrinkles are eliminated and that the flap settles back into its original position, as indicated by realignment of the corneal marks made earlier. The peripheral gutters should be symmetric and even. The physiologic dehydration of the stroma by the endothelial pump will begin to secure the flap in position within several minutes. If a significant epithelial defect is present or a large, loose sheet of epithelium is created, a bandage contact lens should be placed. Once the flap is adherent, the eyelid speculum is removed carefully so as not to move the flap. Most surgeons place varying combinations of antibiotic, NSAID, and corticosteroid drops on the eye at the conclusion of the procedure. The flap is usually rechecked at the slit lamp before the patient leaves to make sure it has remained in proper alignment. A clear shield or protective goggles are often placed to guard against accidental trauma that could displace the flap. Patients are instructed not to rub or squeeze their eyes.

Many surgeons instruct their patients to use topical antibiotics and corticosteroids postoperatively for 5–7 days. When the femtosecond laser has been used, some surgeons use more frequent applications of corticosteroid eyedrops or use them for a more prolonged period. In addition, it is very important that the surface of the flap be kept well lubricated in the early postoperative period. Patients may be told to use the protective shield for 1 day to 1 week when they shower or sleep and to avoid swimming and hot tubs for 2 weeks. Patients are examined 1 day after surgery to ensure that the flap has remained in proper alignment and that there is no evidence of infection or excessive inflammation. In the absence of complications, the next examinations are typically at approximately 1 week, 1 month, 3 months, 6 months, and 12 months postoperatively.

Lui MM, Silas MA, Fugishima H. Complications of photorefractive keratectomy and laser in situ keratomileusis. *J Refract Surg.* 2003;19:S247–S249.

Price FW. LASIK. *Focal Points: Clinical Modules for Ophthalmologists.* San Francisco: American Academy of Ophthalmology; 2000, module 3.

Schallhorn SC, Amesbury EC, and Tanzer DJ. Avoidance, recognition, and management of LASIK complications. *Am J Ophthalmol.* 2006;141:733–739.

Outcomes

LASIK studies vary considerably in the techniques used, the degree of refractive error treated, the postoperative follow-up planned, and the variables analyzed. Consequently, it is often difficult to compare the outcomes of different studies. Some trials separate the results into low, moderate, and high myopia categories; others merge the postoperative visual acuity results for all refractive errors. Furthermore, the definitions of these categories vary among studies.

With the evolution of laser technology, the improvement in visual results has been substantial. A 1999 clinical trial using a conventional laser for myopic astigmatic LASIK yielded postoperative UCVA of 20/20 in 47% of eyes. More recent 2003 clinical trials of wavefront-guided ablation for myopic astigmatic LASIK achieved UCVA of 20/20 in 79%–98% of eyes. The following sections describe LASIK results reported from FDA clinical trials and publications.

Boxer Wachler BS. Effect of pupil size on visual function under monocular and binocular conditions in LASIK and non-LASIK patients. *J Cataract Refract Surg.* 2003;29:275–278.

el Maghraby A, Salah T, Waring GO III, Klyce S, Ibrahim O. Randomized bilateral comparison of excimer laser in situ keratomileusis and photorefractive keratectomy for 2.50 to 8.00 diopters of myopia. *Ophthalmology.* 1999;106:447–457.

Mutyala S, McDonald MB, Scheinblum KA, Ostrick MD, Brint SF, Thompson H. Contrast sensitivity evaluation after laser in situ keratomileusis. *Ophthalmology.* 2000;107:1864–1867.

Pop M, Payette Y. Photorefractive keratectomy versus laser in situ keratomileusis: a control-matched study. *Ophthalmology.* 2000;107:251–257.

Reviglio VE, Bossana EL, Luna JD, Muino JC, Juarez CP. Laser in situ keratomileusis for myopia and hyperopia using the Lasersight 200 laser in 300 consecutive eyes. *J Refract Surg.* 2000;16:716–723.

Low myopia

FDA clinical trials involving patients with low myopia (<–6.00 D) treated with conventional (non–wavefront-guided) LASIK report that 67%–86% of eyes achieved UCVA of 20/20 or better, 93%–100% achieved 20/40 or better, and 94%–100% obtained a postoperative refraction within 1.00 D of the intended refraction. Up to 2.1% of eyes lost 2 or more lines of BCVA.

el Danasoury MA, el Maghraby A, Klyce SD, Mehrez K. Comparison of photorefractive keratectomy with excimer laser in situ keratomileusis in correcting low myopia (from –2.00 to –5.50 diopters): a randomized study. *Ophthalmology.* 1999;106:411–420.

Fernandez AP, Jaramillo J, Jaramillo M. Comparison of photorefractive keratectomy and laser in situ keratomileusis for myopia of –6 D or less using the Nidek EC-5000 laser. *J Refract Surg.* 2000;16:711–715.

Tole DM, McCarty DJ, Couper T, Taylor HR. Comparison of laser in situ keratomileusis and photorefractive keratectomy for the correction of myopia of –6.00 diopters or less. Melbourne Excimer Laser Group. *J Refract Surg.* 2001;17:46–54.

Moderate myopia

Large published series and FDA clinical trials involving patients with moderate myopia (approximately –6.00 to –12.00 D) treated with conventional LASIK report that 26%–71% of eyes achieved an UCVA of 20/20 or better, 55%–100% reached at least 20/40, and

41%–96% were within 1.00 D of intended correction. The percentage of eyes losing 2 or more lines of BCVA ranged from 0% to 4.5%. The poorer outcomes usually reflected earlier studies using older laser technology.

High myopia

High myopia is most often defined as myopia greater than –12.0 D, although several studies report treatment results in patients with up to –29.00 D. Within this range, the predictability of the procedure is markedly reduced, with 26%–65% of eyes achieving at least 20/40 UCVA and 32%–65% attaining a postoperative refraction within 1.00 D of the intended correction. In addition, when such high amounts of myopia were treated, there was a higher incidence of loss of BCVA than in the correction of lower levels of myopia. However, patients with high myopia often gain BCVA after LASIK, probably due to decreased image minification, compared with the BCVA achieved with preoperative spectacles.

As experience with LASIK has accumulated, an increasing number of surgeons have chosen to perform LASIK or surface ablation only rarely, if ever, for corrections above –12.00 D. The required ablation depths for high corrections may leave an inadequate stromal bed (less than 250 μm at a minimum) for long-term structural stability of the cornea. Although some studies have reported no eyes with loss of 2 or more lines of BCVA, other series have reported up to 27% loss of 2 or more lines of BCVA for this range of myopic LASIK. The amount of good high-contrast UCVA that can be achieved is not as predictable when a high level of correction is required. Further, high levels of correction have an unacceptably high number of side effects, including glare, halos, and loss of contrast sensitivity. These difficulties are attributable to the induction of higher-order aberrations, particularly spherical aberration, because of the marked flattening of the central cornea compared with the midperipheral cornea.

Hersh PS, Brint SF, Maloney RK, et al. Photorefractive keratectomy versus laser in situ keratomileusis for moderate to high myopia: a randomized prospective study. *Ophthalmology.* 1998;105:1512–1522.

Kawesch GM, Kezirian GM. Laser in situ keratomileusis for high myopia with the VISX Star laser. *Ophthalmology.* 2000;107:653–661.

Pallikaris IG, Siganos DS. Excimer laser in situ keratomileusis and photorefractive keratectomy for correction of high myopia. *J Refract Corneal Surg.* 1994;10:498–510.

Myopia with astigmatism

Overall, the results for toric LASIK ablations are not as predictable as those for spherical LASIK ablations. Most often, the procedure undercorrects the cylinder, which may simply indicate the need for improved nomograms or may indicate an inaccuracy in the axis ablated. Often it is difficult to determine the outcome of treatment for myopic astigmatism when a large series of patients is reviewed. Some clinical trials summarize the final outcome for all patients and do not distinguish between results for myopia and those for myopic astigmatism.

In FDA clinical trials including patients undergoing LASIK for myopic astigmatism, 43%–87% of eyes achieved UCVA of 20/20 or better and 84%–99% achieved UCVA of 20/40 or better; 82%–92% of eyes were within ±1.00 D of the intended refraction. Up to 1.8% lost 2 or more lines of BCVA.

Casebeer JC, Kezirian GM. Outcomes of spherocylinder treatments in the comprehensive refractive surgery LASIK study. *Semin Ophthalmol.* 1998;13:71–78.

McDonald MB, Carr JD, Frantz JM, et al. Laser in situ keratomileusis for myopia up to –11 diopters with up to –5 diopters of astigmatism with the Summit Autonomous LADARVision excimer laser system. *Ophthalmology.* 2001;108:309–316.

Hyperopia

In contrast to a myopic ablation, where the central cornea is ablated and flattened, a hyperopic ablation steepens the central cornea by ablating a doughnut-shaped area in the midperiphery. Initial problems with hyperopic treatment included decreased predictability and stability compared with myopic treatment, as well as loss of BCVA (partially secondary to decentrations with small optical zones). With enlargement of both the optical zone and the peripheral blend zone, as well as improved centration due to the help of tracking devices, studies of LASIK treatment for hyperopia with longer follow-up periods have shown improved outcomes.

In FDA clinical trials of LASIK for hyperopia up to 6.00 D, 49%–59% of eyes achieved postoperative UCVA of 20/20 or better, 93%–96% achieved postoperative UCVA of 20/40 or better, 86%–87% were within 1.00 D of emmetropia postoperatively, and up to 3.5% of eyes lost 2 or more lines of BCVA. Overall, studies with larger ablation zones have demonstrated good results for refractive errors up to +4.00 for conventional treatments, but predictability and stability are markedly reduced with LASIK treatments for hyperopia that are above this level. Consequently, most refractive surgeons do not treat up to the highest levels of hyperopia that have been approved by the FDA for conventional treatments.

Davidorf JM, Eghbali F, Onclinx T, Mahoney RK. Effect of varying the optical zone diameter on the results of hyperopic laser in situ keratomileusis. *Ophthalmology.* 2001;108:1261–1265.

Tabbara KF, El-Sheikh HF, Islam SM. Laser in situ keratomileusis for the correction of hyperopia from +0.50 to +11.50 diopters with the Keracor 117C laser. *J Refract Surg.* 2001; 17:123–128.

Hyperopic astigmatism

Several FDA clinical trials of hyperopic astigmatic correction report that 37%–65% of eyes achieved postoperative UCVA of 20/20 or better, 91%–99% had UCVA of 20/40, 87%–91% were within 1.00 D of emmetropia, and 3.8%–5.8% lost 2 or more lines of BCVA. Efficacy was decreased with higher refractive errors.

Salz JJ, Stevens CA; LADARVision LASIK Hyperopia Study Group. LASIK correction of spherical hyperopia, hyperopic astigmatism, and mixed astigmatism with the LADARVision excimer laser system. *Ophthalmology.* 2002;109:1647–1656.

Mixed astigmatism

Mixed astigmatism is defined as refractive error with cylinder greater than sphere and of opposite sign. LASIK has been approved by the FDA for mixed astigmatism up to 6.00 D of sphere and cylinder. The outcomes of LASIK for mixed astigmatism are similar to the results for hyperopia and hyperopic astigmatism: 46%–62% of eyes had UCVA of 20/20 or better, 93%–99% had postoperative UCVA of 20/40 or better, 88%–96% were within 1.00 D of emmetropia, and up to 2% lost 2 or more lines of BCVA.

Wavefront-guided treatments

Wavefront-guided LASIK coupled with sophisticated eye-tracking systems have greatly improved the accuracy and reproducibility of results, allowing even higher percentages of patients to obtain uncorrected vision of 20/20 and 20/40. In wavefront-guided LASIK for myopic astigmatism, for example, up to about −10.00 to −12.00 D, 79%–95% of patients obtained 20/20 UCVA, and 96%–100% obtained 20/40 UCVA. In wavefront-guided LASIK for hyperopic astigmatism, up to +6.00 D, 55%–59% of patients obtained 20/20 UCVA, and 93%–97% obtained 20/40 UCVA. In wavefront-guided LASIK for mixed astigmatism, up to +5.00 D of cylinder, 56%–61% of patients obtained 20/20 UCVA, and 95% obtained 20/40 UCVA.

See Table 2-1, in Chapter 2, for a list of FDA-approved lasers for refractive surgery.

Re-treatment

Although LASIK reduces refractive error and improves UCVA in almost all cases, some patients have residual refractive errors that require re-treatment. The degree of refractive error that warrants re-treatment varies depending on the patient's lifestyle and expectations. Re-treatment rates also vary, depending on the degree of refractive error being treated, the laser and nomograms used, and the expectations of the patient population. One advantage of LASIK compared with surface ablation is that refractive stability generally occurs earlier, allowing earlier enhancements, typically within the first 3–6 months after LASIK; with surface ablation, the ongoing activation of keratocytes and the risk of haze after enhancement usually requires a wait of at least 6 months before an enhancement surface ablation can be safely performed. Typically, re-treatment rates are higher in hyperopia and in high myopia than in other indications.

One study showed that rates of re-treatment are higher with higher initial correction, with residual astigmatism, and for patients older than 40 years. Re-treatment rates vary from 1% to 11%, based on surgeon experience, patient demands, and the other factors just described. Another study reported the overall re-treatment rate as 10.5% after LASIK for myopia, hyperopia, or astigmatism. Re-treatment is usually performed by lifting the preexisting lamellar flap and applying additional ablation to the stromal bed. In most cases, the flap can be lifted even several years after the original procedure, with reports of successfully lifted flaps 5–6 years after the initial procedure. If, however, a strong Bowman's layer scar has formed, a new flap can be created with a microkeratome. Care must be taken if a new flap is cut for an enhancement, as reports of free slivers of tissue, irregular stromal beds, and irregular astigmatism have been published. The advent of the femtosecond laser, which creates a new flap at a predetermined depth, may reduce some of the potential problems. In eyes that have undergone primary LASIK with the femtosecond laser, however, attempting to lift a flap more than 6 months postoperatively may be difficult due to stronger healing and scarring. In addition, because the femtosecond laser usually creates a thinner flap than the microkeratome, care must be taken to avoid tearing the flap when manipulating and lifting it.

Davis EA, Hardten DR, Lindstrom M, Samuelson TW, Lindstrom RL. LASIK enhancements: a comparison of lifting to recutting the flap. *Ophthalmology*. 2002;109:2308–2313.

Hersh PS, Fry KL, Bishop DS. Incidence and associations of retreatment after LASIK. *Ophthalmology*. 2003;110:748–754.

When a preexisting flap is lifted, it is important to minimize epithelial disruption. A jeweler's forceps, Sinskey hook, or 27-gauge needle can be used to localize the edge of the previous flap. Because the edge of the flap can be seen more easily at the slit lamp than with the diffuse illumination of the operating microscope of the laser, it may be easier to begin a flap lift at the slit lamp and then to complete it at the excimer laser. Alternatively, the surgeon can often visualize the edge of the flap under the diffuse illumination of the operating microscope by applying pressure with a small Sinskey hook or a similar device; the edge of the flap will dimple and disrupt the light reflex (Fig 6-18). A careful circumferential epithelial dissection is performed so that the flap can then be lifted without tearing the epithelial edges. Smooth forceps, iris spatulas, and several instruments specifically designed for dissecting the flap edge (Fig 6-19) can be used to lift the original flap.

Once the ablation has been performed, the flap is repositioned and the interface is irrigated, as in the initial LASIK procedure. Special care must be taken to ensure that no loose epithelium is trapped beneath the edge of the flap that could lead to epithelial ingrowth;

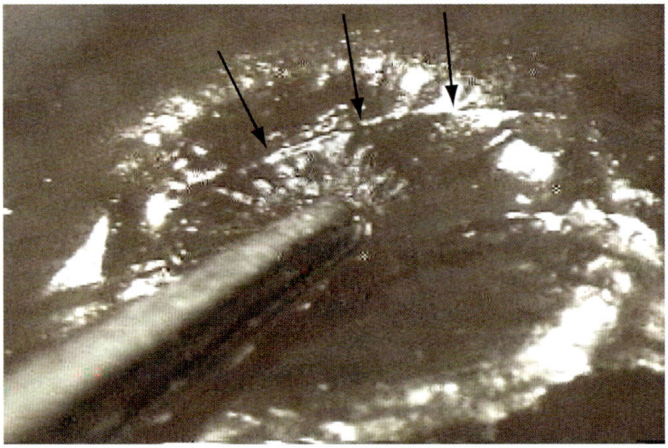

Figure 6-18 Indenting the cornea with forceps to visualize the edge of the flap *(arrows)* through an operating microscope prior to an enhancement procedure. *(Courtesy of Roger F. Steinert, MD.)*

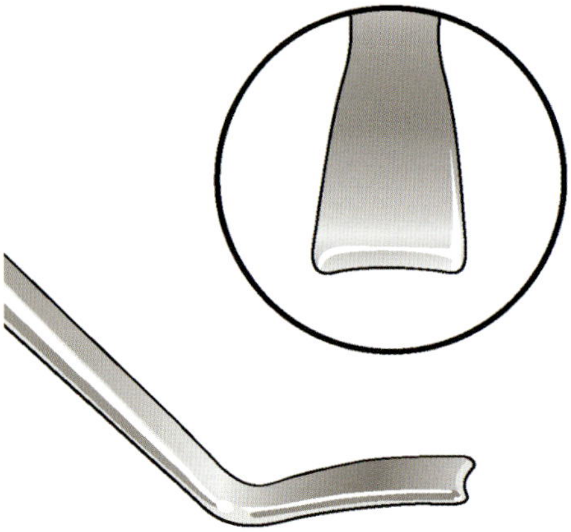

Figure 6-19 Rosenfeld glide dissector. *(Reproduced with permission from Feder RS, Rapuano CJ.* The LASIK Handbook: A Case-based Approach. *Philadelphia: Lippincott Williams & Wilkins; 2007:89, fig 4.2.)*

the risk of epithelial ingrowth is greater after re-treatments than after primary cases. The routine use of a bandage contact lens following enhancements may increase this risk.

Chan CC, Boxer Wachler BS. Comparison of the effects of LASIK retreatment techniques on epithelial ingrowth rates. *Ophthalmology.* 2007;114:640–642.

Surface ablation may be considered to enhance a previous primary LASIK treatment. Surface ablation performed on a LASIK flap carries an increased risk of haze formation and irregular astigmatism, but it is an appealing alternative when the residual stromal bed is insufficient for further ablation, when the LASIK was performed by another surgeon and the flap thickness, or RST, is not known, or with conditions such as a buttonhole or incomplete flap. Care must be taken when removing the epithelium over a flap to avoid inadvertently lifting or dislocating the flap. The procedure should include scraping motions that extend from the hinge toward the periphery. A rotating brush should not be used to remove the epithelium from a LASIK flap. The risk of postoperative haze due to surface ablation over a previous LASIK flap may be prevented or minimized by topical corticosteroids, topical mitomycin C 0.02%, and oral vitamin C (500 mg orally twice a day). A circular cellulose corneal shield soaked in mitomycin C 0.02% is applied to the ablated cornea for anywhere from 12 seconds to 2 minutes, followed by copious irrigation with chilled balanced salt solution. There are no controlled studies comparing the efficacy of the various application times for mitomycin C.

Carones F, Vigo L, Carones A, Brancato R. Evaluation of photorefractive keratectomy retreatments after regressed myopic laser in situ keratomileusis. *Ophthalmology.* 2001;108:1732–1737.

Weisenthal RW, Salz J, Sugar A, et al. Photorefractive keratectomy for treatment of flap complications in laser in situ keratomileusis. *Cornea.* 2003;22:399–404.

The choice of conventional versus wavefront-guided treatment when enhancing patients who have previously undergone conventional LASIK is not yet well established. Some studies report better results in both safety and efficacy with conventional LASIK re-treatment. With the wavefront-guided re-treatments, particularly in the setting of high spherical aberrations, the risk of overcorrection may be greater. Other studies demonstrate the superiority of wavefront-guided re-treatments, especially with regard to reducing lower- and higher-order aberrations. Future studies comparing both techniques should resolve this issue.

Hiatt JA, Grant CN, Boxer Wachler BS. Complex wavefront-guided retreatments with the Alcon CustomCornea platform after prior LASIK. *J Refract Surg.* 2006;22:48–53.

Jin GJ, Merkley KH. Conventional and wavefront-guided myopic LASIK retreatment. *Am J Ophthalmol.* 2006;141:660–668.

Complications

Microkeratome complications

In the past, the more severe complications associated with LASIK were related to problems with the microkeratome, and, in 0.6%–1.6% of cases, it has been reported, a planned LASIK procedure was abandoned because of such problems. Today, advances in microkeratome technology have significantly reduced the incidence of severe, sight-threatening complications. However, it is still imperative that meticulous care be taken in the cleaning and assembly of the microkeratome to ensure that a smooth, uninterrupted keratectomy is performed.

Defects within the blade, poor suction, or uneven progression of the microkeratome across the cornea can produce an irregular, thin, or buttonhole flap (Fig 6-20), which can result in irregular astigmatism with loss of best-corrected vision. A steep corneal curvature is a risk factor for the development of these intraoperative flap complications. If a thin or buttonhole flap is created, or if an incomplete flap does not provide a sufficient-size corneal stromal surface to perform the laser ablation, the flap should be replaced and the ablation should not be performed. Significant visual loss can be prevented if, under such circumstances, the ablation is not performed and the flap is allowed to heal before another refractive procedure is attempted months later. In such a case, a bandage soft contact lens is applied to stabilize the flap, typically for several days to 1 week. A new flap can usually be safely cut after at least 3 months of healing, preferably with a different microkeratome head, one designed to produce a deeper cut; the ablation can be applied at that time. Alternatively, once the defective flap is judged to be healed, some surgeons prefer surface ablation.

Occasionally, a free cap is created instead of a hinged flap (Fig 6-21). In these cases, if the stromal bed is large enough to accommodate the laser treatment, the corneal cap is placed in a moist chamber and the treatment is applied. It is important to replace the cap epithelial side up and to properly position it using the previously placed radial marks. A temporary 10-0 nylon suture can be placed to create an artificial hinge, but the physiologic dehydration of the stroma by the endothelial pump generally will keep the cap secured in proper position. A bandage soft contact lens can help protect the cap. A flat corneal curvature (less than 40.00 D) is a risk factor for developing a free cap because the flap diameter is often smaller than average in flat corneas.

Corneal perforation is a rare but devastating intraoperative complication that can occur if the microkeratome is not properly assembled or if the depth plate in an older-

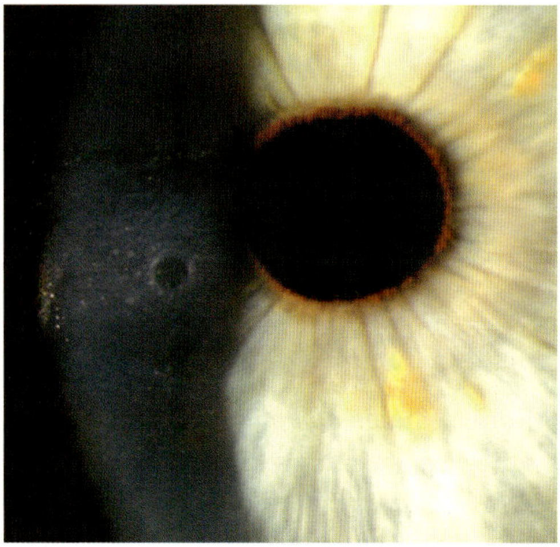

Figure 6-20 LASIK flap with buttonhole. *(Reproduced with permission from Feder RS, Rapuano CJ.* The LASIK Handbook: A Case-based Approach. *Philadelphia: Lippincott Williams & Wilkins; 2007:95, fig 5.1. Photograph courtesy of Christopher Rapuano, MD.)*

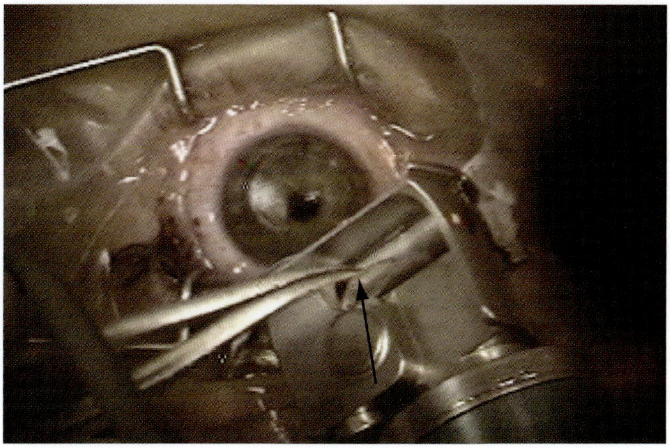

Figure 6-21 A free cap due to transection of the hinge. The cap is being lifted from the microkeratome with forceps *(arrow)*, and care is being taken to maintain the orientation of the epithelial external layer to prevent accidental inversion of the cap when it is replaced. *(Courtesy of Roger F. Steinert, MD.)*

model microkeratome is not properly placed. It is imperative, therefore, that before beginning, the surgeon double-check that the microkeratome has been properly assembled. Most newer microkeratomes are made with a prefixed depth plate, so this source of error is eliminated. Corneal perforation can also occur when LASIK is performed on an excessively thin cornea. Corneal thickness must be measured with pachymetry prior to the LASIK procedure, especially in patients who are undergoing re-treatment. Intraoperative pachymetry should especially be considered during re-treatment of a patient who has had LASIK by another surgeon. In such a case, the surgeon may not know the thickness of the stromal bed after the flap is lifted because he or she may not have information about prior flap thickness. It is important to counsel patients undergoing re-treatment preoperatively that if intraoperative pachymetry reveals an unsafe RST, the procedure may need to be aborted.

Jacobs JM, Taravella MJ. Incidence of intraoperative flap complications in laser in situ keratomileusis. *J Cataract Refract Surg.* 2002;28:23–28.

Lin RT, Maloney RK. Flap complications associated with lamellar refractive surgery. *Am J Ophthalmol.* 1999;127:129–136.

Epithelial erosions

The friction of microkeratome passage across the pressurized cornea may loosen a sheet of epithelium ("epithelial slide") or cause a frank epithelial defect. Although patients with epithelial basement membrane dystrophy are at particular risk, in which case PRK rather than LASIK is advisable, other patients show no preoperative abnormality. The risk of epithelial erosion during LASIK correlates with older age. Also, in bilateral LASIK procedures, the second eye has a greater likelihood of sustaining an epithelial defect (57%) if the first eye developed an intraoperative epithelial defect. Techniques suggested to decrease the erosion rate include limiting toxic topical medications, using chilled proparacaine, minimizing use of topical anesthetic until just prior to the skin prep or to starting the procedure, having the patient keep his or her eyes closed after administration of topical anesthetic, frequent use of corneal lubricating drops, meticulous microkeratome maintenance, and shutting off suction on the microkeratome reverse pass. Recent reports suggest that flap creation with the femtosecond laser may be associated with a reduced incidence of epithelial defects because there is no microkeratome movement across the epithelium. In cases of significant epithelial defects, a bandage soft contact lens is often applied immediately postoperatively and retained until stable re-epithelialization occurs, with subsequent use of intensive lubricants and, occasionally, punctal occlusion. In recalcitrant cases, persistent abnormal epithelium with recurrent erosions or loss of BCVA may require debridement and even superficial phototherapeutic keratectomy (PTK) using the technique employed for treatment of recurrent erosions (see BCSC Section 8, *External Disease and Cornea*). Epithelial defects are associated with an increased incidence of postoperative DLK, infectious keratitis, flap striae, and epithelial ingrowth, and surgeons should watch closely for them.

Tekwani NH, Huang D. Risk factors for intraoperative epithelial defect in laser in-situ keratomileusis. *Am J Ophthalmol.* 2002;134:311–316.

Striae

Flap folds, or striae, are a major cause of decreased visual acuity after LASIK. Some 56% of flap folds occur on the first postoperative day, and 95% occur within the first week. Risk factors for development of folds include excessive irrigation under the flap during LASIK, thin flaps, and deep ablations with flap–bed mismatch.

Although there is no consensus on definitions and treatments for flap folds, there is agreement on certain facts. Flap folds are painless and may be asymptomatic. Recognition of visually significant folds is important because the success rate of treating folds falls dramatically with time. Early intervention is often critical in treating folds that cause loss of BCVA and/or visual distortion.

In evaluating a patient with corneal folds, the first step is determining the BCVA. Folds are not treated if the BCVA and the subjective visual acuity are excellent. In fact, the subjective vision frequently does not correlate with the number and severity of folds. However, visually significant folds often induce irregular astigmatism and may be associated with hyperopic astigmatic refractive errors.

Folds are examined with a slit lamp using direct illumination, retroillumination, and fluorescein staining. Circumferential folds may be associated with high myopia and typically resolve with time. Folds that are parallel and grouped in the same direction may indicate a flap slippage, which requires prompt intervention. Corneal topography is typically not helpful in diagnosing folds.

The challenge for the ophthalmologist is to determine which folds are visually significant and will not resolve with time. These folds should be treated promptly with flap massage at the slit lamp or by stretching the flap with sponges and forceps, with or without lifting. Folds that are visually insignificant cause minimal or no symptoms, are not associated with a loss of BCVA, demonstrate a normal fluorescein staining pattern and normal corneal topography, may resolve with time (eg, circumferential folds after a large myopic ablation), and do not require intervention.

Some ophthalmologists have attempted to use specific clinical characteristics to classify folds into those that involve the entire thickness of the flap, called *macrostriae,* or *macrofolds,* and superficial folds that are mostly in Bowman's layer, called *microstriae,* or *microfolds* (Table 6-2). This classification system can be helpful in guiding treatment. Macrostriae typically require prompt flap repositioning to prevent permanent visual distortion or loss of BCVA. Microstriae may resolve with time and do not require intervention.

Macrostriae represent full-thickness, undulating stromal folds. These folds invariably occur because of initial flap malposition or postoperative flap slippage (Fig 6-22A). Current approaches to smoothing the flap and avoiding striae at the end of the LASIK procedure vary widely. No matter which technique is used, however, the surgeon must carefully examine for the presence of striae once the flap is repositioned. Coaxial and oblique illumination should be used at the operating microscope for this purpose. Checking the patient in the early postoperative period is important to detect flap slippage. A protective plastic shield is often used for the first 24 hours to discourage the patient from touching the eyelids and inadvertently disrupting the flap.

Flap subluxation has been reported to occur in up to 1.4% of eyes. Careful examination should disclose a wider gutter on the side where the folds are most prominent. Flap slippage should be rectified as soon as it is recognized because the folds rapidly become fixed. Under the operating microscope or at the slit lamp, an eyelid speculum is placed, the flap is lifted and repositioned, copious irrigation is used in the interface, and the flap is repeatedly stroked perpendicular to the fold until the striae resolve or improve. Using hypotonic saline or sterile distilled water as the interface irrigating solution swells the flap and may initially reduce the striae, but swelling reduces the flap diameter, which widens the gutter, delays flap adhesion due to prolonged endothelial dehydration time, and may worsen the striae after the flap dehydrates. If the macrostriae have been present for more than 24 hours, reactive epithelial hyperplasia in the valleys and hypoplasia over the elevations of the macrostriae tend to fix the folds into position. In such a case, in addition to refloating the flap, the central 6 mm of the flap over the macrostriae may be de-epithelialized to remove this impediment to smoothing the wrinkles. A bandage soft contact lens should be used to stabilize the flap and to protect the surface until full re-epithelialization occurs. In cases of intractable macrostriae, a tight 360° antitorque running suture or multiple interrupted sutures using 10-0 nylon may be placed for several weeks, but irregular astigmatism may be present after suture removal.

Microstriae are fine, hairlike optical irregularities that are best seen on red reflex illumination or light reflected off the iris (Fig 6-22B, C). They are fine folds in Bowman's layer, and this anterior location accounts for the disruption of BCVA. Computer topographic color maps do not usually show these fine irregularities. Disruption of the surface contour may result in irregularity of the topographer's Placido disk image. In addition, application of dilute fluorescein often reveals so-called negative staining, where the elevated striae disrupt the tear film and fluorescence is lost over them.

Some striae may not be visually significant. In addition, mild loss of visual acuity and other optical symptoms such as ghost images usually improve over time, as the epithelial thickness adjusts to the folds and restores a more regular anterior tear film. Until this occurs, nonpreserved artificial tears should be administered frequently to the ocular surface

Table 6-2 Differentiation of Macrostriae and Microstriae in LASIK Flaps

Characteristic		Macrostriae	Microstriae
Pathology		Large folds involving entire flap thickness	Fine folds, principally in Bowman's layer
Cause		Flap slippage	Mismatch of flap to new bed; contracture of flap
Slit-lamp appearance	Direct illumination	Broad undulations as parallel or radial converging lines; widened flap gutter may be seen	Fine folds, principally in Bowman's layer; gutter usually symmetric
	Retroillumination	Same as above	Folds more obvious on retroillumination
	Fluorescein	Same as above, with negative staining pattern	Often has normal fluorescein pattern
Analogy		Wrinkles in skewed carpet	Dried, cracked mud
Topography		Possible disruption over striae	Color map may be normal or slightly disrupted; Placido disk mires show fine irregularity
Vision		Decreased BCVA and/or multiplopia if central	Subtle decreased BCVA or multiplopia if clinically significant; microstriae masked by epithelium are universal and asymptomatic
Treatment options	Acute	Refloat/reposition flap immediately	Observe; support surface with aggressive lubrication
	Established	Refloat, de-epithelialize over striae, hydrate and stroke, apply traction, or suture	If visually significant, refloat; try hydration, stroking, suturing
		Phototherapeutic keratectomy	Phototherapeutic keratectomy

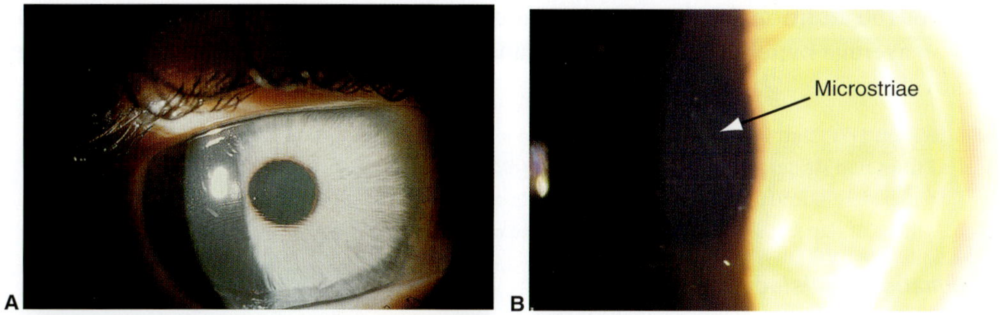

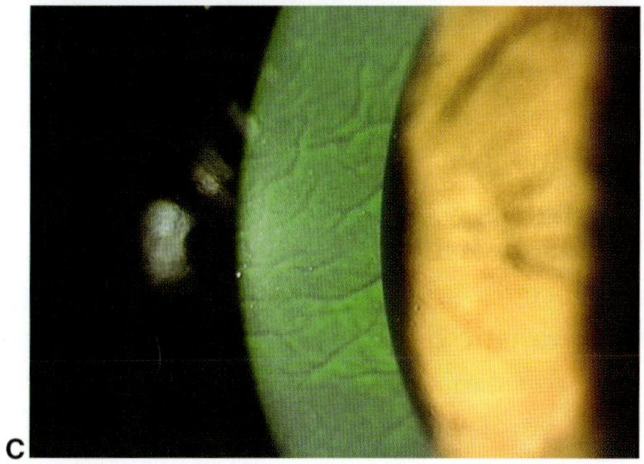

Figure 6-22 **A,** Retroillumination of multiple horizontal parallel macrostriae in the visual axis from mild flap dislocation. **B,** Diffuse illumination of visually insignificant microstriae in the visual axis after LASIK. **C,** Numerous randomly directed microstriae on fluorescein staining. These resemble multiple cracks in a piece of ice, are seen on the first postoperative day after LASIK, and usually resolve without intervention. *(Part A reprinted with permission from* External Disease and Cornea: A Multimedia Collection. *San Francisco: American Academy of Ophthalmology; 2000; part B courtesy of Jayne S. Weiss, MD; part C courtesy of Steven C. Schallhorn, MD.)*

and/or a bandage soft contact lens should be used to encourage remodeling of a smooth corneal surface.

Many interventions for microstriae have been recommended, with variable results. Some surgeons advocate hydration of Bowman's layer. Although hydration eventually occurs with prolonged stroking of the epithelial surface with a moistened surgical spear sponge or irrigating cannula, microstriae also usually disappear within minutes of deliberate de-epithelialization of the area over the microstriae, followed by application of several drops of sterile distilled water. A hypotonic solution applied directly to Bowman's layer also speeds the disappearance of the microstriae. If the striae persist, then the flap should be lifted, the interface irrigated with balanced salt solution, the stromal surface of the flap stroked and stretched perpendicular to the striae, and the flap repositioned. In severe cases, traction with fine-tooth forceps may also be helpful. Care must be taken not to tear the fragile flap. A bandage soft contact lens is then applied and topical antibiotic and corticosteroid drops are prescribed until re-epithelialization is established.

If optically significant microstriae persist, the flap may be sutured in an attempt to reduce the striae through tension. As with macrostriae (discussed earlier), however, suturing has the potential to induce new irregular astigmatism. An alternative procedure is PTK. Pulses from a broad-beam laser, set to a maximal diameter of 6.5 mm, are applied initially to penetrate the epithelium in about 200 pulses. The epithelium acts as a masking agent, exposing the elevated striae before the valleys between the striae. After the transepithelial ablation, additional pulses are applied, and a thin film of medium-viscosity artificial tears is administered every 5–10 pulses, up to a maximum of 100 additional pulses. If these guidelines are followed, little to no haze results and an average hyperopic shift of less than +1.00 D occurs, due to the minimal tissue removal.

Jackson DW, Hamill MB, Koch DD. Laser in situ keratomileusis flap suturing to treat recalcitrant flap striae. *J Cataract Refract Surg.* 2003;29:264–269.

Steinert RF, Ashrafzadeh A, Hersh PS. Results of phototherapeutic keratectomy in the management of flap striae after LASIK. *Ophthalmology.* 2004;111:740–746.

Traumatic flap dislocation

Flap subluxation has been reported to occur in up to 1.4% of eyes. Dislocation of the LASIK flap is not uncommon on the first postoperative day, when dryness and adhesion of the flap to the upper tarsal conjunctiva is sufficient to cause the flap to slip; this is stabilized only by the negative (suction) pressure of the corneal endothelial pump. After the first day, however, the re-epithelialization of the gutter begins the process of increasing flap stability. Within several weeks, keratocytes begin to lay down new collagen at the cut edge of Bowman's layer, and eventually a fine scar is established at the edge of the flap. Minimal healing occurs across the stromal interface for several years, however, allowing flap lifting for enhancement procedures. Late traumatic dislocation from blunt trauma has been reported more than 1 year after LASIK; this can also occur if the shearing force exceeds the strength of the peripheral Bowman's layer–level healing.

Dry eye and corneal sensation

Dry eye is one of the most frequent side effects of LASIK; it has been reported in 60%–70% of all patients, to varying degrees. The surgeon must carefully monitor the patient postoperatively for signs of punctate keratitis or more severe manifestations of neurotrophic epitheliopathy. As patients await the return of innervation, their treatment should include the use of nonpreserved artificial tears, gels, and ointments. To avoid the potential of migration under the flap, however, ointments should not be used in the early postoperative period. More severe or recalcitrant dry eyes may require topical cyclosporine A, topical corticosteroids, oral tetracyclines, oral omega-3 fatty acids, and punctal occlusion. (See also Chapter 10.)

Both the surgeon and the patient must remain aware that many patients seeking laser vision correction do so because of contact lens intolerance, and dry eyes are one of the most common reasons for that intolerance. Such dryness will persist after the treatment and will be transiently worsened during the recovery by the denervation of the flap. The patient may feel that long-term, persistent dryness has worsened and may blame the LASIK procedure. If the patient has known or suspected dry-eye syndrome prior to undergoing LASIK, intensive topical lubrication, topical cyclosporine A, and systemic treatments, as outlined earlier, can be instituted preoperatively to try to improve the condition of the ocular surface. Some studies have reported better surgical and visual outcomes with such prophylactic maneuvers.

Salib GM, McDonald MB, Smolek M. Safety and efficacy of cyclosporine 0.05% drops versus unpreserved artificial tears in dry-eye patients having laser in situ keratomileusis. *J Cataract Refract Surg.* 2006;32:772–778.

Central islands and decentration

See the discussion in Surface Ablation earlier in this chapter. The main difference here is that central islands tend not to resolve as frequently after LASIK as they do after surface ablation.

Diffuse lamellar keratitis

Diffuse lamellar keratitis (DLK) has been referred to as sterile interface inflammation, "sands of the Sahara" (SOS), and—perhaps most accurately—diffuse interface keratitis (Fig 6-23). This syndrome can range from asymptomatic interface haze near the edge of the flap to marked diffuse haze under the flap with diminished BCVA. The condition appears to be a nonspecific sterile inflammatory response to a variety of mechanical and toxic insults. The interface under the flap is a potential space; any cause of anterior stromal inflammation may cause white blood cells to accumulate in that space. DLK has been reported in association with epithelial defects that occur during primary LASIK or during enhancement, or even months after the LASIK procedure from corneal abrasions or infectious keratitis. Other reported inciting factors include foreign material on the surface of the microkeratome blade or motor, meibomian gland secretions, povidone-iodine solution (from the preoperative skin prep), substances produced by laser ablation, contamination of the sterilizer with gram-negative endotoxin, and red blood cells in the interface. The inflammation generally resolves on its own without sequelae, but severe cases can lead to scarring or flap melting.

Diffuse lamellar keratitis is usually classified by the stages described in Table 6-3. Although stages 1 and 2 usually respond to frequent topical corticosteroids, stages 3 and 4 usually require lifting the flap and irrigating, followed by intensive topical corticosteroid

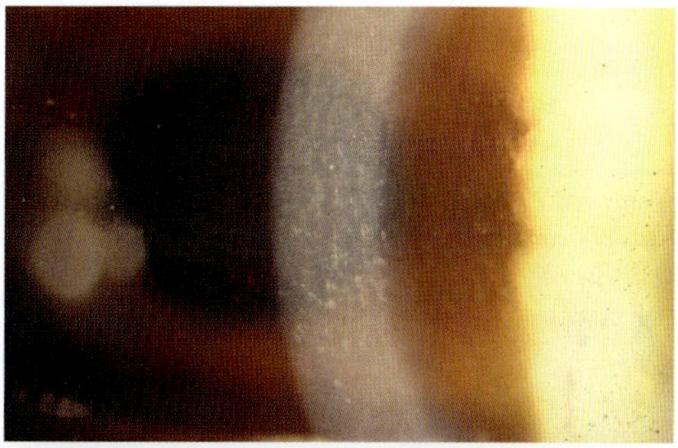
A

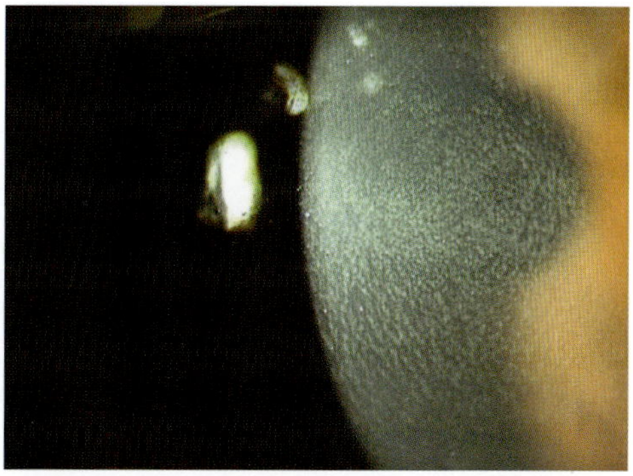
B

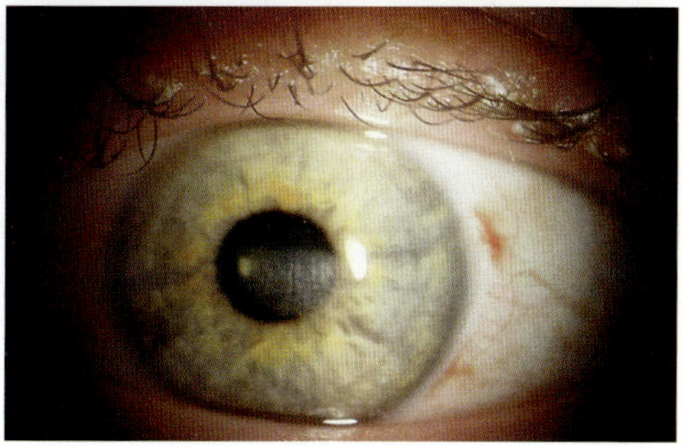
C

Figure 6-23 Diffuse lamellar keratitis. **A,** High magnification of stage 2 DLK (note accumulation of inflammatory cells in the fine ridges created by the oscillating microkeratome blade). **B,** Stage 3 DLK (dense accumulation of inflammatory cells centrally). **C,** Stage 4 DLK with central scar and folds. *(Parts A and B courtesy of Roger F. Steinert, MD; part C courtesy of Jayne S. Weiss, MD.)*

treatment. Systemic corticosteroids may be used adjunctively in severe cases. Some surgeons use topical and systemic corticosteroids in stage 3 DLK instead of lifting the flap. Recovery of vision in DLK is usually excellent if the condition is detected and treated promptly.

A surgeon should have a low threshold for lifting or irrigating underneath the flap in suspected cases of DLK. Lifting the flap allows removal of inflammatory mediators from the interface, corneal cultures to be performed, and direct placement of corticosteroids and NSAIDs to suppress inflammation and collagen necrosis.

Hoffman RS, Fine IH, Packer M. Incidence and outcomes of LASIK with diffuse lamellar keratitis treated with topical and oral corticosteroids. *J Cataract Refract Surg.* 2003;29:451–456.

Holland SP, Mathias RG, Morck DW, Chin J, Slade SG. Diffuse lamellar keratitis related to endotoxins released from sterilizer reservoir biofilms. *Ophthalmology.* 2000;107:1227–1233.

Linebarger EJ, Hardten DR, Lindstrom RL. Diffuse lamellar keratitis: diagnosis and management. *J Cataract Refract Surg.* 2000;26:1072–1077.

Smith RJ, Maloney RK. Diffuse lamellar keratitis: a new syndrome in lamellar refractive surgery. *Ophthalmology.* 1998;105:1721–1726.

Steinert RF, McColgin AZ, White A, Horsburgh GM. Diffuse interface keratitis after laser in situ keratomileusis (LASIK): a nonspecific syndrome. *Am J Ophthalmol.* 2000;129:380–381.

Pressure-induced stromal keratitis Late-onset interface opacity similar to DLK, often with a visible fluid cleft in the interface, has been reported as a result of elevated IOP and has been termed *pressure-induced stromal keratitis (PISK)* (Fig 6-24). The surgeon must be aware of this unusual condition in order to properly diagnose and treat it. The pressure-induced fluid accumulation can appear very similar to DLK and is often associated with prolonged corticosteroid treatment. It is important to measure IOP both centrally and peripherally, possibly with a pneumotonometer or Tono-Pen, because applanation pressure may be falsely lowered centrally by fluid accumulation in the lamellar interface. Treat-

Table 6-3 Staging of Diffuse Lamellar Keratitis

Stage	Findings
1	Peripheral faint white blood cells; granular appearance
2	Central scattered white blood cells; granular appearance
3	Central dense white blood cells in visual axis
4	Permanent scarring or stromal melting

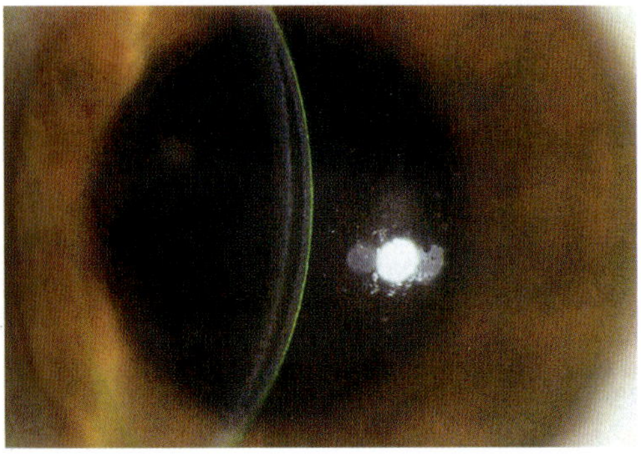

Figure 6-24 An optically clear fluid-filled space is present between the flap and stromal bed that is caused hypothetically by transudation of fluid across the endothelium from a steroid-induced elevation of IOP. *(Reproduced with permission from Hamilton DR, Manche EE, Rich LF, Maloney RK. Steroid-induced glaucoma after laser in situ keratomileusis associated with interface fluid.* Ophthalmology. *2002;109:659–665.)*

ment for PISK involves rapid tapering or cessation of the corticosteroid drops and use of glaucoma medication to lower IOP. Severe glaucomatous visual loss has been reported in undiagnosed cases.

Belin MW, Hannush SB, Yau CW, Schultze RL. Elevated intraocular pressure-induced interlamellar stromal keratitis. *Ophthalmology.* 2002;109:1929–1933.

Hamilton DR, Manche EE, Rich LF, Maloney RK. Steroid-induced glaucoma after laser in situ keratomileusis associated with interface fluid. *Ophthalmology.* 2002;109:659–665.

Infectious keratitis

It is important to differentiate sterile interface inflammation from potentially devastating infectious inflammation. Increased pain and decreased vision are the primary indicators of infection. However, postoperative eye pain is common, so it is difficult for patients to distinguish between normal eye pain and abnormal eye pain. Infection following LASIK is usually associated with redness, photophobia, and decreased vision. Due to the severing of corneal nerves with flap creation, corneal sensation may be reduced, along with the subjective symptom of pain that usually accompanies infection. Several distinct features can help distinguish between DLK and infectious keratitis (Table 6-4). DLK is usually visible within 24 hours of surgery and typically begins at the periphery of the flap. There is usually a gradient of inflammation, with the inflammation being most intense at the periphery and diminishing toward the center of the cornea. In general, the inflammatory reaction seen in DLK is diffusely distributed but localized and confined to the flap interface; it does not extend far beyond the edge of the flap (Fig 6-25). In contrast, post-LASIK infectious keratitis usually begins 2–3 days after surgery and involves a more focal inflammatory reaction that is not confined to the lamellar interface. An anterior chamber reaction may further help to differentiate between an infectious and a sterile process. The inflammatory reaction can extend up into the flap, deeper into the stromal bed, and even beyond the confines of the flap.

Infection within the interface can lead to flap melting, severe irregular astigmatism, and corneal scarring that requires corneal transplantation. If infection is suspected, the flap should be lifted and the interface cultured and irrigated with antibiotics. The most common infections are from gram-positive organisms, followed closely in frequency by

Table 6-4 DLK vs Infectious Keratitis

DLK	Infection
Usually seen within first 24 hours	Usual onset at least 2–3 days postoperatively
Typically begins at flap periphery	Can occur anywhere under flap
More intense inflammation at periphery decreasing toward center	
Inflammation primarily confined to interface	Inflammation extends above and below interface, and beyond flap edge
Diffuse inflammation	Focal inflammation around infection
Flap melts can occur	Flap melts can occur

Used with permission from Culbertson WW. Surface ablation and LASIK patients share similar infection potential. *Refractive Eyecare.* September 2006:12.

those from atypical mycobacteria. A more rapid diagnosis for mycobacteria than that based on culture results may be made by acid-fast and fluorochrome stains (Fig 6-26).

In general, the onset of symptoms may provide a clue as to the etiology of the infection. Infections occurring within 10 days of surgery are typically bacterial, with the preponderance being from gram-positive organisms. Suggested empirical treatment could include tobramycin (14 mg/mL) and vancomycin (25–50 mg/mL) or a fourth-generation fluoroquinolone and cefazolin (50 mg/mL). Infections presenting more than 10 days after surgery are more likely caused by atypical mycobacteria and fungi. Topical clarithromycin (10 mg/mL), oral clarithromycin (500 mg bid), and topical amikacin (8 mg/mL) are recommended for treatment of mycobacterial infections. If a filamentous fungus is identified, natamycin (50 mg/mL) is recommended; amphotericin (1.5 mg/mL) is recommended for yeast infections. If the infection does not respond to treatment, amputation of the flap may be necessary to improve antibiotic or antifungal penetration. The fourth-generation fluoroquinolones gatifloxacin and moxifloxacin have excellent efficacy against the more common bacteria that cause post-LASIK infections, including some atypical mycobacteria; however, monotherapy with them alone may not be sufficient. An infected LASIK flap may occur after a recurrent erosion (Fig 6-27).

Freitas D, Alvarenga L, Sampaio J, et al. An outbreak of *Mycobacterium chelonae* infection after LASIK. *Ophthalmology*. 2003;110:276–285.

Karp CL, Tuli SS, Yoo SH, et al. Infectious keratitis after LASIK. *Ophthalmology*. 2003;110:503–510.

Epithelial ingrowth

Epithelial ingrowth occurs in less than 3% of eyes (Fig 6-28). Isolated nests of epithelial cells in the lamellar interface that are not advancing and are not affecting vision do not need to be treated. However, if the epithelium is advancing toward the visual axis, is associated with irregular astigmatism (Fig 6-29), or triggers overlying flap melting, it

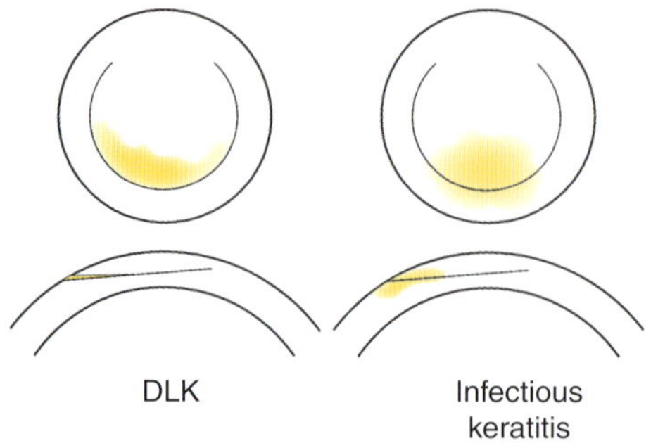

Figure 6-25 Diffuse lamellar keratitis (DLK) is differentiated from infectious keratitis by the confinement of the infiltrate to the interface alone in DLK. *(Reproduced with permission from Culbertson WW. Surface ablation and LASIK patients share similar infection potential.* Refractive Eyecare. *September 2006:12.)*

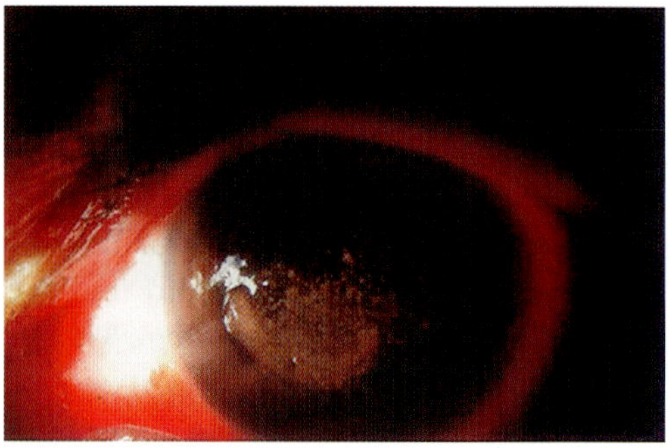

Figure 6-26 *Mycobacterium chelonae* interface infection presenting 3 weeks following LASIK and initially treated as DLK with topical corticosteroids. *(Reproduced with permission from Feder RS, Rapuano CJ.* The LASIK Handbook: A Case-based Approach. *Philadelphia: Lippincott Williams & Wilkins; 2007.)*

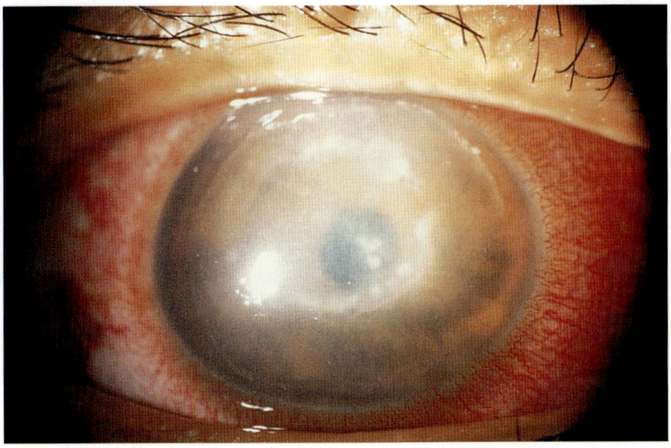

Figure 6-27 Infectious keratitis in a LASIK flap after recurrent epithelial abrasion. *(Courtesy of Jayne S. Weiss, MD.)*

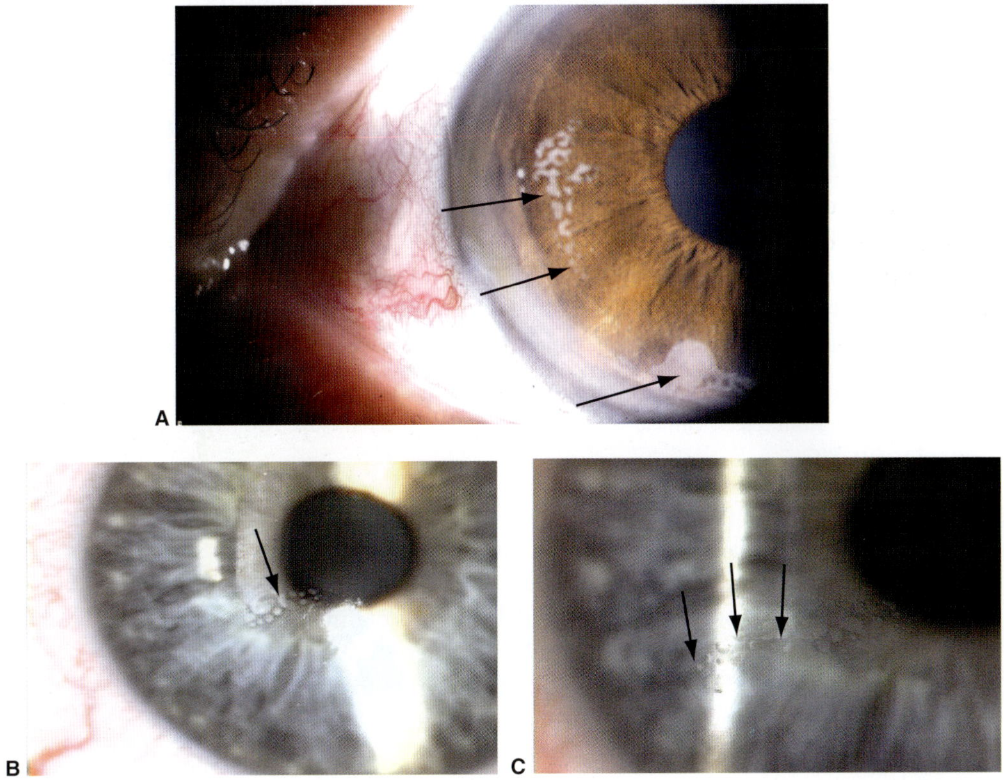

Figure 6-28 Epithelial ingrowth in the interface under a LASIK flap. **A,** Peripheral ingrowth of 1–2 mm *(arrows)* is common and inconsequential and does not require intervention unless it induces melting of the overlying flap. **B,** Central nests of epithelial cells *(arrow)* disrupt the patient's vision by elevating and distorting the flap. The flap must be lifted and the epithelium debrided. **C,** Inspection of the midperiphery shows the track followed by the invading epithelium from the periphery toward the center *(arrows)*. *(Courtesy of Roger F. Steinert, MD.)*

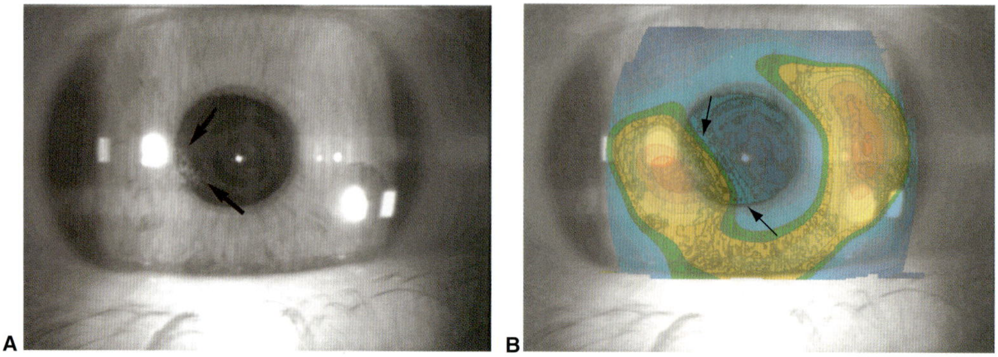

Figure 6-29 **A,** Epithelial ingrowth in visual axis *(arrows).* **B,** Corresponding topographic steepening and irregularity on Orbscan topography. *(Part B courtesy of Jayne S. Weiss, MD.)*

should be removed by lifting the flap and scraping it from both the underside of the flap and the stromal bed and then repositioning the flap. After scraping the inner flap surface and stromal bed, some surgeons remove epithelium from the peripheral cornea as well to allow for flap adherence before the epithelial edge advances up to the flap edge. Recurrent epithelial ingrowth can be treated with repeat lifting and scraping, with or without flap suturing or using fibrin glue at the flap edge.

The incidence of epithelial ingrowth is greater in patients who develop an epithelial defect at the time of the procedure and in those undergoing a re-treatment with lifting of a preexisting flap. In these instances, special care should be taken to ensure that no epithelium becomes caught under the edge of the flap when it is repositioned. Placement of a bandage contact lens at the conclusion of the procedure may also decrease the incidence of epithelial ingrowth for patients at higher risk of developing this complication.

Asano-Kato N, Toda I, Hori-Komai Y, Takano Y, Tsubota K. Epithelial ingrowth after laser in situ keratomileusis: clinical features and possible mechanisms. *Am J Ophthalmol.* 2002; 134:801–807.

Interface debris

Debris in the interface is occasionally seen postoperatively. The principal indication for intervention, with flap lifting, irrigation, and manual removal of debris, is an inflammatory reaction elicited by the foreign material. Small amounts of lint, nondescript particles, or tiny metal particles from stainless steel surgical instruments are usually well tolerated. A small amount of blood that may have oozed into the interface from transected peripheral vessels may also be tolerated; however, a significant amount of blood usually elicits an inflammatory cell response and should be irrigated from the interface at the time of the LASIK procedure (Fig 6-30). Use of a topical vasoconstrictor such as epinephrine to facilitate coagulation when the flap is being replaced helps to minimize this problem. The surgeon should be aware that applying epinephrine prior to laser ablation can result in pupillary dilation and decentration. Blood remaining in the interface typically resolves spontaneously with time.

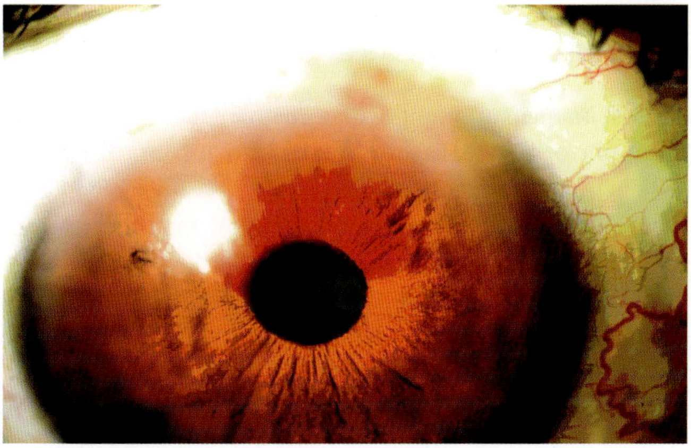

Figure 6-30 Blood in the LASIK interface. *(Courtesy of Jayne S. Weiss, MD.)*

Ectasia

The importance of an adequate residual stromal bed to prevent structural instability and postoperative corneal ectasia is discussed in Patient Selection, earlier in this section. Current standards recommend a minimum residual stromal bed of at least 250 μm after completion of the ablation (see Chapter 3), although there are no controlled studies to confirm this clinical impression. Although keratectasia is usually associated with LASIK performed for higher myopic corrections, in thin corneas, or in patients who have had multiple laser ablations, cases of ectasia have been reported in corrections as low as −4.00 D where the residual stromal bed was believed to be thicker than 250 μm. In many of these cases, later examination showed that the microkeratome created a flap thicker than expected, resulting in a thinner residual stromal bed. In other cases, preoperative forme fruste keratoconus, subtle keratoconus, pellucid marginal degeneration, or other ectasias may have been present. In a retrospective study of 10 eyes from 7 patients who developed corneal ectasia after LASIK, all patients had either preoperative undiagnosed forme fruste keratoconus (88%) or an RST of less than 250 μm (70%). Often, good vision can be restored with a rigid gas-permeable contact lens. The implantation of symmetric or asymmetric intrastromal ring segments (eg, Intacs) to reduce the irregular astigmatism has been successful in selected cases. In extreme cases, corneal transplantation may be required.

In 2003, Binder published a comprehensive review of the literature analyzing 85 cases of post-LASIK corneal ectasia and concluded, "The current literature is unable to define a specific residual corneal thickness or a range of preoperative corneal thickness that would put an eye at risk for developing ectasia." Also, Binder has put out a summary of his 9000 LASIK cases, which includes over 200 cases where patients had RST of <250 μm and did not develop postoperative ectasia. In addition, he reported several cases of postoperative ectasia in patients with RST ≥300 μm. An increasing number of LASIK surgeons believe that post-LASIK ectasia may develop only in eyes with an underlying tendency for keratoconus or pellucid marginal degeneration, a diagnosis that is currently beyond our capabilities in certain cases.

In 2005, a joint statement was issued by the American Academy of Ophthalmology, the International Society for Refractive Surgery, and the American Society of Cataract and Refractive Surgery summarizing current knowledge of corneal ectatic disorders and ectasia after LASIK. Their 8 conclusions were

1. No specific test or measurement is diagnostic of a corneal ectatic disorder.
2. A decision to perform LASIK should take into account the entire clinical picture, not just the corneal topography.
3. Although some risk factors have been suggested for ectasia after LASIK, none are absolute predictors of its occurrence.
4. Because keratoconus may develop in the absence of refractive surgery, the occurrence of ectasia after LASIK does not necessarily mean that LASIK was a causative or contributing factor for its development.
5. Risk factors for ectasia after LASIK may not also predict ectasia after surface ablation.
6. Ectasia is a known risk of laser vision correction.
7. Forme fruste keratoconus is a topographic diagnosis rather than a clinical one. It is not a variant of keratoconus. Rather, forme fruste implies subclinical disease with the potential for progression to clinically evident keratoconus.
8. Although to date no formal guidelines exist and good scientific data for future guidelines are presently lacking, in order to reduce some of the risks of ectasia after LASIK, the groups recommended that surgeons review topography prior to surgery. Intraoperative pachymetry should be used to measure flap thickness and calculate the RST after ablation to ascertain if the RST is near the safe lower limits for the procedure, for that patient.

Binder PS. Ectasia after laser in situ keratomileusis. *J Cataract Refract Surg.* 2003;29:2419–2429.

Binder PS, Lindstrom RL, Stulting RD, et al. Keratoconus and corneal ectasia after LASIK. *J Cataract Refract Surg.* 2005;31:2035–2038.

Fogla R, Rao SK, Padmanabhan P. Keratoectasia in 2 cases with pellucid marginal corneal degeneration after laser in situ keratomileusis. *J Cataract Refract Surg.* 2003;29:788–791.

Ou RJ, Shaw EL, Glasgow BJ. Keratectasia after laser in situ keratomileusis (LASIK): evaluation of the calculated residual stromal bed thickness. *Am J Ophthalmol.* 2002;134:771–773.

Randleman JB, Russell B, Ward MA, Thompson KP, Stulting RD. Risk factors and prognosis for corneal ectasia after LASIK. *Ophthalmology.* 2003;110:267–275.

Ocular aberrations

Several studies have demonstrated that although excimer laser photoablation causes the majority of lower-order aberrations and higher-order aberrations in LASIK surgery, creation of the flap also contributes to lower-order aberrations and higher-order aberrations. Some studies have shown that femtosecond lasers cause little or no change in higher-order aberrations, in contrast to mechanical microkeratomes. Pallikaris showed that flap creation alone, without lifting, caused no significant change in refractive error or visual acuity but did cause a significant increase in total higher-order wavefront aberrations.

Pallikaris IG, Kymionis GD, Panagopoulou SI, Siganos CS, Theodorakis MA, Pellikaris AI. Induced optical aberrations following formation of a laser in situ keratomileusis flap. *J Cataract Refract Surg.* 2002;28:1737–1741.

Porter J, MacRae S, Yoon G, Roberts C, Cox IG, Williams DR. Separate effects of the microkeratome incision and laser ablation on the eye's wave aberration. *Am J Ophthalmol.* 2003;136:327–337.

Tran DB, Sarayba MA, Bor Z, et al. Randomized prospective clinical study comparing induced aberrations with IntraLase and Hansatome flap creation in fellow eyes: potential impact on wavefront-guided laser in situ. *J Cataract Refract Surg.* 2005;31:97–105.

Waheed S, Chalita MR, Xu M, Krueger RR. Flap-induced and laser-induced ocular aberrations in a two step LASIK procedure. *J Refract Surg.* 2005;21:346–352.

Rare complications

Rare complications of LASIK include optic nerve ischemia, premacular subhyaloid hemorrhage, macular hemorrhage associated with preexisting lacquer cracks or choroidal neovascularization, choroidal infarcts, postoperative corneal edema associated with preoperative cornea guttata, and ring scotoma. Diplopia is another rare complication and is related to technical problems, prior need for prisms, aniseikonia, iatrogenic monovision, and improper control of accommodation in patients with strabismus.

Gimbel HV, Anderson Penno EE, van Westenbrugge JA, Ferensowicz M, Furlong MT. Incidence and management of intraoperative and early postoperative complications in 1000 consecutive laser in situ keratomileusis cases. *Ophthalmology.* 1998;105:1839–1848.

Kushner BJ, Kowal L. Diplopia after refractive surgery: occurrence and prevention. *Arch Ophthalmol.* 2003;121:315–321.

Stulting RD, Carr JD, Thompson KP, Waring GO III, Wiley WM, Walker JG. Complications of laser in situ keratomileusis for the correction of myopia. *Ophthalmology.* 1999;106:13–20.

Sugar A, Rapuano CJ, Culbertson WW, et al. Laser in situ keratomileusis for myopia and astigmatism: safety and efficacy. A report by the American Academy of Ophthalmology. *Ophthalmology.* 2002;109:175–187.

Conclusion

Although LASIK is the most popular refractive surgery procedure performed today, it does have limitations. Many surgeons will not use LASIK to treat to the full extent of the FDA parameters, including higher levels of myopia (≤–14.00 D) and hyperopia (≤+6.00 D), because of poorer predictability and the increased possibility of complications.

Although LASIK has rapidly surpassed PRK in popularity for treating many refractive errors, visual results of the 2 procedures are actually very similar. A study of patients treated for myopia of –1.00 to –9.50 D showed equal refractive outcomes. Another study of treatment of myopia between –6.00 and –15.00 D showed a slightly decreased incidence of postoperative optical symptoms in LASIK compared with PRK. However, in a randomized bilateral comparison of LASIK and PRK in patients with –2.50 to –8.00 D, almost twice as many were highly satisfied with their LASIK eye compared with their PRK eye 1 year after treatment. In addition to having less postoperative pain and more rapid visual recovery, the LASIK eyes were more likely to achieve UCVA of 20/20 or better and less likely to have postoperative topographic irregularities.

The incidence of complications in LASIK decreases with surgeon experience and, as with any surgical procedure, it is preferable to optimize surgical technique in order to try to avoid complications. When recognized and properly treated, however, most complications will not result in loss of BCVA. Irregular astigmatism, for example, is a common cause of decreased BCVA; often, though, epithelial hyperplasia and hypoplasia occur, smoothing the corneal surface over time, reducing the irregular astigmatism, and improving visual acuity. If significant symptoms persist, however, the patient may benefit from selective surface treatments.

Technological advances will continue to improve visual outcomes. Wavefront-guided laser ablation, also discussed in Chapter 1, offers the potential to improve visual quality. Surface ablation is increasing in popularity in conjunction with the wavefront-guided lasers because surface ablation avoids the higher-order aberrations induced by the corneal flap in LASIK. However, a recent review of FDA study reports and indexed, peer-reviewed literature failed to demonstrate that wavefront-guided refractive surgery outperformed conventional LASIK that incorporated newer technological refinements such as broad ablation zones, smoothing to the periphery, and eye trackers. Future advances in laser technology may eventually afford true custom ablation, including treatment of such entities as irregular astigmatism for which there is currently no effective refractive surgical procedure.

McColgin AZ, Steinert RF. LASIK. In: Tasman W, Jaeger EA, eds. *Duane's Clinical Ophthalmology*. Philadelphia: Lippincott Williams & Wilkins; 2001.

Netto MV, Dupps W Jr, Wilson SE. Wavefront-guided ablation: evidence for efficacy compared to traditional ablation. *Am J Ophthalmol.* 2006;141:360–368.

Wavefront-Guided Surface Ablation and LASIK

Background

Conventional excimer laser ablation treats lower-order, or spherocylindrical, aberrations such as myopia, hyperopia, and astigmatism. These lower-order aberrations constitute approximately 90% of all aberrations. Higher-order aberrations make up the remainder; these aberrations cannot be treated with spectacles. We are still learning about the visual impact of higher-order aberrations in the normal population; the small amounts found in this population may not adversely affect vision. Higher-order aberrations are also a by-product of excimer laser ablation. Some can cause symptoms, such as loss of contrast sensitivity and nighttime halos and glare, that decrease the quality of vision. The aberration most commonly associated with these visual complaints is spherical aberration.

In an effort to reduce preexisting aberrations and reduce the induction of new aberrations, wavefront-guided ablation creates ablation profiles that are customized for individual patients. In addition to addressing higher-order aberrations, wavefront-guided treatments can correct the lower-order aberrations of spherical error and astigmatism.

When compared with conventional excimer laser ablation, wavefront-guided ablation appears to offer better contrast acuity and induces fewer postoperative higher-order aberrations. However, although improvements in aberrometry and registration systems have led to improved outcomes, patients undergoing the procedure may still have more higher-order aberrations postoperatively than they did preoperatively.

Wavefront-guided ablation is not suitable for all patients and may not be appropriate for use after cataract surgery, particularly that involving multifocal IOLs. In addition, wavefront data may be impossible to obtain in very irregular corneas or with smaller pupillary diameters. In the future, patients with very irregular corneas that cannot be treated with wavefront technology may be treated with topography-based ablations. In general, wavefront-guided ablation removes more tissue than conventional ablation.

The technology is still evolving and may lead to further expansion of refractive surgical indications and additional improvements in postoperative results. (See also the discussion in Chapter 1.)

Nuijts RM, Nabar VA, Hament WJ, Eggink FA. Wavefront-guided versus standard laser in situ keratomileusis to correct low to moderate myopia. *J Cataract Refract Surg.* 2002;28: 1907–1913.

Instrumentation

Wavefront mapping systems are unique to the specific wavefront-guided laser used. FDA-approved wavefront-guided excimer lasers include the Alcon CustomCornea, the VISX IR WaveScan, the Bausch & Lomb Zyoptix, Nidek, and the WaveLight Allegretto WAVE systems. Calibration should be performed according to the manufacturer's specifications.

Preoperative Preparation

Preoperative wavefront analysis is performed first. Some systems require pupillary dilation to capture wavefront data, whereas others do not. The wavefront refraction indicated on wavefront analysis is then compared with the manifest refraction and should differ by no more than 0.75 D; in cases where the difference exceeds 0.75 D, both the manifest refraction and the wavefront analysis should be repeated. If the wavefront refraction is more myopic than the manifest refraction, the patient may be accommodating, and reassurance and oral diazepam may be required to obtain the correct treatment. If the wavefront refraction is more hyperopic than the manifest refraction, the wavefront refraction is generally correct. Higher-order aberrations such as spherical aberration may masquerade as myopia, and coma may masquerade as cylinder, so although the wavefront refraction may not match the manifest refraction, the wavefront refraction is often correct. Monovision may be adjusted into the wavefront treatment. The data are either electronically transferred to the laser or downloaded to a disk and then transferred to the laser. Unlike a conventional excimer laser, where the manifest or cycloplegic refraction is used to program the laser, the wavefront-guided laser uses programmed wavefront data to create a custom ablation pattern.

The accuracy of the wavefront analysis may depend somewhat on the experience of the examiner obtaining the data. Wavefront analysis may not be possible in patients with extremely irregular corneas, such as corneas with prior PKP or corneal scars, and these patients are not candidates for wavefront-guided ablation.

CHAPTER 7

Collagen Shrinkage Procedures

History

The idea of using heat to alter the shape of the cornea was first proposed by Lans, a Dutch medical student, in 1898. When Lans used electrocautery to heat the corneal stroma, he noticed astigmatic changes in the cornea. Two years later, in 1900, Terrien reported the use of cautery to correct the severe astigmatism associated with Terrien marginal degeneration, and in 1928, Knapp used cautery to improve the visual acuity of patients with keratoconus.

In 1975, Gasset and Kaufman proposed a modified technique known as *thermokeratoplasty* to treat keratoconus. They theorized that the hot cautery used in prior reports caused collagen necrosis, leading to tissue destruction and corneal melting. Their goal was to measure the heat applied to the cornea and control its application, in order to shrink collagen fibers without causing necrosis. The cornea was reportedly heated to 115°C in the region of the cone, which resulted in an overall flattening of the cornea. They performed the procedure on eyes requiring penetrating keratoplasty in which the vision was not correctable with spectacles or contact lenses. Vision improved to 20/30 or better in most eyes, and penetrating keratoplasty was avoided in 95% of their 59 patients. Similar attempts by others during the 1970s proved less successful, and complications, such as delayed epithelial healing, recurrent epithelial erosions, corneal neovascularization, aseptic stromal necrosis and melting, stromal scarring, iritis, and hypopyon, were encountered.

It is now known that the optimal temperature for avoiding stromal necrosis while still obtaining collagen shrinkage is approximately 60°–65°C, much lower than that used by Gasset and Kaufman. Human collagen fibrils can shrink by almost two thirds when exposed to temperatures in this range, as the heat disrupts the hydrogen bonds in the supercoiled structure of collagen. In the cornea, the maximal shrinkage is approximately 7%. When higher temperatures are reached (>78°C), tissue necrosis occurs.

Various other approaches to heating the cornea have been proposed, none of which has met with long-term acceptance. In an attempt to reduce possible complications, Rowsey and co-workers in 1981 introduced an alternative method for heating the cornea using diathermy (radiofrequency current). This was thought to be more predictable, and it delivered less total energy. They used the Los Alamos keratoplasty unit, in which the probe treated an area between 200 and 400 µm below the corneal epithelium. Although immediate corneal changes were noted, marked regression occurred over time with this technique.

In 1984, Fyodorov introduced a technique of radial thermokeratoplasty using a handheld heated nichrome needle designed for deeper thermokeratoplasty. The handheld probe contained a retractable 34-gauge wire heated to 600°C. A motor advanced the wire to a preset depth of 95% of the corneal pachymetry for a duration of 0.3 second. Fyodorov used different patterns to treat hyperopia and astigmatism. However, excessive heating of the cornea resulted in necrosis and corneal remodeling, and regression of treatment and unpredictability limited its success.

Neumann AC, Fyodorov S, Sanders DR. Radial thermokeratoplasty for the correction of hyperopia. *Refract Corneal Surg.* 1990;6:404–412.

Laser Thermokeratoplasty

In the 1990s, multiple lasers were tested for use in laser thermokeratoplasty (LTK), including CO_2, cobalt-magnesium-fluoride, erbium:glass, and holmium:yttrium-aluminum-garnet (Ho:YAG). Only the Ho:YAG laser reached commercial production and FDA approval. The Ho:YAG laser produces light in the infrared region at a wavelength of 2100 nm and has corneal tissue penetration to approximately 480 to 530 μm. Two different delivery systems were investigated: a contact system and a noncontact laser.

The contact laser was originally developed as part of the integrated Summit workstation. The contact Ho:YAG handheld probe emitted a 300-μsec pulse at a repetition rate of 15 Hz and a pulse power of approximately 19 mJ. Laser applications were placed in a set pattern around the corneal periphery. High degrees of regression and induced astigmatism were noted. The system never received FDA approval for the correction of hyperopia and is no longer commercially available.

The noncontact Sunrise Hyperion system was approved by the FDA in 2000. This laser used a slit-lamp delivery system to deliver 8 simultaneous spots at a wavelength of 2.1 μm at a frequency of 5 Hz and a pulse duration of 250 μsec. The system was approved for the temporary correction of 0.75 to 2.5 D of hyperopia with less than 1.0 D of astigmatism. Few, if any, units remain in clinical use.

Because the Ho:YAG lasers heat the surface of the cornea and rely on passive conduction of heat, it is not possible to heat the cornea evenly. The surface of the cornea has to be heated above 65°C to obtain an adequate temperature rise in the midstroma. However, this temperature leads to epithelial necrosis, initial patient discomfort, and inadequate heating of the deeper layers of the cornea. Strong initial interest in LTK has waned, partly because of the visual fluctuations and refractive regression and partly because of the high purchase price of the equipment. LTK has largely been superseded by conductive keratoplasty.

Conductive Keratoplasty

In recent years, radiofrequency has again emerged as a method of heating the cornea. In 2002, the FDA approved the ViewPoint CK system (Refractec, Bloomington, MN) for the temporary treatment of mild to moderate hyperopia (+0.75 to +3.25 D) with astigmatism of 0.75 D or less. In 2004, conductive keratoplasty (CK) received FDA approval for treatment of presbyopia in the nondominant eye of a presbyopic patient with an endpoint of −1.00 to −2.00 D. For both treatments, patients are typically 40 years of age or older and have had a stable refraction for at least 12 months.

Conductive keratoplasty is a nonablative, collagen-shrinking procedure. It is based on the delivery of radiofrequency energy through a fine conducting tip that is inserted into the peripheral corneal stroma (Fig 7-1). Because of its electrolytic properties, the cornea conducts radiofrequency energy. As the current flows through the tissue surrounding the tip, resistance to the current creates localized heat. Collagen lamellae in the area surrounding the tip shrink in a controlled fashion and form a column of denatured collagen. The ViewPoint CK system consists of a portable console, an eyelid speculum that acts as the electrical return path, and a handpiece that holds the 450-µm-long and 90-µm-wide metal Keratoplast tip (Fig 7-2).

For hyperopia treatment, the surgeon first marks the cornea in a set pattern and then inserts the tip into the stroma in a ring pattern around the peripheral cornea (Fig 7-3) according to the supplied nomogram (Table 7-1). The CK unit delivers a set power and

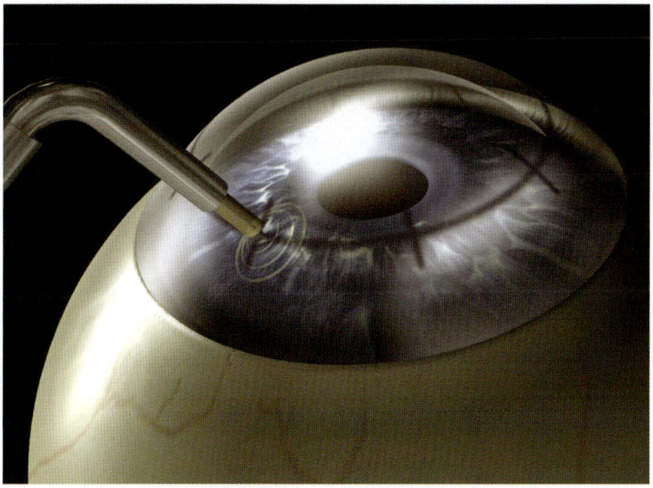

Figure 7-1 Conductive keratoplasty delivers radiofrequency energy to the cornea through a handheld probe that is inserted into the peripheral cornea. *(Courtesy of Refractec, Inc.)*

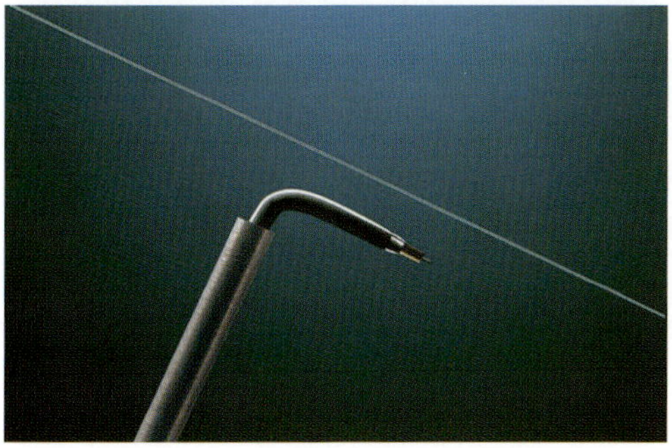

Figure 7-2 The CK probe (displayed next to a 10-0 nylon suture for comparison) consists of a thin conductive wire, 450 µm long and 90 µm wide. *(Courtesy of Refractec, Inc.)*

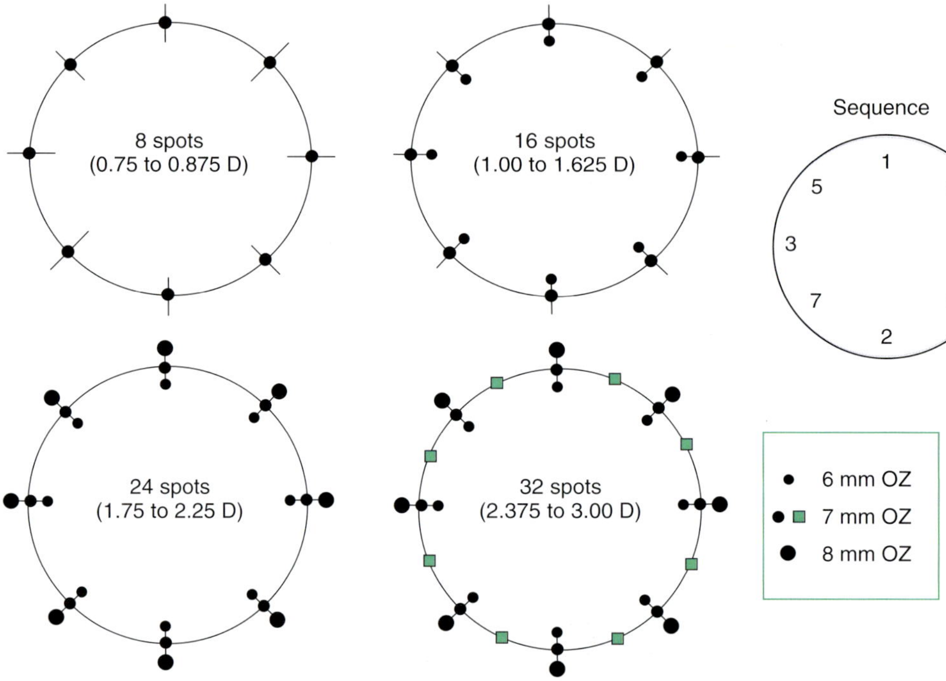

Figure 7-3 In CK, radiofrequency energy is delivered in a series of spots to the corneal periphery. More circles of spots are used for higher hyperopic corrections. When 32 spots are applied, the last 8 spots are placed in the intermediate areas (between existing spots) of the 7.0 mm ring. *(Courtesy of Refractec, Inc.)*

Table 7-1 Application Nomogram for Conductive Keratoplasty

Spherical Equivalent	Number of Spots	Treatment Diameter
0.75 to 0.875 D	8	7.0 mm
1.00 to 1.625 D	16	6.0 mm; 7.0 mm
1.75 to 2.25 D	24	6.0 mm; 7.0 mm; 8.0 mm
2.375 to 3.00 D	32	6.0 mm; 7.0 mm; 8.0 mm; intermediate 7.0 mm

duration (0.6 second) when the foot pedal is depressed (for equipment sold internationally, both power and duration can be adjusted by the surgeon). The number and location of spots determines the amount of refractive change, with an increasing number of spots and rings used for higher amounts of hyperopia. The CK procedure is performed under topical anesthesia and typically takes less than 5 minutes. The collagen shrinkage leads to visible striae between the treated spots, which fade with time (Fig 7-4). The shortening of the collagen fibrils creates a band of tightening that increases the curvature of the central cornea.

Patient Selection and Results

The Refractec system is approved for the temporary reduction of spherical hyperopia in patients 40 years or older with a spherical equivalent of +0.75 to +3.25 D and ≤0.75 D of astigmatism. The clinical trial consisted of 12-month data in 401 eyes, with a mean cohort

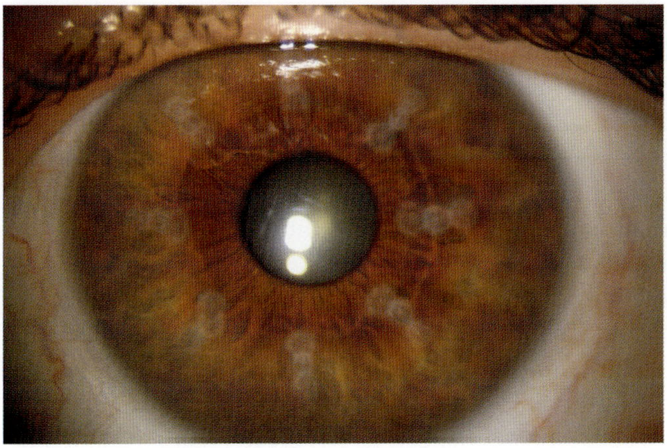

Figure 7-4 A month after a 24-spot CK treatment in a patient with +2.0 D hyperopia, the spots are beginning to fade. Three sets of 8 spots were applied at a 6.0-mm, 7.0-mm, and 8.0-mm optical zone. *(Courtesy of Refractec, Inc.)*

age of 55.3 years (range: 40.2–73.9 years). The mean cycloplegic spherical equivalent was +1.86 ± 0.63 D. By 12 months postoperatively, 92% of study patients had achieved uncorrected visual acuity (UCVA) of 20/40 or better, 74% were 20/25 or better, and 54% were 20/20 or better. By 24 months postoperatively, 93% of study patients had achieved UCVA of 20/40 or better, 76% were 20/25 or better, and 52% were 20/20 or better. There was a slow continued drift toward increasing hyperopia, with regression of +0.21 D and +0.48 D at 12 and 24 months, respectively. Overall, there was a 20% loss of effect after 2 years. This "loss of effect" is probably a combination of true regression and the normal hyperopic drift that is seen as patients age. The results in the FDA CK trial for presbyopia were similar. The clinical trial consisted of 12-month data with 126 eyes included in the study. The treatment goal of the study was monovision correction. Preoperatively, 0% were Jaeger type 1 (J1) or better and 5% (5 eyes) were Jaeger type 3 (J3) or better. At 1 year postoperatively, 35% (37 eyes) were J1 or better and 77% were J3 (82 eyes) or better uncorrected.

Hersh PS. Optics of conductive keratoplasty: implications for presbyopia management. *Trans Am Ophthalmol Soc.* 2005;103:412–456.

McDonald MB. Conductive keratoplasty: a radiofrequency-based technique for the correction of hyperopia. *Trans Am Ophthalmol Soc.* 2005;103:512–536.

Conductive keratoplasty is not FDA approved for use in patients who have undergone radial keratotomy or in those with keratoconus, ectatic disorders, or significant irregular astigmatism. The upper limit of +3.25 D (spherical equivalent) appears to be the current treatment ceiling for this technology, and multiple applications over time or more spots do not seem to enhance or increase that limit.

Safety

Although the efficacy results for CK appear to be similar to those of LASIK and LTK, the safety variables are superior. In the principal FDA clinical trial, no patient was worse than 20/40 and no patient lost more than 2 lines of vision. One patient out of 391 had >2.0 D of induced cylinder, and no patient with a preoperative best-corrected visual acuity of ≥20/20 had <20/25 at 1 year. Although induced cylinder of >2.0 D is an FDA safety variable, smaller amounts of induced cylinder were apparent. At 1 year, 6% of patients had >1.0 D of induced cylinder. The magnitude of the induced cylinder decreases with time. No central corneal haze was noted at 12 months and endothelial cell counts were similar before and after the study.

Despite initial reports of refractive stability, long-term follow-up has revealed regression and/or lack of adequate effect with CK. It has been theorized that significant corneal compression by the probe pushed away the deep corneal stroma, leading to less effect and greater variability. The "Light Touch" technique modification was introduced to minimize tissue compression. With this technique, the initial compression seats the probe. Pressure on the probe is then released until almost no corneal distortion is noted. Reports suggest an enhanced effect, greater stability, and a decreased number of spots to achieve the desired result. The "Light Touch" nomogram (Table 7-2) uses fewer spots and larger optical zones than the original (corneal compression) nomogram (see Table 7-1) Currently, the major clinical use of CK is in the treatment of presbyopia in emmetropic patients.

Other Applications

A number of potential off-label uses also exist for CK. In overcorrected myopic LASIK and myopic PRK, CK can be used to correct hyperopia. In these cases, CK obviates the need to lift or cut another flap. In one report, CK was used to treat both keratoconus and post-LASIK ectasia. Although corneal irregularities improved immediately, with some visual improvement, some cases showed regression of effect at 1 month. Larger studies with additional follow-up are needed.

In postcataract or postkeratoplasty patients with astigmatism, CK can be used to steepen the flat axis, because each spot is individually placed. The overall effect is still a myopic shift, so CK is particularly useful when the spherical equivalent is hyperopic. In a study of 16 patients who had CK for hyperopia after cataract surgery, 1-year data showed that CK for low to moderate postcataract hyperopia was effective and safe.

Conductive keratoplasty appears to have advantages both in cost and in allowing flexible (off-label) treatment patterns because the tip can be placed anywhere on the cornea. More experience and long-term data will be required to determine how impor-

Table 7-2 Sample Application Nomogram for Conductive Keratoplasty *"Light Touch"*

Spherical Equivalent	Number of Spots	Treatment Diameter
1.00 D	8	8.0 mm
1.75 D	8	7.0 mm
2.50 D	16	7.0 mm and 8.0 mm

tant CK will be in the refractive surgeon's armamentarium. Currently, however, its use remains fairly limited.

Alió JL, Ramzy MI, Galal A, Claramonte PJ. Conductive keratoplasty for the correction of residual hyperopia after LASIK. *J Refract Surg.* 2005;21:698–704.

Claramonte PJ, Alió JL, Ramzy MI. Conductive keratoplasty to correct residual hyperopia after cataract surgery. *J Cataract Refract Surg.* 2006;32:1445–1451.

Kolahdouz-Isfahani AH, McDonnell PJ. Thermal keratoplasty. In: Brightbill FS, ed. *Corneal Surgery: Theory, Technique, and Tissue.* 3rd ed. St. Louis: CV Mosby; 1999.

CHAPTER 8

Intraocular Surgery

In its first 2 decades, refractive surgery was synonymous with corneal refractive surgery, which compensates for refractive error by altering the contour of the anterior surface of the eye. Several factors expanded the range of refractive surgery to include intraocular surgery. Ophthalmologists became accustomed to cataract patients not only expecting to see clearly after their operation but also becoming less dependent on glasses as a consequence of intraocular lens (IOL) surgery. Technology has helped to achieve this goal. Small-incision cataract surgery with self-sealing, astigmatism-neutral wounds has all but eliminated the high postoperative astigmatism that was previously common. Improved biometry (eg, immersion A-scan and IOL Master), new power calculation formulas, and new software have made IOL power selection more accurate. Foldable IOLs, multifocal IOLs, toric IOLs, and accommodating IOLs are now a reality. These technological advances have led to a renewed interest in clear lens surgery, particularly for correction of hyperopia in the presbyopic patient.

Phakic IOLs (PIOLs) represent a new category of IOL that expands the range of keratorefractive surgery, offering surgeons and their patients new options for vision correction. The combination of corneal and intraocular refractive surgery, or *bioptics,* may ultimately allow patients at the extremes of refractive error to achieve predictable outcomes by combining the advantages of the PIOL in treating large corrections with the adjustability of a keratorefractive technique. In addition, the optical quality may be improved by dividing the refractive correction between 2 different locations.

This chapter discusses the intraocular surgical techniques that are now or are soon expected to be within the armamentarium of the refractive surgeon.

Phakic Intraocular Lenses

Background

The history of the PIOL to correct refractive error began in Europe in the 1950s with Strampelli, Dannheim, and Barraquer each separately attempting to design a PIOL that would be well tolerated in the eye. The lack of modern IOL-manufacturing capabilities and microsurgical techniques, as well as the lack of knowledge about the fragility of anterior segment structures, resulted in a high incidence of corneal edema, iritis, cataract, and glaucoma in these initial attempts at PIOL implantation. Ultimately, many of these early IOLs were removed, and by the late 1960s, interest in PIOL implantation had waned.

In the middle 1980s, interest in PIOLs was renewed. Improvements in IOL manufacturing, the development of modern microsurgical techniques, increased viscoelastic and topical corticosteroid availability, and improved understanding of the corneal endothelium and anterior segment structures led to greater success with PIOL surgery. Worst modified his aphakic, iris-fixated "claw" IOL to correct both myopia and hyperopia. Baikoff worked on variations of the open-loop, flexible anterior chamber IOL to correct myopia, and Fyodorov experimented with a plate-haptic IOL for use in the posterior chamber.

Different PIOL designs were associated with different types of complications. Early versions of the Baikoff anterior chamber PIOLs were associated with significant endothelial cell loss. The PIOL placed in the ciliary sulcus over a clear lens was associated with pupillary block and cataract. Refinements in IOL design have reduced the incidence of complications, which has resulted in the increasing popularity of these PIOLs outside the United States. Within the United States, 2 PIOLs are currently FDA approved for myopia. A posterior chamber PIOL is distributed as the Visian ICL (Implantable Collamer Lens) by STAAR (Monrovia, CA). The PIOL designed by Worst, which is iris-supported, is marketed as Verisyse by AMO (Advanced Medical Optics, Santa Ana, CA). The Verisyse PIOL is known outside the United States as the Artisan lens and is distributed by Ophtec (Groningen, Netherlands). Representative lenses in each category (Table 8-1) are discussed in the following sections.

Advantages

PIOLs have the advantage of treating a much larger range of myopic and hyperopic refractive errors than can be safely and effectively treated with corneal refractive surgery. The skills required for insertion are, with a few exceptions, similar to those used in cataract surgery. The equipment is significantly less expensive than an excimer laser, and most or all of it is already used for cataract surgery.

The PIOL is removable; therefore, the refractive effect should theoretically be reversible. However, any intervening damage caused by the PIOL would most likely be permanent.

When compared with clear lens extraction (discussed later in this chapter), the PIOL has the advantage of preserving natural accommodation and may have a lower risk of postoperative retinal detachment because of the preservation of the crystalline lens and the lack of vitreous destabilization.

Disadvantages

PIOL insertion is an intraocular procedure with all the potential risks associated with intraocular surgery. Each PIOL style has its own set of associated risks. In the case of PIOLs with polymethylmethacrylate (PMMA) optics, insertion requires a larger wound, which may result in unintended postoperative astigmatism. There is less flexibility than with LASIK for fine-tuning the refractive outcome. If a patient eventually develops a visually significant cataract, the PIOL will have to be explanted at the time of cataract surgery, possibly through a larger-than-usual wound. Although PIOLs for hyperopia are being investigated, there is less enthusiasm for these lenses because the anterior chamber tends

Table 8-1 Phakic IOLs

Position	Model	Available Power	Optic Size/Effective Diameter	Length	Material	Manufacturer
Angle-supported	NuVita MA20 (myopia)	–7.00 to –20.00 D	5.0 mm/4.5 mm	12.0, 12.5, 13.0, 13.5 mm	PMMA (foldable in early trials)	Bausch & Lomb
	Vivarte/GBR (myopia)	–7.00 to –22.00 D	5.5 mm	12.0, 12.5, 13.0 mm	Acrylic optic; PMMA haptics	ZEISS-IOLTech
	(multifocal)	–5.00 to +5.00 D				
	(near add)	+2.50				
	ZSAL-4 Plus (myopia)	–6.00 to –20.00 D	5.5 mm/5.0 mm	12.0, 12.5, 13.0 mm	PMMA	Morcher (Stuttgart, Germany)
	AcrySof ACP-IOL (myopia)	–8.00 to –16.00 D	5.5 mm	12.5, 13.0, 13.5 mm	Acrylic	Alcon
	Phakic 6 H2 (myopia)	–4.00 to –20.00 D	5.5–6.0 mm	11.5–14.0 mm	PMMA	Ophthalmic Innovations International (O.I.I.; Ontario, CA)
	(hyperopia)	+2.00 to +10.00 D				
	Kelman Duet (myopia)	–6.00 to –20.00 D	6.3 mm/5.5 mm	12.0, 12.5, 13.0, 13.5 mm	Silicone optic PMMA haptics	Tekia (Irvine, CA)
	I-CARE (myopia)	–3.00 to –20.00 D	6.3 mm/5.5 mm	12.0, 12.5, 13.0, 13.5 mm	Acrylic	Corneal (Pringy, France)
	(hyperopia)	+3.00 to +10.00 D				

(Continued)

Table 8-1 *(continued)*

Position	Model	Available Power	Optic Size/Effective Diameter	Length	Material	Manufacturer
Iris-supported*	Verisyse model VRSM5US (myopia)	–3.00 to –15.50 D	5.0 mm	8.5 mm	PMMA	AMO
	Verisyse model VRSM6US (myopia)	–3.00 to –23.50 D	6.0 mm	8.5 mm	PMMA	AMO
	Artisan model 203 (hyperopia)	+3.00 to +12.00 D	5.0 or 6.0 mm	8.5 mm	PMMA	Ophtec
	Artisan toric IOL	Custom	5.0 or 6.0 mm	8.5 mm	PMMA	Ophtec
	Artiflex/Veriflex (foldable) (myopia)	–3.00 to –23.50 D	5.0 or 6.0 mm	8.5 mm	Polysiloxane	Ophtec
Sulcus-supported†	Visian ICL (myopia)	–3.00 to –23.00 D	4.65–5.50 mm	12.1, 12.6, 13.2, 13.7 mm	Collamer	STAAR
	Visian ICL (hyperopia)	+3.00 to +12.00 D		11.5–13.2 mm	Collamer	STAAR
	Toric ICL	Up to +2.50 Custom to +4.00 D	4.75–5.50 mm	11.5–13.2 mm	Collamer	STAAR
	Sticklens (myopia)	–7.00 to –25.00 D	6.5 mm	11.5 mm	Acrylic	IOLTech (La Rochelle, France)
	Sticklens (hyperopia)	+4.00 to +7.00 D	6.5 mm	11.5 mm	Acrylic	IOLTech

*The Artisan lens (Ophtec), marketed as the Verisyse lens (AMO), has been FDA approved for use in the lens power range of –5.00 to –20.00 D.

†The Visian ICL (STAAR) posterior chamber phakic IOL has received FDA approval to correct myopia in the range of –3.00 to –20.00 D.

Adapted in part from Lovisolo CF, Reinstein DZ. Phakic intraocular lenses. *Surv Ophthalmol.* 2005;50:549–587.

to be shallower, and progressive shallowing may occur with advancing age. This can be associated with pupil ovalization, angle closure, and increased endothelial cell loss. No PIOLs currently available in the United States treat astigmatism, but toric versions are under investigation.

Patient Selection

Indications

Patients who are near or beyond the FDA-approved limits for laser vision correction may be candidates for a PIOL. Although the programmable upper limit of myopic excimer laser treatment is as high as −14.00 D, some surgeons have reduced the upper limit of LASIK and surface ablation in their refractive practices because of the reduced predictability, high rate of regression, increased incidence of microstriae, and night-vision problems that can occur with treatment of a patient with high myopia. Similarly, LASIK and surface ablation for hyperopia above +4.00 D and astigmatism correction above 4.00 D of cylinder are less accurate than at lower corrections. If surgeons become comfortable with the use of PIOLs, it is possible they may choose to implant them for refractive powers significantly lower than the programmable excimer laser limits.

Most PIOLs for myopia can correct up to −20.00 D (see Table 8-1). In the United States, for example, the 6-mm optic Verisyse iris-fixation PIOL corrects up to −23.50 D and the 5-mm optic lens corrects up to −15.50 D. All 3 categories of PIOL are available outside the United States for correcting hyperopia of at least +10.00 D. AMO, STAAR, and CIBA Vision (Duluth, GA) are conducting clinical trials of toric PIOLs.

PIOLs can be an attractive alternative if surface ablation or LASIK is contraindicated. LASIK surgery is contraindicated if the resultant residual corneal stromal bed thickness would be <250 μm, as this could increase the risk of developing corneal ectasia. PIOLs may be used off-label in eyes with irregular topographies from forme fruste keratoconus and even frank keratoconus, and they may induce less dry eye than corneal refractive procedures. Because extremes of corneal curvature lead to induced aberrations and degradation of optical quality, a final corneal curvature flatter than 34.00 D in myopic corrections or steeper than 50.00 D in hyperopic corrections is also undesirable. More sophisticated measurement and treatment planning based on wavefront analysis may refine these limits.

Contraindications

PIOLs have specific contraindications. They should not be used if there is preexisting intraocular disease such as a compromised corneal endothelium, iritis, significant iris abnormality, rubeosis iridis, cataract, or glaucoma.

The anterior chamber diameter, anterior chamber depth, and pupil size must be appropriate for the specific PIOL being considered. (The anatomical requirements for the placement of each style of IOL are discussed in the next section.)

Patient evaluation

A thorough preoperative evaluation is necessary, as detailed in Chapter 3. One area that has not been well investigated is the importance of IOL optic size relative to scotopic pupil size. Pupil size larger than optic size may be associated with edge glare.

Informed consent

As with any refractive procedure, an informed consent written specifically for this procedure should be obtained prior to surgery. The patient should be informed about both the potential short-term and long-term risks of the procedure and about any available alternatives. With some of the newer technologies, long-term risks and results may not yet be known. The surgeon must make sure the patient has realistic expectations about the surgical outcome of the procedure.

Ancillary tests

Specular microscopy and corneal pachymetry are both helpful for evaluating the health of the corneal endothelium. In addition, anterior chamber depth should be carefully assessed because adequate depth is critical for the safe implantation of a PIOL. If the anterior chamber depth is <3.0 mm, the risk of endothelial and iris or angle trauma from the placement of an anterior chamber, iris-fixated, or posterior chamber PIOL is increased. Anterior chamber depth can be estimated at the slit lamp by using measured central corneal thickness as a reference. Anterior chamber depth can also be measured by ultrasound or anterior segment OCT, slit-beam topography (eg, Orbscan [Bausch & Lomb, Rochester, NY]) or Scheimpflug photography (eg, Pentacam [Oculus, Lynnwood, WA]; Galilei [Ziemer, Port, Switzerland]), if available. The phakic eye has a shallower anterior chamber than the aphakic eye.

Methods for IOL power selection are specific to each PIOL and manufacturer. Some manufacturers provide software for IOL power calculation. As with any IOL implant, novice surgeons should follow the guidelines prescribed by manufacturers and experienced, trusted surgeons and then modify the formulas as they gain their own experience.

Surgical Technique

Topical anesthesia with an intracameral supplement is appropriate if the patient can cooperate and the PIOL can be inserted through a small incision. If the patient cannot cooperate for topical anesthesia or if a large incision is required, peribulbar anesthesia is preferable. Retrobulbar anesthesia should be used with caution in patients with a high axial length because of the increased risk of perforation. Pupil dilation may occur after anesthetic injection, which may be undesirable in the case of anterior chamber PIOL and iris-fixated PIOL insertion. Topical pilocarpine 1% or 2% administered preoperatively can block this dilation effect but may decenter the pupil.

A peripheral iridotomy is recommended for each of the PIOL categories to reduce the risk of pupillary block and angle closure. A laser iridotomy can be performed 7–14 days prior to the PIOL surgery, or the iridotomy can be performed as part of the implant procedure. Preoperative laser iridotomy is preferable when small-incision implant surgery is performed (eg, with foldable anterior chamber or posterior chamber PIOLs). Both iridotomy and iridectomy are technically more difficult to perform through a beveled clear corneal incision. Viscoelastic should be meticulously removed at the conclusion of surgery to prevent postoperative elevation of IOP.

Angle-supported anterior chamber phakic intraocular lens

Several angle-supported anterior chamber phakic intraocular lenses (ACPIOLs) are now in FDA trials. An ACPIOL can be inserted through a temporal clear corneal wound or a superior scleral pocket. The larger the incision, the greater the likelihood of induced astigmatism. The wound size depends on the diameter of the ACPIOL optic. The effective optical diameter for some ACPIOLs is small—for example, the 4.5-mm NuVita (Bausch & Lomb) and the 5.0-mm 93A (Morcher, Stuttgart, Germany). Small diameter size minimizes the wound size required for insertion but increases the potential for edge glare in patients with larger pupils. The Vivarte ACPIOL (IOLTech, La Rochelle, France) has an acrylic optic that is 5.5 mm and foldable and can be inserted through a 3.2-mm clear corneal incision (Fig 8-1).

Sizing the ACPIOL ACPIOLs are generally available in lengths between 12.0 and 14.0 mm, in 0.5-mm increments. The proper length is usually estimated by measuring the white-to-white diameter with calipers between the 3 and 9 o'clock meridians. Some computerized corneal topography devices such as the slit-beam topography system can provide a white-to-white measurement. High-frequency ultrasound biomicroscopy, anterior segment OCT, or the Scheimpflug photography systems may ultimately provide more accurate measurements for ACPIOL implantation. Apple and colleagues have examined autopsy eyes and found the white-to-white measurement to be an imprecise approximation of anterior chamber diameter. It is important to remember that the white-to-white measurement in the 12 o'clock meridian is significantly less than the same measurement between 3 and 9 o'clock. Consequently, an ACPIOL length based on the horizontal measurement may be too large for the anterior chamber if the IOL is oriented vertically. Proper sizing is critical to reduce the risk of problems such as pupil ovalization, lens decentration, chronic inflammation, and secondary glaucoma.

Iris-fixated PIOL

The iris-fixated PIOL is generally inserted through a superior limbal incision. The long axis of the PIOL is ultimately oriented perpendicular to the axis of the incision. A side port incision is made approximately 2 clock-hours on either side of the center of the incision. A 12 o'clock incision requires side port incisions at 10 and 2 o'clock. The "claw" haptics

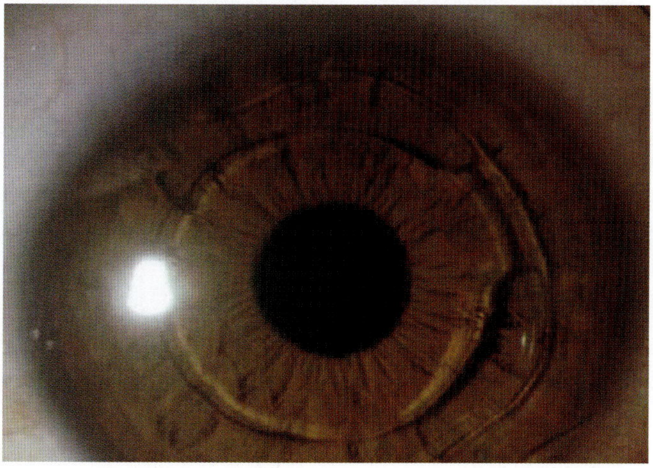

Figure 8-1 Vivarte ACPIOL 3 months after implantation. *(Courtesy of IOLTech.)*

are fixated to the iris by a process called *enclavation.* After the PIOL has been carefully centered over the pupil, it is stabilized with a forceps while a specially designed enclavation needle is introduced through one of the side port incisions and a knuckle of iris is brought up into the "claw" haptic. This is repeated on the other side. If adjustment of the PIOL position becomes necessary after fixation, the iris must be released before the PIOL is moved. Careful wound closure helps minimize surgically induced astigmatism.

The Verisyse (AMO) is currently FDA approved for myopia of −5.00 to −20.00 D, with recommendations for minimal preoperative endothelial cell count dependent on age.

Sizing the iris-fixated PIOL Because this PIOL is fixated to the midperipheral iris, not the angle or sulcus, the iris-fixated PIOL has the advantage of having a one-size-fits-all length. It is 8.5 mm in length, with a 5.0- or 6.0-mm PMMA optic (Fig 8-2). An iris-fixated PIOL with a flexible optic that can be inserted through a small wound is currently under investigation. Once approved, it will be marketed by AMO in the United States as the Veriflex IOL.

Posterior chamber phakic intraocular lens

The smaller incision used for foldable posterior chamber phakic intraocular lenses (PCPIOLs) offers the advantage of decreased astigmatism. The available plate-haptic PCPIOLs are made of flexible materials. The Implantable Collamer Lens, or Visian ICL (Fig 8-3), is made of a hydrophilic material known as collamer, which is a copolymer of hema (99%) and porcine collagen (1%). The optic of the PCPIOL is vaulted both to avoid contact with the crystalline lens and to allow aqueous to flow over the crystalline lens. This vaulting can be seen with ultrasound biomicroscopy or Scheimpflug photography (Fig 8-4). The lens manufacturers suggest that an acceptable amount of vaulting of the PCPIOL optic over the crystalline lens is 1.0 ± 0.5 corneal thicknesses.

To perform the implantation, the pupil is dilated preoperatively to 8.0 mm with tropicamide 1% and phenylephrine 2.5%. A 3.0- to 3.2-mm temporal clear corneal incision is then made, and a paracentesis is made superiorly and inferiorly to aid in positioning the PCPIOL. The PCPIOL is inserted using a cohesive viscoelastic and, after the lens unfolds, the haptics are manipulated under the iris (Fig 8-5). The surgeon should avoid contact with the central 6.0 mm of the lens because it might cause damage. Positioning instruments should be inserted through the paracenteses and should be kept peripheral to this central

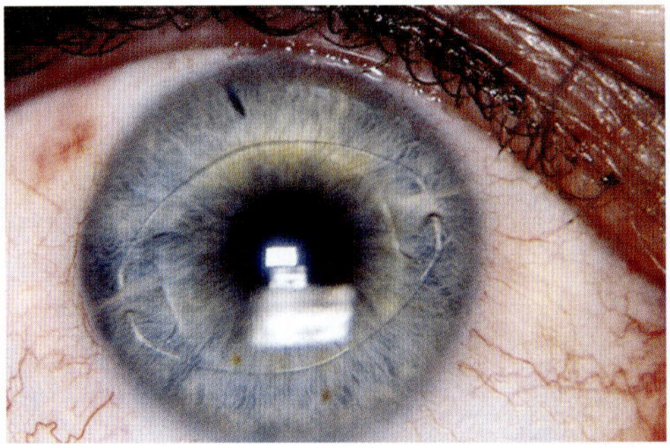

Figure 8-2 Verisyse, iris-fixation PIOL for myopic correction. *(Courtesy of AMO.)*

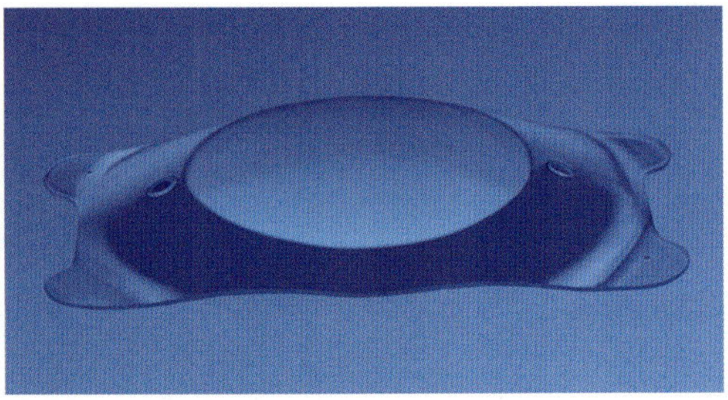

Figure 8-3 Side view of the Visian ICL PCPIOL. *(Courtesy of STAAR.)*

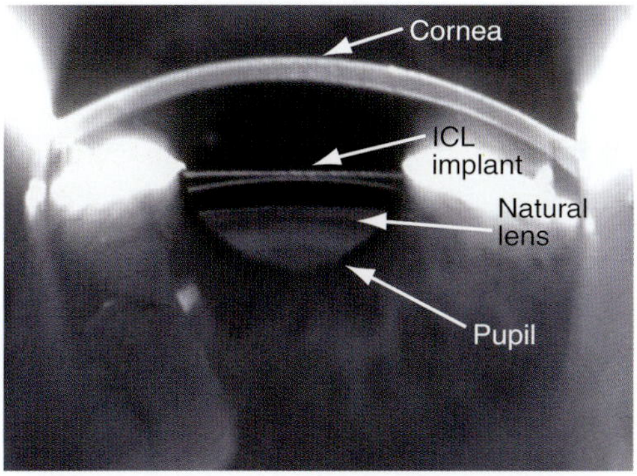

Figure 8-4 Visian ICL PCPIOL within the posterior chamber, as seen with Scheimpflug photography. *(Courtesy of STAAR.)*

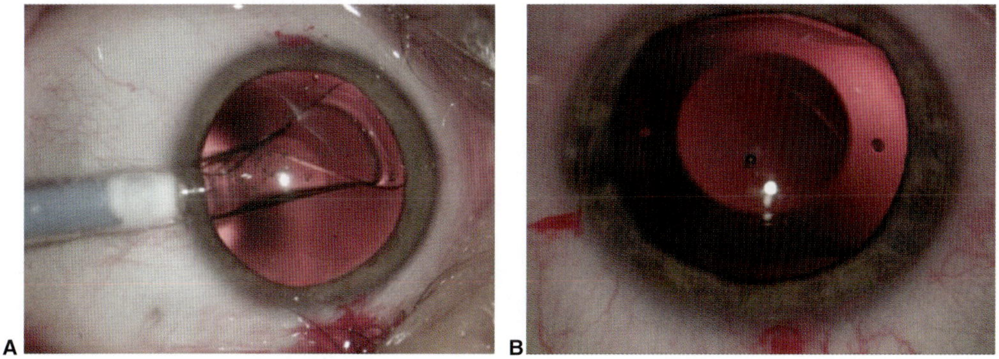

Figure 8-5 **A,** Visian ICL PCPIOL unfolds in the anterior chamber after placement with the IOL inserter. **B,** Visian ICL PCPIOL unfolded and in position in the posterior chamber anterior to the crystalline lens. *(Courtesy of STAAR.)*

area. The pupil is then constricted with an intracameral miotic agent such as acetylcholine chloride (eg, Miochol). Viscoelastic should be removed at the conclusion of the case.

Sizing the PCPIOL The correct IOL length is selected by using the white-to-white caliper measurement between the 3 and 9 o' clock meridians. Alternative methods for sizing the IOL include high-frequency ultrasound, OCT, slit-beam or Scheimpflug imaging, and laser interferometry. To date, no one technique has shown clear superiority over the others.

Outcomes

The outcomes and complications of surgery with various PIOLs are analyzed in several studies (Tables 8-2, 8-3). With improved methods for determining power, outcomes have steadily improved. Significant postoperative gains in lines of BCVA over the preoperative levels are likely due to a reduction in the image minification that is present with spectacle correction of high myopia. A loss of BCVA is rare. Also, the loss of contrast sensitivity noted after LASIK for high myopia does not occur after PIOL surgery. In fact, contrast sensitivity increases in all spatial frequencies when compared with preoperative contrast sensitivity with best spectacle correction.

Table 8-2 Results With Phakic IOLs

Study	PIOL Model	Number of Eyes	Mean Preoperative Spherical Equivalent (Range)	Postoperative Result Within ±0.50 D of Emmetropia	Postoperative Result Within ±1.00 D of Emmetropia	Uncorrected Visual Acuity 20/40 or Better	Gain ±2 Lines Best-Corrected Visual Acuity	Loss ±2 Lines Best-Corrected Visual Acuity
ACPIOL								
Baikoff (1998)	ZB5M	134	−12.50 D (−7.00 to −18.80 D)	32%	58.8%	57%	50.7%	8.3%
Leccisotti (2005)	ZSAL-4 IOL	190	−14.37 D ± 4.40 D	19.0%	40%	~60%		
Allemann (2000)	NuVita	21	−18.95 D		Mean spherical equivalent −1.93 D		65%	0%
Iris-fixated IOL								
Menezo (1998)	Iris claw lens	111	−14.81 D (−8.00 to −20.00 D)		82.9%	36.3%	77%	
Budo (2000)	Verisyse	249	−12.95 D ± 4.35 D	57.1%	78.8%	76.8%	63.3% in > −15.00 D group 23.5% in −5.00 to 15.00 D group	1.2%
FDA clinical trial (2004)	Verisyse	684	-5.00 to 20.00 D	71.7% at 3 years	94.7% at 3 years	92% at 3 years		0.3% at 3 years n=591
PCPIOL								
FDA clinical trial (2005)	ICL	526	-3.00 to −20.00 D	70.0% at 3 years n=363	89.3% at 3 years n=363	94.7% at 3 years n=189		0.8%
Zaldivar (1998)	ICL	124	−13.38 D (−8.50 to −18.65 D)	44%	69%	68%	36%	0.8%
Arne (2000)	ICL	58	−13.85 D (−8.00 to −19.25 D)	Mean spherical equivalent −1.22 D	56.9%	Mean postoperative acuity 20/50	77.6% gained ≥1 line	3.4%
Vukich (2003)	ICL	258	−10.05 D (−3.00 to −20.00 D)	57.4% at 2 years	80.2% at 2 years	92.5% at 1 year	10.9%	1.2%
Davidorf (1998)	ICL (for hyperopia)	24	+6.51 D (+3.75 to +10.50 D)	58%	79%	63%	8%	4%

Table 8-3 Incidence of Complications With Phakic IOLs

Study	PIOL Model	Number of Eyes	Glare/Halos	Pupil Ovalization	Mean Endothelial Cell Loss	Cataract	Pigment Dispersion	IOP Elevation
ACPIOL								
Alio (1999)	ZB5M/MF/ ZSAL-4	263	20% at 1 year 10% at 7 years	5.9%	8.4% at 7 years			
Baikoff (1998)	ZB5M	134 35	18.8% at 1 year 12.5% at 3 years	9.9% at 1 year 27.5% at 3 years	4.6% at 3 years			
Leccisotti (2005)	ZSAL-4	190	18% 12–24 months	11% 12–24 months	6.2% at 1 year			
Iris-fixated IOL								
FDA clinical trial (2004)	Verisyse	662	18.2% n=472	hyphema 0.2%	4.75% at 3 years n=353	5.2% (12/232)	Iritis 0.5%	None
Budo (2000)	Artisan	518	8.8% at 3 years n=249	No pupil change Rare hyphema resolved	9.4% cumulative, but stabilized over 3 years n=129	None reported		Rare, transient IOP elevation
PCPIOL								
Vukich (2003)	ICL	257			No corneal edema from 1 to 24 months	6.7% anterior subcapsular cataract at 2 years		
Arne (2000)	ICL	58	54.3%		<3.9% at 1 year	3.4% anterior subcapsular cataract	15.5%	3.4%
FDA clinical trial (2005) (5-year specular microscopy data [2007])	ICL	526	3 years glare: worse 9.7%; better 12.0% halos worse 11.4%; better 9.1%		Cumulative loss of 12.8% approaching stability at 5 years	Visually significant ASC 0.4%; NS 1.0%		0.4% No cases of visual field loss or nerve damage
Zaldivar (1998)	ICL	124	2.4%			2.4%		11.3%

Alió JL, de la Hoz F, Pérez-Santonja JJ, Ruiz-Moreno JM, Quesada JA. Phakic anterior chamber lenses for the correction of myopia: a 7-year cumulative analysis of complications in 263 cases. *Ophthalmology.* 1999;106:458–466.

Allemann N, Chamon W, Tanaka HM, et al. Myopic angle-supported intraocular lenses: two-year follow-up. *Ophthalmology*. 2000;107:1549–1554.

Arne JL, Lesueur LC. Phakic posterior chamber lenses for high myopia: functional and anatomical outcomes. *J Cataract Refract Surg.* 2000;26:369–374.

Baikoff G, Arne JL, Bokobza Y, et al. Angle-fixated anterior chamber phakic intraocular lens for myopia of –7 to –19 diopters. *J Refract Surg.* 1998;14:282–293.

Budo C, Hessloehl JC, Izak M, et al. Multicenter study of the Artisan phakic intraocular lens. *J Cataract Refract Surg.* 2000;26:1163–1171.

Davidorf JM, Zaldivar R, Oscherow S. Posterior chamber phakic intraocular lens for hyperopia of +4 to +11 diopters. *J Refract Surg.* 1998;14:306–311.

Jiménez-Alfaro I, Gómez-Telleria G, Bueno JL, Puy P. Contrast sensitivity after posterior chamber phakic intraocular lens implantation for high myopia. *J Refract Surg.* 2001;17:641–645.

Leccisotti A, Fields SV. Clinical results of ZSAL-4 angle-supported phakic intraocular lenses in 190 myopic eyes. *J Cataract Refract Surg.* 2005;31:318–323.

Lovisolo CF, Reinstein DZ. Phakic intraocular lenses. *Surv Ophthalmol.* 2005;50:549–587.

Sanders DR, Vukich JA, Doney K, Gaston M; Implantable Contact Lens in Treatment of Myopia Study Group. U.S. Food and Drug Administration clinical trial of the Implantable Contact Lens for moderate to high myopia. *Ophthalmology*. 2003;110:255–266.

United States Food and Drug Administration. Summary of Safety and Effectiveness Data. Artisan Phakic Lens. PMA: P030028. Date of approval: 9/10/04.

United States Food and Drug Administration. Summary of Safety and Effectiveness Data. STAAR Visian ICL (Implantable Collamer Lens). PMA: P030016. Date of approval: 2/22/05.

Zaldivar R, Davidorf JM, Oscherow S. Posterior chamber phakic intraocular lens for myopia of –8 to –19 diopters. *J Refract Surg.* 1998;14:294–305.

Complications

Most manufacturers continue to modify the design of their PIOLs to improve results and minimize complications. Older studies do not necessarily reflect the complication rate associated with more recently developed PIOLs. When experienced surgeons implant these PIOLs, the incidence of sight-threatening complications is quite low. However, because the PIOLs are used in young, active individuals, longer follow-up is needed to accurately determine their safety. Many of the most important potential complications of PIOLs, such as cataract, endothelial cell loss, and retinal detachment, may not manifest for many years. Both the patient and the surgeon need to recognize this current inability to accurately assess the incidence of PIOL complications.

Anterior chamber PIOLs

The most frequent complications reported for ACPIOLs are nighttime glare and halos, pupil ovalization, and endothelial cell loss (see Table 8-3). Ovalization of the pupil is more likely when the ACPIOL is too large, whereas movement of an ACPIOL that is too small can cause endothelial damage and decentration. The risk of pupillary block is low because iridotomies have become part of the surgical protocol. Because complications such as endothelial cell loss and pupil ovalization may take years to develop, the true frequency of these complications can be assessed only after a follow-up of many years. A stated rate of endothelial cell loss at a particular postoperative interval is the equivalent of a snapshot view. Whether cell loss continues or the endothelium stabilizes can only be determined with long-term follow-up, and any reported complication rate should be critically evaluated with these considerations in mind (see Table 8-3). Further, direct comparison of studies of varying size using different IOL models within a given PIOL category may have limited value.

Glare and halos, the most commonly reported symptoms following ACPIOL insertion, occur in 18.8%–20% of patients, but these symptoms appear to decrease by as much as 50% over a postoperative period of 7 years. The incidence is significantly reduced with a larger ACPIOL optic. Endothelial cell loss 1–7 years after ACPIOL insertion ranges from 4.6% to 8.4%. Pupil ovalization can occur because of iris tuck during ACPIOL insertion, or it can occur over time due to chronic inflammation and fibrosis around the haptics within the anterior chamber angle. The incidence of pupil ovalization ranges from 5.9% to 27.5% and is directly related to the postoperative interval studied.

ACPIOL rotation was frequently observed in one study, but not in others. Acute postoperative iritis occurred in 4.6% of cases, and retinal detachment occurred in 3%.

Iris-fixated PIOLs

At a 1-year follow-up in the FDA clinical trials of 662 patients who had the Verisyse (Artisan) iris-fixation PIOL implanted for myopia, 1 patient had a hyphema, 5 had IOL dislocations, and 3 had iritis. Surgical reintervention was required in 28 patients. The incidence of retinal detachment was 0.6%. Cumulative endothelial cell loss over a 3-year period was 5.6% with 111 patients studied. Cell loss was highest when the anterior chamber depth was less than 3.2 mm. The change in glare, starbursts, and halos from the preoperative to postoperative state was assessed by questionnaire. The incidence of these symptoms developing after surgery was 13.5%, 11.8%, and 18.2% , respectively. However, improvement in these symptoms occurred in 12.9%, 9.7%, and 9.8%, respectively. In general, nighttime symptoms were worse in patients with larger pupil diameters. Cataract is a rare complication of the iris-fixated PIOL.

Pop M, Payette Y. Initial results of endothelial cell counts after Artisan lens for phakic eyes: an evaluation of the United States Food and Drug Administration Ophtec Study. *Ophthalmology.* 2004;111:309–311.

Posterior chamber PIOLs

In addition to nighttime glare and halos and the potential to cause endothelial damage, as seen in other types of PIOLs, the placement of a PCPIOL may increase the risk of cataract formation and pigmentary dispersion. If the PCPIOL is too small, the vaulting will decrease, but the risk of cataract may increase; if the PCPIOL is too large, iris chafing with pigmentary dispersion could result. The concern over cataract formation was confirmed by a series published in 1999, where cataract formation was reported in 53% of eyes (9/17) at 3 months to 2 years after insertion of a silicone PCPIOL of a Fyodorov design. The majority of these cataracts were anterior subcapsular. It is not currently known whether the mechanism of cataract formation is mechanical or metabolic. If a visually significant cataract develops, it is possible to remove the PCPIOL, perform cataract surgery, and implant a PCIOL.

Brauweiler PH, Wehler T, Busin M. High incidence of cataract formation after implantation of a silicone posterior chamber lens in phakic, highly myopic eyes. *Ophthalmology.* 1999;106:1651–1655.

In Zaldivar's report of 124 eyes implanted with the Visian ICL, mean follow-up was 11 months. Glare was present in only 2.4% of eyes (3/124). The incidence of nighttime visual symptoms was around 10% in the FDA clinical trial for the Visian ICL, but interestingly, a similar percentage had an improvement in these symptoms following surgery. After 2 years of follow-up on 58 eyes, Arne reported a 54.3% incidence of halos and night-driving disturbance, which were less frequent when a larger optic was used. Lens opacities occurred in 2.4% (3/124) to 3.4% (2/58). The incidence of visually significant cataract in the FDA clinical trial (see the Sanders et al, 2003, reference earlier in the chapter) was 0.4% for anterior subcapsular cataracts and 1% for nuclear sclerotic cataracts. Jiménez-Alfaro studied fluorophotometry after PCPIOL insertion and showed a steady reduction in crystalline lens transmittance over a 2-year period, with a decrease of 2.24% at the second postoperative year. Aqueous flare increased to nearly 50% in the first month after surgery and was still 27% above normal 2 years following surgery.

The most frequent complication in Zaldivar's study was PCPIOL decentration, with <1 mm decentration in 14.5% of eyes (18/124) and visually significant decentration of >1 mm in 1.6% of eyes (2/124). In one case, recentration was performed and in the other the PCPIOL was removed (Fig 8-6). A case of inverted PCPIOL also occurred. No eye had an endothelial cell loss of >3.8% at 1 year. Cumulative endothelial cell loss at 3 years was 8% in the Visian FDA evaluation; however, 5-year data showed a 12.8% loss of endothelial cells. Cell loss between year 4 and year 5 was 2.1%, the lowest interval rate of cell loss. A declining coefficient of variation and an increasing percent of hexagonal cells seem to indicate that the endothelium is stabilizing at 5 years.

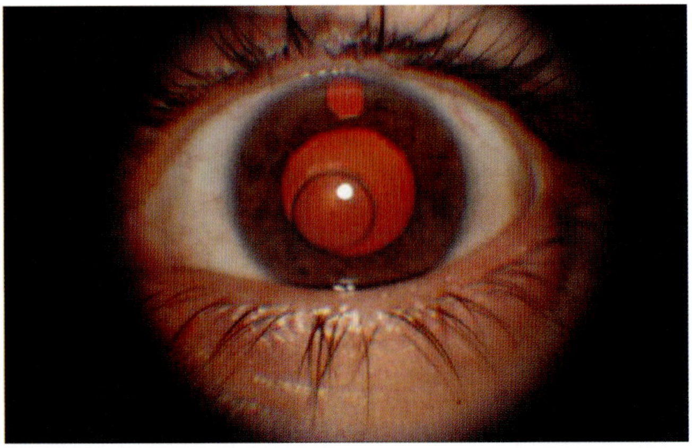

Figure 8-6 Patient with inferiorly decentered PCPIOL. *(Courtesy of Jayne S. Weiss, MD.)*

The incidence of retinal detachment after PCPIOL insertion is very low. In a recent series of 16 eyes, surgical reattachment was achieved in 100%, with a mean follow-up of 35.25 months (range 12–67 months) and a mean postoperative best spectacle-corrected visual acuity of 20/28.

Arne JL, Lesueur LC. Phakic posterior chamber lenses for high myopia: functional and anatomical outcomes. *J Cataract Refract Surg.* 2000;26:369–374.

Jiménez-Alfaro I, Benítez del Castillo JM, García-Feijoó J, Gil de Bernabé JG, Serrano de La Iglesia JM. Safety of posterior chamber phakic intraocular lenses for the correction of high myopia: anterior segment changes after posterior chamber phakic intraocular lens implantation. *Ophthalmology.* 2001;108:90–99.

Martínez-Castillo V, Boixadera A, Verdugo A, Elies D, Coret A, García-Arumi J. Rhegmatogenous retinal detachment in phakic eyes after posterior chamber phakic intraocular lens implantation for severe myopia. *Ophthalmology.* 2005;112:580–585.

STAAR Surgical Company. US Clinical Study. Specular Microscopy: 5-year Cumulative Data on Visian ICL. Submitted to FDA 2-7-07.

United States Food and Drug Administration. Summary of Safety and Effectiveness Data. STAAR Visian ICL (Implantable Collamer Lens). PMA: P030016. Date of approval: 2/22/05.

Zaldivar R, Davidorf JM, Oscherow S. Posterior chamber phakic intraocular lens for myopia of −8 to −19 diopters. *J Refract Surg.* 1998;14:294–305.

Bioptics

Bioptics is a term suggested by Zaldivar in the late 1990s to describe the combination of PCPIOL implantation followed at a later time with LASIK to treat patients with extreme myopia and/or residual astigmatism. Because of the limitations of the individual procedures, the concept of first inserting a PIOL to reduce the amount of myopia correction required and then refining the residual spherical and astigmatic correction with LASIK has gained appeal. LASIK is typically performed approximately 1 month after the PIOL surgery.

Another term, *adjustable refractive surgery (ARS),* is also used to describe combined intraocular and corneal refractive surgery. Güell and colleagues have described ARS, which involves creating a corneal flap just prior to inserting an iris-fixated PIOL and then, at a later time, lifting the flap and performing the laser procedure. This 2-stage modification avoids the potential for endothelial trauma by an iris-fixated PIOL or an ACPIOL during the microkeratome pass. Microkeratomes were later shown to be safe in performing LASIK following iris-fixated PIOLs. In addition, the femtosecond laser distorts the anterior segment less than a microkeratome and is also safe to use in bioptics procedures. If in doubt, bioptics with surface ablation is also a reasonable alternative. The bioptics concept has been used to correct high hyperopia as well. As new treatment options are developed, the possibilities for other combinations of refractive surgery will likely increase.

The ability to successfully combine refractive procedures further expands the limits of refractive surgery. The predictability, stability, and safety of LASIK may increase if a smaller refractive error is treated with the corneal surgery. In addition, there is usually sufficient corneal tissue to maximize the treatment zone diameter without exceeding the limits of ablation depth. The LASIK procedure provides the feature of adjustability to the overall refractive operation. These benefits must be balanced with the combined risks of performing 2 surgeries rather than 1 surgery.

Outcomes

In the initial reports of bioptics and ARS, the range of treatment for myopia was −18.75 to −35.00 D and −16.00 to −23.00 D, respectively (Table 8-4). If the long-term results of PIOLs prove acceptable, the use of bioptics may expand to the treatment of smaller refractive errors because of the advantages of superior optical performance and greater accuracy of refractive correction.

Güell JL, Vázquez M, Gris O. Adjustable refractive surgery: 6-mm Artisan lens plus laser in situ keratomileusis for the correction of high myopia. *Ophthalmology.* 2001;108:945–952.

Güell JL, Vázquez M, Gris O, De Muller A, Manero F. Combined surgery to correct high myopia: iris claw phakic intraocular lens and laser in situ keratomileusis. *J Refract Surg.* 1999;15:529–537.

Zaldivar R, Davidorf JM, Oscherow S, Ricur G, Piezzi V. Combined posterior chamber phakic intraocular lens and laser in situ keratomileusis: bioptics for extreme myopia. *J Refract Surg.* 1999;15:299–308.

Clear Lens Extraction (Refractive Lens Exchange)

Patient Selection

Indications

The indications for refractive lensectomy with IOL implantation are evolving. Refractive lensectomy with IOL implantation is usually considered only if alternative refractive procedures are not feasible and there is a strong reason why spectacles or contact lenses are unacceptable alternatives. If the cornea is too thin, too flat, or too steep, or the refractive error exceeds the limit of excimer laser treatment, clear lens extraction and PIOL implantation are options. Refractive lens exchange may be preferable to a PIOL in the presence of a lens opacity that is presently visually insignificant but that may eventually progress and cause visual loss. Clear lens exchange for refractive correction is generally not considered medically necessary and is usually not a covered expense.

Informed consent

Potential candidates must be capable of understanding the short-term and long-term risks of clear lens extraction. They must understand that performing the surgery on both eyes sequentially rather than simultaneously is recommended to decrease the potential of a devastating complication such as bilateral endophthalmitis. Patients must understand that unless they are left with a degree of myopia or a multifocal or accommodating IOL is implanted, they will incur the loss of near vision. Intraocular lens implantation following removal of a clear lens represents an off-label use of the IOL; this should be explained to the prospective patient. A consent form developed specifically for this surgery should

Table 8-4 Results of Bioptics and Adjustable Refractive Surgery

Study	Number of Eyes	Mean Preoperative Spherical Equivalent (Range)	Postoperative Result Within ±0.50 D of Emmetropia	Postoperative Result Within ±1.00 D of Emmetropia	Uncorrected Visual Acuity 20/40 or Better	Gain ≥2 Lines Best-Corrected Visual Acuity	Loss ≥2 Lines Best-Corrected Visual Acuity
Zaldivar (1999) Bioptics	67	–23.00 D (–18.75 to –35.00 D)	67%	85%	69%	76%	0%
Güell (2001) Adjustable refractive surgery	26	–18.42 D (–16.00 to –23.00 D)	80.7%	100%	77%	42%	0%
Chayet (2001) ICL/LASIK or PRK	37	–17.74 D (–9.75 to –28.00 D)	83.7%	97.2%	89.1%	64.8%	3%

be given to the patient prior to surgery to allow ample time for review and signature. A sample consent form for refractive lens exchange for the correction of hyperopia and myopia is available from the Ophthalmic Mutual Insurance Company (OMIC) at www.omic.com.

Myopia

In addition to all the risks associated with cataract surgery, the surgeon must specifically inform the patient about the substantial risk of retinal detachment associated with removal of the crystalline lens. Myopia is already a significant risk factor for retinal detachment in the absence of lens surgery, and this risk rises with increased axial length. The risk in eyes with up to 3.00 D of myopia may be as much as 4 times as great as it is in emmetropic eyes. In eyes with greater than 3.00 D of myopia, the risk of retinal detachment may be as high as 10 times the risk in emmetropia. In the absence of trauma, more than 50% of retinal detachments occur in myopic eyes.

Preferred Practice Patterns Committee, Retina Panel. *Posterior Vitreous Detachment, Retinal Breaks, and Lattice Degeneration.* San Francisco: American Academy of Ophthalmology; 2003.

Wilkinson CP. Retinal implications of refractive lensectomy and phakic IOLs. *Subspecialty Day Program 2001.* San Francisco: American Academy of Ophthalmology; 2001.

Hyperopia

As patients approach presbyopic age, moderate and high hyperopia become increasingly bothersome. The perceived accelerated onset of presbyopia occurs because some accommodation is expended in an effort to clarify distance vision. Many hyperopic patients have significant chronic accommodative spasm.

If the amount of hyperopia is beyond the range of alternative refractive procedures, clear lens extraction with IOL insertion might be the only available surgical option. As is the case with myopia, the patient must be informed about the risks of intraocular surgery. A patient with a shallow anterior chamber from a thickened crystalline lens or small anterior segment would not be a candidate for a PIOL and could benefit from a reduced risk of angle-closure glaucoma following clear lens extraction. The hyperopic patient has a lower risk of retinal detachment than the myopic patient.

Surgical Planning and Technique

Although refractive lensectomy has similarities to cataract surgery, there are some special considerations for planning and performing the procedure. It is important to determine if the source of myopia is a steep cornea or an increased axial length. If the cornea is quite steep, corneal topography should be performed to rule out an ectatic corneal condition. Keratoconus and pellucid marginal degeneration induce irregular astigmatism, which can affect the immediate visual outcome and can have long-term implications. When astigmatism is present in the refraction, keratometry and corneal topography will help the surgeon determine whether the astigmatism is lenticular or corneal in origin. Only the corneal component of astigmatism will remain postoperatively. The patient should be informed if substantial astigmatism is expected to be present after surgery and, to optimize the visual outcome, a plan should be devised to correct it. Small amounts of corneal astigmatism (<1.00 D) may be reduced if the incision is placed in the steep meridian. Superior clear corneal incisions are occasionally associated with large unpredictable astigmatic shifts, possibly because of the reduced distance from the superior limbus—as compared with the temporal limbus—to the center of the cornea. Some surgeons believe that scleral pocket incisions are preferable when a superior incision site is required.

Limbal relaxing incisions may be used to correct larger amounts of corneal astigmatism (see Chapter 4). Toric IOLs are another option. Supplemental surface ablation or LASIK could also be considered (see the preceding discussion of bioptics). Although glasses or contact lenses are an alternative for managing residual astigmatism, refractive surgery patients often reject this option.

All patients should have a dilated fundus examination prior to surgery, but the high axial myopic patient should also have a detailed evaluation of the peripheral retina because of the increased risk of retinal detachment. If relevant pathology is discovered, appropriate treatment or referral to a retina specialist is warranted. If the patient has high axial myopia, retrobulbar injections should be avoided due to the risk of perforating the globe. Peribulbar, sub-Tenon, topical, and intracameral anesthesia are alternative options. In determining the preferred route of anesthetic administration, the surgeon should keep in mind that younger patients are often more anxious than older cataract patients.

An excessively deep anterior chamber may develop during surgery on a patient with high axial myopia. A deep anterior chamber impairs surgical visualization and instrument manipulation. The patient may complain of pain, particularly when the eye is anesthetized with topical and intracameral anesthetic only. An excessively deep chamber can be minimized by avoiding a viscoelastic overfill and by lowering the irrigation bottle at the start of the operation. Finally, the small-incision bimanual phacoemulsification technique may enable the surgeon to maintain a more stable anterior chamber during lens removal.

In hyperopia, a small cornea may be more prone to surgical trauma, the lens may be located more anteriorly, and the crowded anterior chamber may make surgical maneuvers more difficult. In a highly hyperopic eye with an axial length of less than 18 mm, the diagnosis of nanophthalmos should be considered. These eyes are prone to uveal effusion syndrome and postoperative choroidal detachment (see BCSC Section 11, *Lens and Cataract*).

Careful and complete hydrodissection is essential for facilitating lens mobilization. In younger patients, the nucleus is too soft to turn easily with a nucleus rotator if cortical adhesions persist. The soft nucleus is likely to partially prolapse out of the capsular bag during hydrodissection and can be repositioned with viscoelastic. To protect the posterior capsule, some surgeons prefer to leave the lens nucleus in the anterior chamber.

The younger the patient, the more likely the lens can be aspirated with the phacoemulsification tip with vacuum and little to no ultrasound. No matter how soft, a nucleus can only rarely be aspirated through a 0.3-mm irrigation/aspiration tip. If the lens cannot easily be aspirated, necessitating the use of ultrasound, the power should be reduced to the lowest level needed to remove the lens. The surgeon must carefully guard against capsular rupture, as the softer lens material may aspirate abruptly, creating surge and sudden anterior chamber shallowing. Techniques such as "divide and conquer" and "phaco chop" are not possible if the lens is very soft.

Many surgeons believe that an IOL should always be used after clear lens extraction in a patient with high myopia, even when little to no optical power correction is required. Plano IOL power is available if indicated. The IOL acts as a barrier to anterior prolapse of the vitreous, maintaining the integrity of the aqueous–vitreous barrier, in the event that Nd:YAG laser posterior capsulotomy is required. Some IOL models also reduce the rate of posterior capsule opacification.

IOL Calculations in Refractive Lensectomy

High patient expectations for excellent UCVA make accurate IOL power determination even more critical here than in cataract surgery. However, IOL power formulas are less accurate at higher levels of myopia and hyperopia. In addition, in high myopia, a posterior staphyloma can make the axial length measurements less reliable. Careful fundus examination and B-scan ultrasound can identify the position and extent of staphylomas. The SRK/T formula is generally considered to be the most accurate in moderate and highly myopic patients, whereas the Hoffer Q formula is more accurate for moderate and highly hyperopic eyes. The Haigis formula can be used in patients with short or long eyes but requires a large surgeon-specific patient base with varied axial lengths for optimal utility. It is best to use several formulas to determine IOL power for a refractive patient. Software programs now available can give the surgeon IOL predictions calculated by several formulas. The subject of IOL power determination is covered in detail in BCSC Section 11, *Lens and Cataract.*

Hill WE, Byrne SF. Complex axial length measurements and unusual IOL power calculations. *Focal Points: Clinical Modules for Ophthalmologists.* San Francisco: American Academy of Ophthalmology; 2004, module 9.

In the case of a patient with high hyperopia, biometry may suggest that an IOL power beyond what is commercially available is required. The upper limit of available IOL power is now +40.00 D. A special-order IOL of a higher power may be available or may be designed, but acquiring or designing such a lens usually requires the approval of the institutional review board at the hospital or surgical center, which delays the surgery. Another option is a “piggyback” IOL system, in which 2 posterior chamber IOLs are inserted. One IOL is placed in the capsular bag, and the other is placed in the ciliary sulcus. The Holladay 2, Hoffer Q, and Haigis formulas can be used to calculate piggyback IOL power. When piggyback IOLs are used, the combined power should be increased +1.50 to +2.00 D to compensate for the posterior shift of the posterior IOL. One serious complication of a piggyback IOL is the potential for developing an interlenticular opaque membrane. These membranes cannot be mechanically removed or cleared with the Nd:YAG laser; the IOLs must be removed. Interlenticular membranes have occurred most commonly between 2 acrylic IOLs, especially when both IOLs are placed in the capsular bag, which is why this type of piggyback IOL implantation should be avoided. Piggyback IOLs may also shallow the anterior chamber and increase the risk of iris chafing.

Masket S. Refractive lensectomy for correction of hyperopia. *Subspecialty Day Program 2001.* San Francisco: American Academy of Ophthalmology; 2001.

Complications

The incidence of retinal detachment in 49 clear lens exchange patients with greater than −12.00 D of myopia was reported to be 2% at 4 years, increasing to 8.1% at 7 years. It is not known if the risk continues to increase with even longer follow-up; long-term follow-up is needed before this question can be answered. In this study population, 61% of patients required Nd:YAG laser posterior capsulotomy. Laser capsulotomy increased the risk of detached retina from 5.3% to 10% over a 7-year period. Retinal detachment was also significantly more common in males than in females. The effectiveness of prophylactic laser treatment to the retina to prevent detachment is unproven. Limiting incision size with small-incision techniques may have an impact on reducing complications in clear lens exchange.

Colin J, Robinet A, Cochener B. Retinal detachment after clear lens extraction for high myopia: seven-year follow-up. *Ophthalmology*. 1999;106:2281–2285.

Advantages

Clear lens extraction with IOL implantation has the advantage of greatly expanding the range of refractive surgery beyond what can be achieved with currently available methods. The procedure retains the normal corneal contour, which may enhance vision quality, and may treat presbyopia as well as refractive error with the use of multifocal and/or accommodative IOLs.

Disadvantages

The disadvantages of clear lens extraction include the risks associated with any intraocular surgery, including endophthalmitis and choroidal hemorrhage. Although retinal detachment is a significant concern in a myopic eye, it is less of a risk in a hyperopic eye. Patient expectations for excellent UCVA are much higher in this surgery than in cataract surgery, which increases the need for a thorough preoperative discussion, as well as increased attention to detail preoperatively and intraoperatively and treatment of residual refractive error postoperatively.

Toric Intraocular Lenses

Corneal astigmatism of ≥1.50 D is present in 15%–29% of cataract patients. Methods of corrective surgery include arcuate keratotomy or limbal relaxing incisions during or after cataract surgery, excimer laser ablation by either LASIK or surface ablation after adequate healing of the incision, or, for small amounts of cylinder, placing the incision in the axis of plus cylinder. Alternatively, a toric IOL can incorporate the astigmatic correction into the spherical IOL power. Toric IOL placement after clear lens extraction has not been well studied.

Instrumentation

The STAAR toric IOL (Fig 8-7) is an FDA-approved, single-piece, plate-haptic, foldable silicone IOL designed to be placed in the capsular bag using an injector through a 3-mm incision. Once in the eye, it must be oriented with its long axis precisely in the steep meridian. The 6-mm optic is biconvex with a spherocylindrical anterior surface and a spherical posterior surface. The optic has a mark at either end to indicate the axis of plus cylinder. The IOL is available in a length of 10.8 mm or 11.2 mm. A 1.15-mm fenestration located at the end of each haptic is designed to maximize capsular fixation. The IOLs are available in the range of +10.00 to +28.00 D spherical powers, with a choice of cylindrical powers of 2.00 D and 3.50 D. The toric surface corrects less astigmatism when measured at the corneal plane; STAAR states that the 2.00 D IOL corrects 1.40 D of corneal astigmatism and the 3.50 D IOL corrects 2.30 D.

The Alcon AcrySof toric IOL (Fig 8-8) is a recently FDA-approved lens implant, which is built on the same platform as the standard AcrySof posterior chamber lens implant. This toric IOL has a 6.0-mm biconvex acrylic toric optic, available in the range of +10.00 to +30.00 D. The lens is available in the following 3 astigmatism powers: +1.50 D, +2.25 D, and +3.00 D, which correct +1.03 D, +1.55 D, and +2.06 D, respectively, at the spectacle plane. The axis of plus cylinder is marked on the lens optic.

Patient Selection

The toric IOL is appropriate for cataract patients with moderate regular corneal astigmatism. Patients with astigmatism in amounts exceeding the upper correction limits of these lenses require additional measures to obtain full correction. In addition to understanding the risks associated with intraocular surgery, a patient must be capable of understanding the limitations of this IOL. The patient should be informed that implantation of a toric IOL will not eliminate the need for reading glasses (unless monovision is planned). The patient also needs to be informed that the IOL may rotate in the capsular bag shortly after surgery and that a secondary intraocular surgery may be required to reposition it. Because

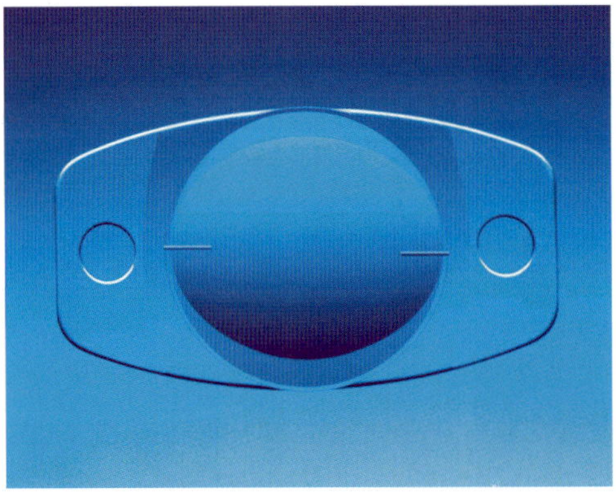

Figure 8-7 STAAR toric IOL. Note the 2 horizontal marks; these should be aligned with the axis of (+) cylinder in the cornea. *(Courtesy of STAAR.)*

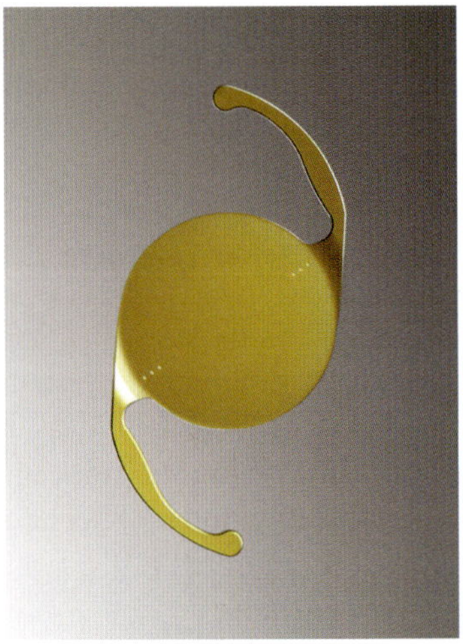

Figure 8-8 AcrySof toric IOL. Note the 2 sets of 3 dots; these are aligned with the axis of (+) cylinder in the cornea. *(Courtesy of Alcon.)*

the STAAR toric IOL is available only in silicone, it would not be appropriate for patients who may require silicone oil for retinal detachment repair in the future. The acrylic Alcon AcrySof toric IOL would be a more appropriate choice in these patients.

Planning and Surgical Technique

The amount and axis of the astigmatism should be measured accurately with a keratometer and confirmed if possible with corneal topography. The axis of astigmatism from the refraction should not be used because it is in part due to lenticular astigmatism, which will be eliminated with cataract surgery. The axis of astigmatism should be marked on the cornea with the patient in an upright position; in this way, any misalignment resulting from the torsional globe rotation that sometimes occurs with movement to a supine position is avoided. Cataract surgery with a wound that is astigmatism-predictable is necessary to achieve the intended benefit of a toric lens.

After the IOL is injected into the capsular bag, the viscoelastic material behind the IOL is aspirated and the IOL is rotated into position on the steep meridian. If the IOL is too short for the capsular bag diameter, it may rotate when balanced salt solution is used to re-form the anterior chamber. Some surgeons choose to insert the STAAR toric IOL with the spherocylindrical surface facing the posterior capsule in an effort to minimize the risk of postoperative lens rotation. According to data available from the FDA on the safety of the Alcon toric IOL, the incidence of postoperative surgical intervention for IOL rotation was only 0.4% (1/244).

When a plate-haptic toric IOL is used, the surgeon should take care when performing Nd:YAG capsulotomy. If the capsulotomy is too large, a plate-haptic IOL may prolapse posteriorly. Capsular fixation around the fenestrations helps to stabilize this IOL. This is not an issue with the AcrySof toric IOL.

Outcomes

In clinical trials with the STAAR toric IOL, a UCVA of ≥20/40 following implantation occurred in 48%–84% of patients. Data provided by the FDA reveal an uncorrected acuity of ≥20/40 in 93.8% of 198 patients implanted with Alcon AcrySof toric IOLs (all sizes combined). Postoperative astigmatism was <0.50 D in 48% of patients and <1.00 D in 75%–81% of patients with the plate-haptic IOLs and 61.6% and 87.7%, respectively, for the Alcon toric IOL.

Complications

The major disadvantage of toric IOLs is the possibility of IOL rotation resulting in a misalignment of the astigmatic correction. Full correction is not achieved unless the IOL is properly aligned in the axis of astigmatism. According to STAAR, a 10° off-axis rotation of the lens reduces the correction by approximately one third, a 20° off-axis rotation reduces the correction by two thirds, and an off-axis correction of greater than 30° can actually increase the cylindrical refractive error. In the FDA clinical trials, 76% of patients were reportedly within 10° of preoperative alignment, and 95% were within 30° degrees. Till and colleagues found that 14% of 100 consecutive STAAR toric IOLs inserted had rotated postoperatively by more than 15°. According to data on the Alcon toric IOL available from the FDA, the degree of postoperative rotation in 242 implanted eyes was 5° or less in 81.1% and 10° or less in 97.1%. None of the eyes exhibited postoperative rotation greater than 15°.

Typically, a misaligned IOL is recognized within days of the surgery; it should be repositioned before permanent fibrosis occurs within the capsular bag. However, waiting 1 week for some capsule contraction to occur may ultimately help stabilize this IOL.

Ruhswurm I, Scholz U, Zehetmayer M, Hanselmayer G, Vass C, Skorpik C. Astigmatism correction with a foldable toric intraocular lens in cataract patients. *J Cataract Refract Surg.* 2000;26:1022–1027.

Sun XY, Vicary D, Montgomery P, Griffiths M. Toric intraocular lenses for correcting astigmatism in 130 eyes. *Ophthalmology.* 2000;107:1776–1781.

Till JS, Yoder PR, Wilcox TK, Spielman JL. Toric intraocular lens implantation: 100 consecutive cases. *J Cataract Refract Surg.* 2001;28:295–301.

Multifocal Intraocular Lenses

A multifocal IOL has the advantage of providing the patient with functional vision at near, intermediate, and remote distances. Careful patient selection and counseling, along with preoperative measurement, are critically important for achieving patient satisfaction postoperatively.

Instrumentation

The Array (AMO) multifocal silicone PCIOL was the first multifocal IOL to be granted FDA approval in the United States. It has since been replaced with the second-generation ReZoom lens (AMO), 1 of the 2 currently available approved multifocal IOLs in the United States. The ReZoom (Fig 8-9) lens is a flexible acrylic, distance-dominant zonal refractive IOL that can be inserted through a 2.8-mm clear corneal incision. The lens has 5 expanded refractive zones within the 6.0-mm optic and produces 2.80 D of near power. The pupil must be at least 2.0 mm to achieve the near effect. The newer design has resulted in less glare and fewer halos and starbursts than with the Array lens.

The AcrySof ReSTOR (Alcon) (Fig 8-10) is also a foldable acrylic IOL designed for insertion following small-incision cataract surgery, but in contrast, it is an apodized diffractive lens, which is built on the central 3.6 mm of the optic of the AcrySof PCIOL platform. The effective near power is 3.50 D and the near acuity is less sensitive to pupil diameter than is the ReZoom lens. Diffractive optic multifocal IOLs are also available outside the United States (Tecnis multifocal IOL, AMO) and are currently in FDA trials.

Patient Selection

Patients likely to be successful with a multifocal IOL after cataract surgery are adaptable, relatively easygoing people who place a high value on reducing dependence on glasses or contact lenses. They should have good potential vision. The best candidates are currently dependent on glasses with more than –2.00 D of myopic correction (or more than +1.00 D of preoperative hyperopic correction). They generally have less than 1.00 D of preexisting

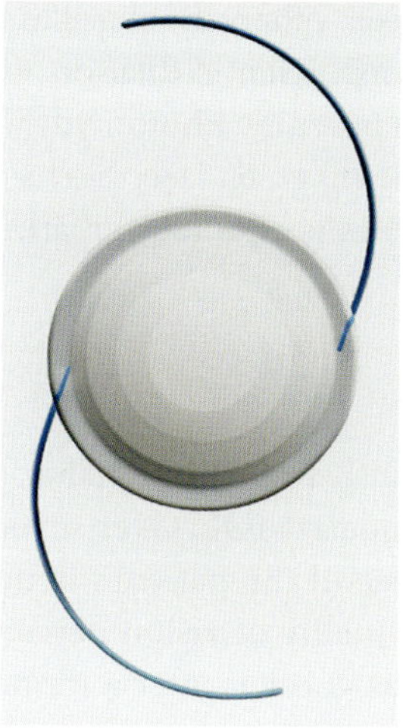

Figure 8-9 ReZoom multifocal IOL. Note the circular zones of refractive correction shown in lens optic. *(Courtesy of AMO.)*

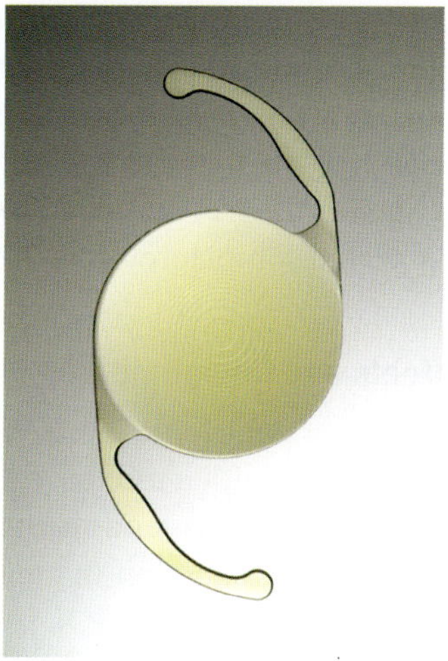

Figure 8-10 ReSTOR multifocal IOL. Note the apodized diffractive changes on the lens optic. *(Courtesy of Alcon.)*

corneal astigmatism. Patients generally adapt to the multifocal effect more quickly after cataract surgery on both eyes.

Multifocal IOLs have been used for presbyopic refractive lensectomy, in which clear lens extraction is performed and then a multifocal IOL is inserted. This may be of particular benefit to the hyperopic patient with presbyopia who has inadequate uncorrected visual function at near and distance. Accommodative IOLs (eg, Crystalens [Eyeonics, Aliso Viejo, CA]; see the discussion later in the chapter) can also be used in this setting. As with any refractive surgery procedure, careful patient selection, education, and expectation management are essential to the success of the procedure.

Surgical Technique

The surgical technique for multifocal IOL insertion is the same as that used in standard small-incision cataract surgery with a foldable acrylic IOL. Optimal refractive effects depend on good IOL centration. If the posterior capsule is not intact, IOL decentration is more likely and an accommodative IOL should not be used; adequate fixation for a multifocal IOL should be evaluated. If adequate centration is not ensured, a multifocal lens should also not be used, and a monofocal IOL should be used instead.

Outcomes

Patients are most likely to achieve independence from glasses following implantation of multifocal IOLs bilaterally. Both of the currently available lenses can allow patients to achieve good distance vision function. The ReSTOR lens provides better unaided visual acuity at near; the ReZoom lens performs better at midrange. A reduction in contrast sensitivity is likely to occur with both lenses. Also, best spectacle-corrected visual acuity may be less than 20/20 with both types of lenses.

As patients age, the pupillary diameter may decrease. When the pupillary diameter falls below 2.0 mm, unaided reading ability may diminish. Gentle dilation with topical mydriatic agents or laser photomydriasis may restore near acuity. Photomydriasis may be performed with an argon or dye photocoagulator, by placing green laser burns circumferentially outside the iris sphincter, or with a Nd:YAG photodisruptor, by creating approximately 4 partial sphincterotomies.

Side Effects and Complications

A patient with a multifocal IOL is likely to have significantly more glare, halos, and ghosting than a patient with a monofocal IOL or an accommodative IOL. Over several months the complaints of halos tend to subside, perhaps because of the patient's neural adaptation. Because of a reduction in contrast sensitivity, the quality of vision perceived by the patient following multifocal IOL insertion may not be as good as after a monofocal IOL implantation. The trade-off of accepting reduced vision quality to reduce one's dependence on glasses must be fully discussed with the patient preoperatively. Intermediate vision is generally weaker with multifocal IOLs than with the accommodative Crystalens. Some surgeons adjust IOL power intended for the nondominant eye to ensure a full range of visual function; others use different models of IOLs to maximize the range of visual function—for example, Crystalens or ReZoom in the dominant eye and ReSTOR in the nondominant eye.

For a more detailed discussion of the surgical treatment of presbyopia, see Chapter 9 of this book.

Fine IH. Refractive lensectomy with multifocal IOL. In: Durrie DS, O'Brien TP, eds. Refractive surgery: back to the future. *Subspecialty Day Program 2002.* San Francisco: American Academy of Ophthalmology; 2002.

Javitt JC, Steinert RF. Cataract extraction with multifocal intraocular lens implantation: a multinational clinical trial evaluating clinical, functional, and quality-of-life outcomes. *Ophthalmology.* 2000;107:2040–2048.

Javitt JC, Wang F, Trentacost DJ, Rowe M, Tarantino N. Outcomes of cataract extraction with multifocal intraocular lens implantation: functional status and quality of life. *Ophthalmology.* 1997;104:589–599.

Wallace RB III. Multifocal and accommodating lens implementation. *Focal Points: Clinical Modules for Ophthalmologists.* San Francisco: American Academy of Ophthalmology; 2004, module 11.

Accommodating Intraocular Lenses

Single-Optic IOLs

The Crystalens (see Fig 9-7) is currently the only accommodating IOL approved by the FDA for improvement of near, intermediate, and distance vision, although other accommodating IOLs are being investigated. The Crystalens is a silicone PCIOL with plate haptics that end in a unique polyamide portion for added capsular fixation. The IOL has a hinge on either side of the optic that allows the lens to flex anteriorly upon accommodation, thus increasing the effective lens power. The optic is available in both a 4.5-mm and a 5.0-mm diameter, the larger being available only for the more commonly used dioptric powers. The major advantages of this lens compared with multifocal IOLs are superior acuity (especially intermediate acuity) and better night vision—benefits that are independent of pupil size. A disadvantage compared with multifocal IOLs is that near acuity may not be as strong. The manufacturer recommends a slightly increased power for the nondominant eye to increase the range of binocular visual acuity. Another disadvantage is a possible unanticipated anterior shift of the lens that increases its effective refractive power. This appears to be more likely to occur with the 4.5-mm optic in patients with axial myopia; the manufacturer has now developed a nomogram in which IOL power is decreased as the axial length increases.

Meticulous cortical removal is essential to prevent a Z-shaped deformity in the IOL. Should this Z-shaped deformation occur, the Nd:YAG laser can be used in a manner prescribed by the manufacturer to release the capsule contracture responsible. If laser posterior capsulotomy becomes necessary, a large opening should be avoided to prevent a posterior shift in the IOL optic and a consequent reduction in effective IOL power.

BioComFold Type 43E (Morcher), 1 CU (HumanOptics, Erlangen, Germany), and TetraFlex (Lenstec, St Petersburg, FL) are other examples of the single-optic IOL designed to simulate accommodation.

Dual-Optic IOLs

The Synchrony IOL (Visiogen, Irvine, CA) is a dual-optic accommodating lens system designed to correct distance and near vision. The 2 silicone optics are connected by a system of springlike struts that push the lenses apart. A +34.0 D anterior lens is paired with an appropriate minus-powered posterior lens, yielding a suitable net effective power for a specific patient. During accommodation, the lens system confined within the capsular bag undergoes an adjustment in the separation of the 2 optics, resulting in an increase in effective lens power. The lens can be injected into the eye through a 3.5-mm incision. The lens is currently undergoing FDA clinical trials in the United States. The Sarfarazi Elliptical Accommodating IOL (Bausch & Lomb) is another example of a dual-optic IOL.

Deformable IOLs

The concept behind the Smart IOL (Medennium, Irvine, CA) is injection of a material that will change into a lens shape upon reaching body temperature. The hydrophobic acrylic material is chemically bonded to wax, which melts inside the eye and allows the predetermined shape and power of the material to emerge. Theoretically, compression of this pliable lens by the capsular bag would allow adjustment of its effective power in a manner similar to the way the crystalline lens adjusts. The lens is not presently ready for clinical trials. Other examples of deformable IOLs that are also in the preliminary stages of development are FlexOptic (AMO), FluidVision IOL (PowerVision, Belmont, CA), and NuLens (NuLens, Herzliya Pituach, Israel). See Chapter 9 for additional discussion.

Hoffman RS, Fine IH, Packer M. Accommodating IOLs: current technology, limitations, and future designs. *Current Insight.* San Francisco: American Academy of Ophthalmology. Available at http://aaophp.aao.org/current_insight/accommodating_IOLs.

Wallace BR III. Multifocal and accommodating lens implantation. *Focal Points: Clinical Modules for Ophthalmologists.* San Francisco: American Academy of Ophthalmology; 2004, module 11.

Wavefront-Designed Intraocular Lenses

The clear crystalline lens in young adults compensates for the spherical aberrations that occur in the average cornea. These aberrations increase with advancing age, and the lens loses the ability to correct for them. As a result, blurred vision, reduced contrast sensitivity, and decreased night vision can occur. The wavefront-designed IOL optic is intended to reestablish this correction following cataract surgery. The Tecnis PCIOL (AMO) is available with either an acrylic or silicone optic and has a modified prolate anterior surface. It has been approved by the FDA for use with cataract surgery to reduce spherical aberration and improve functional vision. Compared with the residual aberrations of other commonly used monofocal IOLs, those measured postoperatively with the Tecnis lens are significantly lower. Also, the lens has been shown to improve night-driving simulator performance over what can be achieved with an acrylic monofocal lens.

The IOL power is based on biometric measurement of each patient. In contrast to wavefront-guided LASIK, however, the wavefront design is not customized for an individual patient. The wavefront design is standardized and based on an average cornea eye model. These lenses should generally not be implanted in patients who have undergone previous wavefront-guided laser refractive surgery to correct hyperopia.

The AcrySof IQ (Alcon) is another aspheric IOL with added negative spherical aberration, designed to compensate for the positive spherical aberration found in the cornea. It is on the same platform as the AcrySof Natural lens. The third aspheric IOL available in the United States is the SofPort AO IOL (Bausch & Lomb). The ReSTOR and Tecnis multifocal IOLs also have added negative spherical aberration to increase contrast sensitivity.

Light-Adjustable Intraocular Lenses

The Light-Adjustable Lens, or LAL (Calhoun Vision, Pasadena, CA), currently under investigation, is a 3-piece silicone-optic IOL in which the silicone matrix has been embedded with silicone subunits called "macromers." When the IOL is irradiated with ultraviolet light through a slit-lamp delivery system, the macromers polymerize and are depleted. Macromers from the nonirradiated part of the IOL optic are in higher concentration and, because of the induced osmotic gradient, diffuse toward the area of irradiation, causing the IOL to swell in this region. The light is thus able to induce a change in the shape of the IOL (Fig 8-11). For myopia, irradiation of the IOL periphery causes a reduction in the central thickness of the IOL. For hyperopia, irradiation of the center of the IOL causes it to swell. Correction of astigmatism can be achieved through a toric exposure pattern. Nomograms have been developed that reportedly can correct hyperopia, myopia, and astigmatism over a 5.00 D range. Once the desired power has been achieved, the IOL optic is diffusely irradiated in a subsequent session within 1–2 weeks postoperatively. This causes

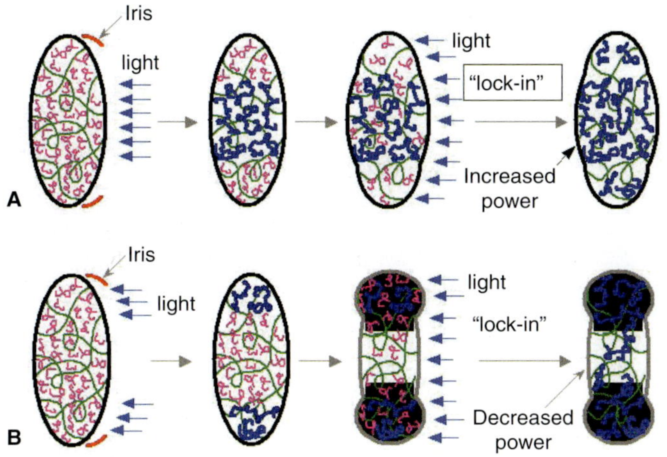

Figure 8-11 Light-adjustable IOL. **A,** When the IOL is treated with light in the center, polymerization occurs and macromers move to the center, increasing the IOL power. **B,** When the IOL is treated with light in the periphery, macromers move to the periphery, decreasing the IOL power. *(Courtesy of Calhoun Vision.)*

all remaining macromers to polymerize in their current location, stopping further diffusion and "locking in" the IOL shape. After that step, the power change becomes irreversible and is no longer adjustable.

Theoretically, the effect of the initial irradiation is reversible to a limited degree. If, for example, an overcorrection of residual myopia occurred and the patient became hyperopic, the previously untouched IOL center could be irradiated in a second procedure prior to the final locking-in step.

This system could hypothetically be used to induce a reversible monovision state that could be adjusted if the patient failed to adapt to it in the first week after surgery. In laboratory studies, multifocal patterns have been placed in the IOL optic and could possibly be designed for specific pupil diameters. In principle, it may be possible to induce a wavefront correction on the IOL that could correct higher-order aberrations.

This IOL is foldable and is reportedly biocompatible in the rabbit model. The system has accurately induced intended power changes at specific irradiation levels in in vitro models. At the time of this writing, human trials have begun outside the United States.

One disadvantage of this IOL system is the need to protect the IOL from sunlight exposure between implantation and the locking-in treatment. Further, it seems possible that if an error occurs in the irradiation treatment related to centration or improper data entry, irreversible changes to the IOL could occur that could affect visual function, potentially requiring IOL exchange surgery. (See also Chapter 9.)

Schwartz DM, Jethmalani J, Sandstedt C, et al. Adjustable IOLs. In: Durrie DS, O'Brien TP, eds. Refractive surgery: back to the future. *Subspecialty Day Program 2002.* San Francisco: American Academy of Ophthalmology; 2002.

CHAPTER 9

Accommodative and Nonaccommodative Treatment of Presbyopia

Introduction

Presbyopia, the normal progressive loss of accommodation, affects all individuals regardless of any underlying refractive error. As bothersome as myopia, hyperopia, and astigmatism are, nothing compares with the relentless loss of near vision and the dependency on glasses that an individual with 20/15 emmetropia feels as middle age approaches. The possibility of "curing" or reducing the effects of presbyopia remains the "Holy Grail" of refractive surgery.

A number of procedures intended to increase the amplitude of accommodation are being investigated. Some of these techniques rely on various types of "scleral expansion." Others involve IOLs capable of anteroposterior movement, with a subsequent change in effective lens power. Still others involve the creation of a multifocal cornea or a multifocal IOL. Some procedures were initially based, in part, on the rejection of the long-accepted Helmholtz theory of accommodation. Because several proposed types of surgery for presbyopia are based on new theories of accommodation, we begin by examining the different theories of accommodation.

Theories of Accommodation

We do not yet have a complete understanding of the relationship between the effect of ciliary muscle contraction and zonular tension on the equatorial lens. In addition, a few markedly different anatomical relationships have been described between the origin of the zonular fibers and the insertion of these fibers into the lens.

The Helmholtz hypothesis, or "capsular theory," of accommodation states that during distance vision, the ciliary muscle is relaxed and the zonular fibers that cross the circumlental space between the ciliary body and the lens equator are under a "resting" tension. With accommodative effort, circumferential ciliary muscle contraction releases this tension on the zonules. There is also an anterior movement of the ciliary muscle annular ring during accommodation. The reduced zonular tension allows the elastic capsule of the lens to contract, causing a decrease in equatorial lens diameter and an increase in the curvatures of the anterior and posterior lens surfaces. This "rounding up" of the lens yields a corresponding increase in its dioptric power that is necessary for near vision (Fig 9-1).

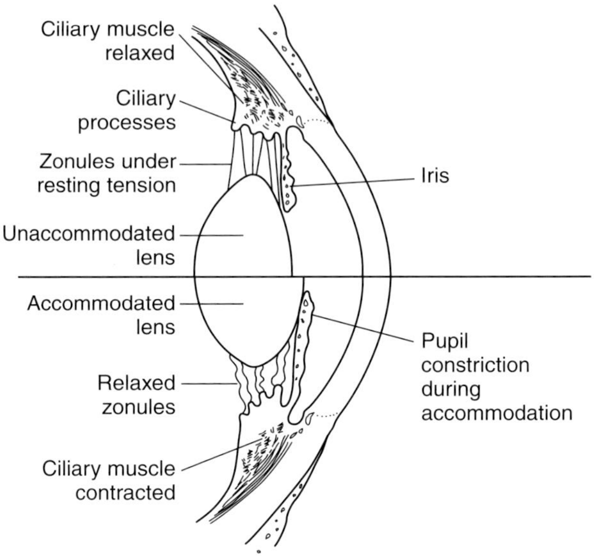

Figure 9-1 In the Helmholtz theory of accommodation, contraction of the ciliary muscle leads to a relaxation of the zonular fibers. The reduced zonular tension allows the elastic capsule of the lens to contract, causing an increase in the anterior and posterior lens curvature. *(Illustration by Jeanne Koelling.)*

When the accommodative effort ceases, the ciliary muscle relaxes and the zonular tension on the lens equator rises to its resting state. This increased tension on the lens equator causes a flattening of the lens, a decrease in the curvature of the anterior and posterior lens surfaces, and a decrease in the dioptric power of the unaccommodated eye.

In the Helmholtz theory, the equatorial edge of the lens moves away from the sclera during accommodation and toward the sclera when accommodation ends. In this theory, all zonular fibers are relaxed during accommodation and all are under tension when the accommodative effort ends. According to Helmholtz, presbyopia results from the loss of lens elasticity with age. When the zonules are relaxed, the lens does not change its shape to the same degree as the young lens; therefore, presbyopia is an aging process that can only be reversed by changing the elasticity of the lens or its capsule.

Southall JPC, ed. *Helmholtz's Treatise on Physiological Optics*. Translated from the 3rd German ed. New York: Dover Publications; 1962.

Diametrically opposed to Helmholtz is the Schachar theory of accommodation. Schachar suggests that during accommodation, ciliary muscle contraction leads to a selective increase in equatorial zonular tension—rather than to the uniform decrease (anterior, equatorial, and posterior) proposed by the Helmholtz theory—with a subsequent pulling of the equatorial lens outward toward the sclera (Fig 9-2). Schachar postulates that accommodation occurs through the direct effect of zonular tension (as opposed to the passive effect proposed by Helmholtz), causing an increase in lens curvature. In this theory, the loss of accommodation with age is a result of the continued growth of the lens, and thus increasing lens diameter, and a decrease in the lens–ciliary body distance, which results in a loss of zonular tension. Anything that increases resting zonular tension (eg, scleral expansion) should restore accommodation.

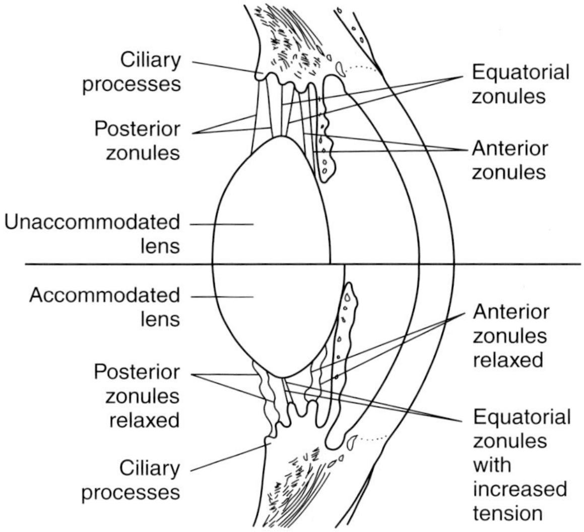

Figure 9-2 Schachar proposes that only the equatorial zonules are under tension during accommodation and that the anterior and posterior zonular fibers serve solely as passive support structures for the lens. *(Illustration by Jeanne Koelling.)*

Schachar proposes that the mechanism for functional lens shape change is equatorial stretching by the zonules; this decreases the peripheral lens volume and increases the central volume, thus producing the central steepening of the anterior central lens capsule (Fig 9-3). During accommodation and ciliary muscle contraction, tension on the equatorial zonular fibers increases, whereas tension on the anterior and posterior zonules is reduced. These actions allow the lens to maintain a stable position at all times, even as it undergoes changes in shape. Schachar suggests that the anterior and posterior zonules serve as passive support structures for the lens, whereas the equatorial zonules are the active components in determining the optical power of the lens.

Schachar RA. Cause and treatment of presbyopia with a method for increasing the amplitude of accommodation. *Ann Ophthalmol.* 1992;24:447, 452.

Evidence from recent studies on both human and nonhuman primates disputes Schachar's theories on accommodation and presbyopia. Investigations in human tissues and with scanning electron microscopy reveal no zonular insertions (equatorial or otherwise) at the iris root or anterior ciliary muscle. Various imaging techniques consistently indicate that the diameter of the crystalline lens *decreases* with accommodation. In vitro laser scanning imaging shows that the crystalline lens does not change focal length when increasing and decreasing radial stretching forces are applied. This runs contrary to Schachar's proposal that the lens remains pliable with age and that presbyopia is due solely to lens growth and crowding that prevents optimum ciliary muscle action.

Glasser A, Kaufman PL. The mechanism of accommodation in primates. *Ophthalmology.* 1999;106:863–872.

A variant of the Schachar theory is one by Strenk and colleagues. Using magnetic resonance imaging studies of the lens, ciliary body, and circumlental space, they have

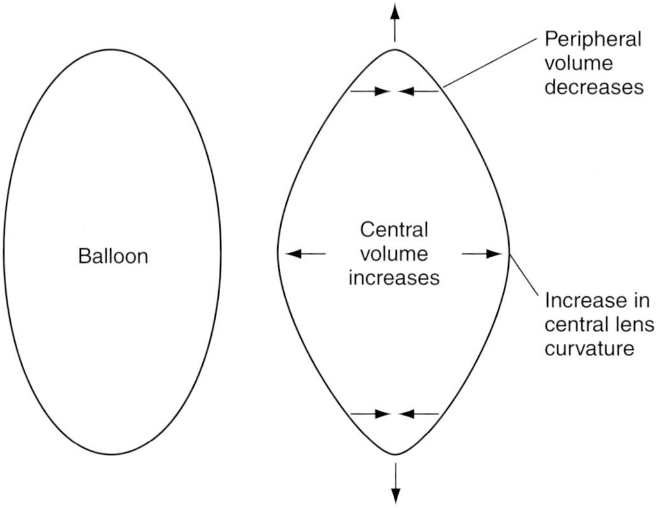

Figure 9-3 Schachar proposes that the increase in equatorial zonular tension causes a decrease in peripheral lens volume and an increase in central lens volume, thus producing an increase in central lens curvature. *(Illustration by Jeanne Koelling.)*

shown that the lens equator remains stable, but the ciliary body moves inward (toward the lens equator) with advancing age and thereby reduces the circumlental space. This evidence lends some support to Shachar's theory that accommodation results from a loss of tension in the zonules, although Strenk has shown that the loss occurs from an enlarging ciliary body.

Strenk SA, Strenk LM, Koretz JF. The mechanism of presbyopia. *Prog Retin Eye Res.* 2005; 24:379–393.

The catenary, or hydraulic support, theory proposed by Coleman and Fish suggests that the lens, zonules, and anterior vitreous form a functional diaphragm between the anterior and posterior chambers of the eye. Contraction of the circular ciliary muscle generates a pressure gradient between the anterior and posterior chambers, causing anterior movement of this lens–zonule diaphragm and, thus, steepening the anterior central lens curvature. Studies done by Coleman with differential IOP transducers in nonhuman primate eyes have revealed a rise in posterior chamber IOP relative to that in the anterior chamber during accommodation. The catenary model shares with the Helmholtz theory the concept that zonular fibers are under tension in the unaccommodated eye and are relaxed in the accommodated state. The lax zonular fibers during accommodation may allow for some of the forward translational movement of the lens during accommodation that is proposed by this theory.

In this model, presbyopia is due to lens volume that increases with age and causes a reduced response of the anterior lens curvature to the posterior chamber pressure gradient generated by ciliary body contraction. Of note, decreased strength/contractility of the ciliary muscle with age is not implicated in this theory.

Coleman DJ, Fish SK. Presbyopia, accommodation, and the mature catenary. *Ophthalmology.* 2001;108:1544–1551.

The premise of "vitreous support" and the lens–zonule diaphragm role in accommodation is important in the theoretical functioning of some of the new IOL models developed to reduce presbyopia, which will be discussed later. None of the 3 theories just discussed fully accounts for all the physiologic and optical events that occur during accommodation. A complete understanding of the process of accommodation and presbyopia remains elusive.

Agarwal A. *Presbyopia: A Surgical Textbook.* Thorofare, NJ: Slack Publishing; 2002.

Nonaccommodative Treatment of Presbyopia

Monovision

Currently in the United States, presbyopia modification in phakic individuals is primarily limited to monovision, in which the refractive power of 1 eye is adjusted to improve near vision (see also Chapter 3). Monovision may be accomplished with contact lenses, LASIK, surface ablation, conductive keratoplasty, or even cataract surgery. The process involves intentionally undercorrecting a myopic patient, overcorrecting a hyperopic patient, or inducing mild myopia in an emmetropic individual. Historically, the term *monovision* was typically applied to patients who wore a distance contact lens in 1 eye and a near contact lens in the other. Often the power difference between the 2 eyes was significant (1.25 to 2.50 D), because the patient always had the option of replacing the near lens with a distance lens when the activity demanded. This obviously is not possible with refractive surgery, so many refractive surgeons routinely target mild myopia (–0.50 to –1.50 D) for the near eye in the presbyopic and peripresbyopic population. The term *modified monovision* is probably more appropriate for this lower level of myopia. Although not affecting accommodative amplitude, this level of myopia is associated with only a mild decrease in distance vision, retention of good stereopsis, and a significant increase in the intermediate zone of functional vision. The intermediate zone is where many activities of daily life occur (eg, looking at a computer screen, store shelves, or a car dashboard). Patients retain good distance vision in their distance eye and experience an increase in near and intermediate vision in their near eye. For many patients, this compromise between good distance vision in both eyes and a loss of near vision versus good distance vision in 1 eye and an increase in near visual function is an attractive alternative to constantly reaching for a pair of reading glasses. Selected patients who expect better near vision may prefer higher amounts of monovision correction (–1.50 to –2.50 D) despite the accompanying decrease in distance vision and stereopsis.

Patient selection

Appropriate patient selection is important in determining the overall success of monovision treatment. The monovision correction can be demonstrated with trial lenses in the examination room, but often a contact lens trial is useful. Patients who are not presbyopic or approaching presbyopia are typically not good candidates for modified monovision. A 25-year-old myopic patient will not appreciate the long-term benefit of mild myopia in 1 eye. Young myopic individuals are usually looking for the best possible distance vision in both eyes.

The best candidates for modified monovision are myopic patients over the age of 40 who, because of their refractive error, retain some useful near vision. This group is able to understand the importance of near vision, and these patients have always experienced adequate near vision simply by removing their glasses. Patients who do not have useful uncorrected near vision preoperatively (myopia >4.50 D, high astigmatism, or contact lens wearers) may be more accepting of the need for reading glasses when their refractive error is treated. In addition, for most patients to function free of spectacles, a minimum of 20/25 or better uncorrected visual acuity (UCVA) is required. Individuals whose correction is high have a decreased likelihood of achieving that level of UCVA. It is typically better to attempt to obtain distance correction in both eyes in order to increase the chance of obtaining adequate distance vision. Finally, most hyperopic patients are typically bothered by their loss of near vision (this is why they seek refractive surgery), and a planned overcorrection in their nondominant eye should be considered.

Many refractive surgeons routinely aim for mild myopia (−0.50 to −0.75 D) in the nondominant eye. Other surgeons may demonstrate monovision with trial lenses or give the patient a trial with contact lenses to ascertain patient acceptance and the degree of near vision desired. Although higher amounts of ametropia (>1.50 D) are not typically used, some patients are willing to accept a decrease in stereopsis and depth perception for the greater improvement in near vision.

In carefully selected patients, monovision has a high degree of acceptance and affords the potential of greater spectacle-free functional vision.

Conductive Keratoplasty

As discussed earlier (see Chapter 7), conductive keratoplasty (CK) is a nonablative, collagen shrinkage procedure approved for the correction of low levels of hyperopia (+0.75 to +3.25 D). Conductive keratoplasty is based on the delivery of radiofrequency energy through a fine conducting tip inserted into the peripheral corneal stroma. The procedure is now FDA approved for the treatment of presbyopia in hyeropic and emmetropic individuals. The treatment does not restore accommodation but instead induces mild myopia (modified monovision) in 1 eye. Relative to the degree of near visual gain, the decrease in distance vision is relatively mild. Initial data reported that 79% of patients could read Jaeger type 2 (J2), 94% could read J3, and 95% maintained >20/25 binocular distance vision. The gain in near vision appears to be greater than expected for the amount of myopia induced and may be caused by the multifocal nature of the post-CK cornea. Conductive keratoplasty is a relatively simple, minimally invasive procedure that spares the central corneal visual axis and has an excellent safety profile. Although it does not increase accommodative amplitude, CK for presbyopia is capable of increasing the range of functional vision in the presbyopic population.

IOL Implants

The IOL options for patients undergoing cataract surgery have increased in recent years. Individuals undergoing cataract surgery can have a traditional monofocal IOL with a refractive target of emmetropia, mild myopia, or monovision (1 eye distance, 1 eye near), or they can choose a multifocal or an accommodating IOL for greater range of focus.

The Array lens (Advanced Medical Optics [AMO], Santa Ana, CA) was the first FDA-approved multifocal IOL. The Array lens is a distance-dominant multifocal lens that simulates accommodation by allowing pseudophakic patients to visualize images at different focal distances without relying on capsular mechanics or ciliary body function. The lens is a zonally progressive, flexible, silicone posterior chamber IOL with 5 concentric zones on its anterior surface. The central 2.1 mm of the optic provides most of the distance refraction, and the surrounding concentric zones alternate between relative distance and near focus, with each zone designed for different lighting conditions and focal distances. It has a 6.0-mm silicone optic and 13-mm-diameter polymethylmethacrylate (PMMA) haptics; the IOL can be placed through a 3.25-mm incision. The aspheric design allows for 100% of the incoming light to be used: 50% for distance, 30% for near, and 20% for intermediate. The Array lens has an effective add of approximately +2.50 D at the corneal plane. Although patients noted loss of contrast sensitivity and had an increased perception of halos with the Array lens as compared with monofocal IOLs, for many, the improved near and distance vision was an acceptable trade-off. In addition, when Array IOLs were placed and tested bilaterally, patients reported that many of the visual phenomena were reduced. In 2005, the FDA approved, and AMO released, an updated multifocal IOL known as the ReZoom lens, which was based on the Array design. The ReZoom lens is a 3-piece acrylic optic, also with 5 refractive zones (Fig 9-4). The first 3 optical zones are blended, and zones 4 and 5 have been modified to reduce the incidence of halos and improve near acuity.

Another multifocal IOL, the AcrySof ReSTOR (Alcon Laboratories, Ft Worth, TX) was also approved by the FDA in 2005. The ReSTOR is either a 1- or a 3-piece foldable diffractive lens that, similar to the other multifocal lenses, simultaneously focuses light from both distance and near targets. The lens, however, is apodized and gradually tapers its diffractive step heights to allow an even distribution of light, which theoretically makes for a smoother transition among images from distance, intermediate, and near targets. The lens also distributes the appropriate amount of light to near and distant focal points, independent of the lighting situation. To do this, the ReSTOR IOL gradually reduces and

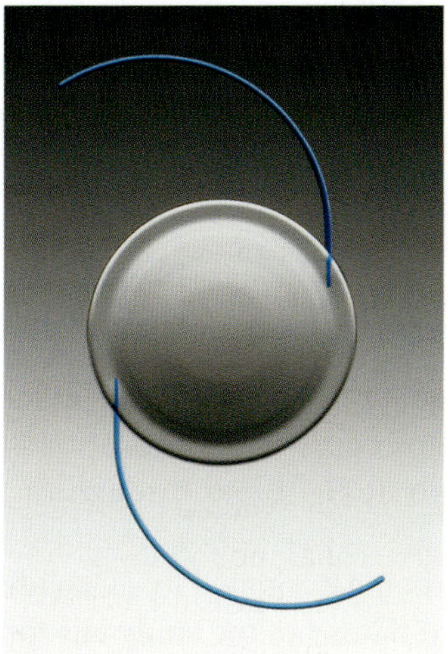

Figure 9-4 AMO ReZoom multifocal IOL showing the 5 concentric refractive zones. *(Courtesy of AMO.)*

blends the step heights of its 3.6-mm diffractive area from 1.3 μm centrally to 0.2 μm peripherally. The peripheral lens area outside the diffractive zone is used mainly for distance vision, whereas the central area of the lens is mainly for near work. Depending on pupil size, there is a loss of 6%–19% of light, which can adversely affect contrast sensitivity, especially in patients with smaller pupils.

Some preliminary studies indicate that freedom from reading glasses may be better achieved with a ReSTOR in 1 eye and a ReZoom in the fellow eye, which allows improved focus at near and intermediate distances, respectively.

Capsular opacification is of greater concern with multifocal IOLs because minimal peripheral changes in the capsule can cause early deterioration in vision. Although capsular opacification is infrequent, future changes in IOL design (eg, edge design) will attempt to reduce the incidence of lens epithelial migration/ingrowth, with the objective of limiting posterior capsular opacification. The ReZoom lens, for example, now has a square posterior edge that improves posterior capsular contact and reduces the incidence of posterior capsular opacities.

Multifocal IOLs cause an increased incidence of glare and halos around lights at night, although the newer multifocal IOLs incorporate technology that significantly reduces such light phenomena. In addition, most of these symptoms are found to decrease over time, and they can be further reduced when nighttime driving glasses are used or topical brimonidine drops are instilled to reduce scotopic pupil size (see also Chapter 8). Nevertheless, careful selection of motivated, well-informed patients is prudent.

Custom or Multifocal Ablations

The approach used with the excimer laser to treat presbyopia is to create a multifocal cornea rather than to restore accommodation. This is the same approach used with CK and corneal inlays (see the following section). The potential for improving near vision without significantly compromising distance vision was investigated after it was noted that, following myopic and hyperopic surface ablation or LASIK, the uncorrected near vision of many patients improved more than was expected. Hyperopic ablations induce central steepening in a relatively small optical zone and have a large peripheral blend zone (Fig 9-5).

Attempts to correct both distance and near vision use a variation of this multifocal approach. A number of ablation patterns are being evaluated and include the following:

- a small central steep zone, where the central portion of the cornea is used for near and the midperiphery is used for distance
- an inferior near-zone ablation pattern
- an inferiorly decentered hyperopic ablation
- a central distance ablation with an intermediate/near midperipheral ablation

Some of these patterns rely on simultaneous vision (similar to patterns used by some bifocal contact lenses or the Array IOL); others use the pupil constriction that occurs with the near reflex (accommodative convergence) to concentrate light rays through the steeper central ablation.

The safety and efficacy of multifocal ablations is being evaluated in a Canadian multicenter trial at the University of Ottawa Eye Institute. Thus far, the study has found that multifocal correction for presbyopia has not compromised the accuracy of distance cor-

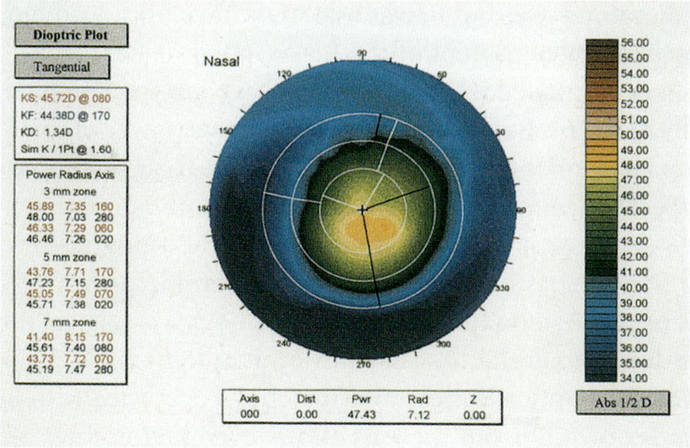

Figure 9-5 Multifocal ablation. Corneal topographic map showing a multifocal pattern after hyperopic LASIK in a 62-year-old with preoperative hyperopia of +4.00. Postoperatively, the UCVA at distance is $20/25^{-2}$ and the UCVA at near is J1. Manifest refraction of –0.25 +0.75 × 20 yields 20/20. Corneal topography demonstrates central hyperopic ablation *(green)* with relative steepening in the lower portion of the pupillary axis *(orange)*, which provides the near add for reading vision. *(Courtesy of Jayne S. Weiss, MD.)*

rection. According to preliminary results, at 12 months, uncorrected distance vision was 20/20 or better in 57% and 20/40 or better in 98% and near vision was J1 in 67% and J5 in 97% of the 75 eyes of 47 patients studied. Contrast sensitivity was initially reduced postoperatively but returned to baseline in the 50- to 75-year age group.

Some investigators approach multifocal ablation for presbyopia by correcting the central optical zone for distance and the successive concentric zones for intermediate and near. These ablations use a 10-mm optical zone under a very large flap but supposedly result in a final overall aspheric curvature to the cornea.

Although the data are limited, the excimer laser offers some potential advantages over other methods for managing presbyopia. The procedure is less invasive than scleral expansion or an accommodating IOL, although more invasive than a corneal inlay, which can be removed. It can concomitantly correct the near and distance refractive error. Continued improvement of the multifocal pattern, using computer modeling that considers a patient's pupil size, treatment diameter, and corneal shape, along with data from long-term studies, may further improve this treatment.

Corneal Inlays

Originally, experimental intracorneal lenses were placed deep in the stroma. These lenses relied on the intrinsic refractive power of the insert for their effect, as there was little or no change in the anterior corneal curvature. The lenses had a high index of refraction and were made of materials such as polysulfone. These materials, however, were not permeable to water and metabolites, and opacification and corneal necrosis were major complications. (See also Chapter 5, under Alloplastic Corneal Inlays.)

The further development of intracorneal lenses has depended on the use of permeable polymer materials that are able to transmit both fluid and nutrients from the aqueous through the endothelium and corneal stroma to the epithelium. Hydrogels have a long history of ophthalmic use, and newer materials have improved biocompatibility and optical properties. The water content of the newer polymers exceeds 70%, so clarity and permeability are both improved. Hydrogel inlays have a refractive index nearly identical to that of the cornea (1.376). Because they lack refractive power of their own, these lenses rely on altering the anterior corneal curvature to induce their refractive effect. Long-term animal studies have confirmed the safety and biocompatibility of this material, and early human trials have demonstrated stable induced corneal topographic changes, although inlay decentrations and intrastromal deposits remain problematic.

The PresbyLens (ReVision Optics, Lake Forest, CA) is a corneal inlay constructed of a microporous hydrogel material that has physical and chemical properties that mimic those of the cornea. It is optically clear and matches the cornea with 78% water content and a refractive index of 1.376, but the lens allows even higher rates of fluid and glucose diffusion. Central thickness depends on the inlay power and type, but all lenses have an edge of about 5.0 μm. The inlay is currently undergoing FDA clinical trials.

Although intracorneal lens implants are currently used principally to correct hyperopia, multifocal versions are in development that offer hope for presbyopia correction. Most of the newer implants are placed in the corneal stroma beneath a planar microkeratome flap (similar to that made for LASIK). The implant acts as a refractive prosthesis and yields a refractive power change to the eye by changing the anterior curvature of the cornea. The degree of curvature change, and thus the refractive power, is partly dependent on the predictability of the flap dimensions (both diameter and thickness).

Another approach being used to obtain a multifocal or bifocal effect with the intracorneal inlay lens is the center-surround or bull's-eye optic. The patient uses the outer portion of the pupillary area for distance vision and a small, round, central optical area for near vision. This concentric design has been used previously in contact lenses and IOLs. The AcuFocus ACI 7000 (AcuFocus, Irvine, California) corneal inlay is a fenestrated 10-μm-thick disk with a clear central zone and opaque peripheral ring. The disk is inserted into the cornea under a LASIK flap. It is made of an opaque biocompatible polymer. When focusing in the distance, the patient's pupil dilates beyond the borders of the inlay to permit the entry of more peripheral light rays. At near, the device is able to increase depth of field as the fenestrations effectively reduce pupillary size, and any unfocused light that may interfere with near vision is eliminated. Preliminary monocular 9-month data in 57 patients show mean uncorrected distance vision of 20/20 and uncorrected near vision of J1+.

A key advantage with all corneal inlays is that essentially no tissue is removed to obtain the refractive correction. Because the implants are removable, the effect is theoretically reversible or modifiable if results are less than satisfactory. Because of the small optical zone, however, problems exist with lens centration, lens movement after insertion, and quality of vision.

Accommodative Treatment of Presbyopia

Scleral Surgery

A number of scleral surgical procedures have been evaluated for the reversal of presbyopia. They all share the objective of attempting to increase zonular tension by weakening or altering the sclera over the ciliary body to allow for its passive expansion. Thornton first proposed weakening the sclera by creating 8 or more scleral incisions over the ciliary body (anterior ciliary sclerotomy, or ACS). Results were mixed and any positive effect appeared short-lived, but numerous studies to advance the technique and understand its effect continue. A prospective study of ACS using a 4-incision technique was discontinued because of significant adverse events, including anterior segment ischemia. In 2001, the American Academy of Ophthalmology stated that ACS was ineffective and a potentially dangerous treatment for presbyopia.

Hamilton DR, Davidorf JM, Maloney RK. Anterior ciliary sclerotomy for treatment of presbyopia: a prospective controlled study. *Ophthalmology.* 2002;109:1970–1977.

Another method involves the placement of scleral expansion bands. Although scleral expansion bands have received mixed results with regard to safety, patient satisfaction, and results, clinical trials are ongoing for these devices. PresVIEW scleral expansion bands (Refocus Group, Dallas, TX) are small polymethylmethacrylate (PMMA) bands, 5.5 mm × 1.3 mm, that are placed in scleral tunnels over the ciliary body parallel to the limbus in the 4 oblique quadrants (Fig 9-6). The bands act as stents, pulling on the sclera and actively expanding the space between the ciliary body and the lens equator. This procedure has been shown to temporarily improve near vision in some patients; it has an improved safety profile compared with previous scleral expansion techniques. Phase 3 trials of the implants are ongoing, and preliminary results show that a majority of patients reported their near vision to be better or significantly better than it was before surgery.

A
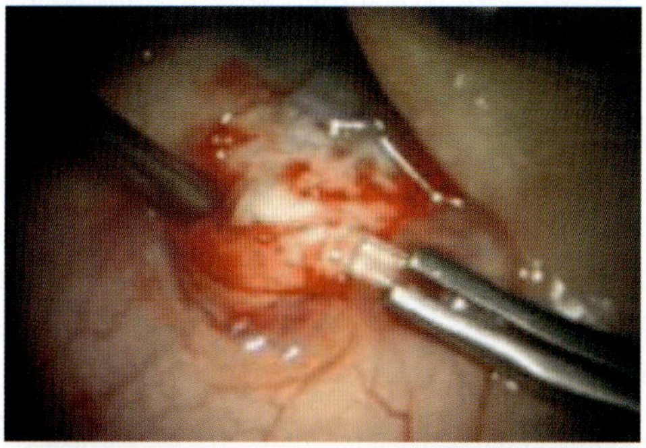

B
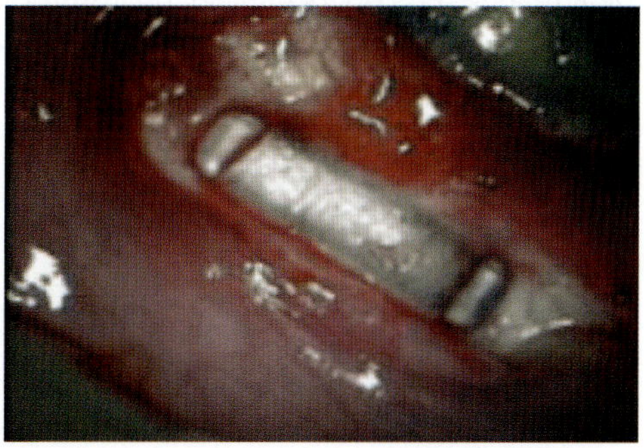

C
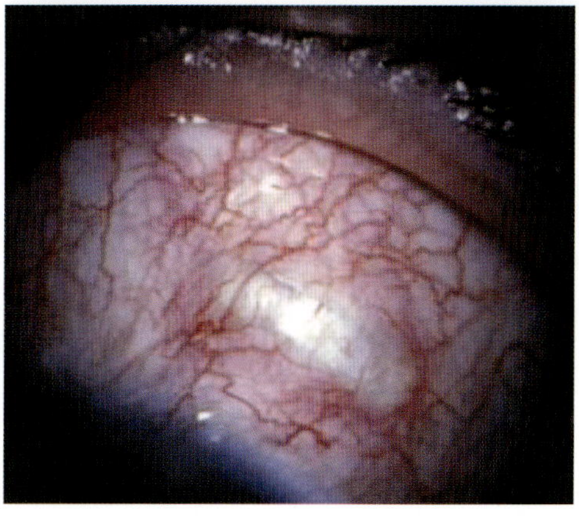

Figure 9-6 A, The scleral expansion band is inserted in a scleral tunnel over the ciliary body parallel to the limbus. **B,** The appearance of the band after placement, prior to conjunctival closure. **C,** The appearance of a well-healed band. *(Courtesy of Refocus Group.)*

Other efforts at scleral expansion have been attempted with an erbium:YAG infrared laser (OptiVision, SurgiLight, Orlando, FL). Using a fiberoptic handpiece, the surgeon makes 4 incisions (400–500 µm) radially in the oblique quadrants over the ciliary body at a depth of 80% of scleral thickness.

Despite some encouraging results in recent FDA trials, it is still unclear whether any of these "expansion" procedures produce real and lasting results with an acceptable safety profile. Specifically, any temporal improvement in near vision has not been shown to result from a restoration of true accommodation of the lens. Although the basis for the surgical procedures may be dubious, it does not necessarily follow that the surgery is ineffective. Indeed, some type of "pseudoaccommodation" may be responsible. Multiple alternative theories have been suggested for the improvement in near acuity. It has been suggested, for example, that scleral expansion surgery may produce anterior displacement of the crystalline lens with myopic shift and, as a result, improve near vision.

Mathews S. Scleral expansion surgery does not restore accommodation in human presbyopia. *Ophthalmology*. 1999;106:873–877.

Further investigations are needed to determine the clinical applications of scleral expansion (including a possible reduction of IOP in glaucoma patients).

Accommodating IOLs

Although scleral expansion surgery is designed for phakic patients, the accommodating IOL attempts to restore a significant amount of true accommodation to a patient with surgically induced pseudophakia. Accommodating IOLs were designed after it was observed that some patients, when fitted with a silicone-plate IOL, reported a return of their near vision beyond what would be expected from their refractive result. Investigations found that during ciliary muscle contraction, a forward displacement of the IOL led to an increase in the effective power of the IOL and an increase in near vision. (Anterior chamber IOLs have lower A-constants than posterior chamber IOLs for the same reason.) Studies have questioned the amplitude of true accommodation that can be expected based solely on anterior displacement of the IOL optic. Other factors, such as pupil size, with-the-rule astigmatism, and mild myopia, may also contribute to unaided near visual acuity.

Findl O, Kiss B, Petternel V, et al. Intraocular lens movement caused by ciliary muscle contraction. *J Cataract Refract Surg*. 2003;29:669–676.

Langenbucher A, Huber S, Nguyen NX, Seitz B, Gusek-Schneider GC, Kuchle M. Measurement of accommodation after implantation of an accommodating posterior chamber intraocular lens. *J Cataract Refract Surg*. 2003;29:677–685.

An IOL that uses this accommodative approach is the Crystalens (Eyeonics, Aliso Viejo, CA). The Crystalens is a modified silicone, plate-haptic lens. The lens has a biconvex optic that is 4.5 or 5.0 mm in diameter. It is constructed with a hinge at the junction of the haptic and optic to facilitate forward movement of the optic. The Crystalens is approved by the FDA to improve near, intermediate, and distance vision after cataract extraction (Fig 9-7).

The Crystalens was designed to maximize its anterior movement. Although the exact cause of the movement is unclear, it appears to be a combination of posterior chamber pressure on the back surface of the IOL and ciliary body pressure on the IOL haptics that

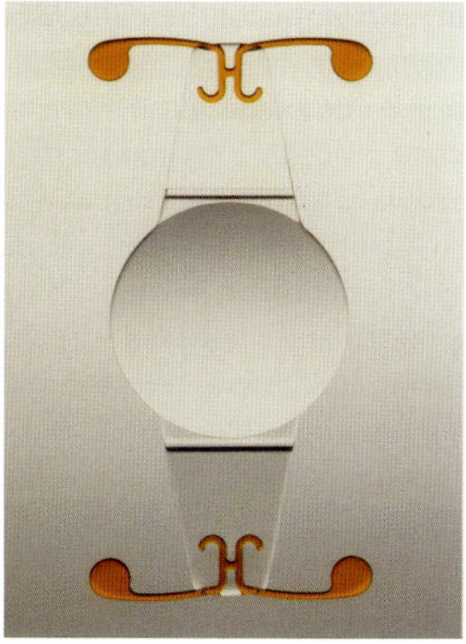

Figure 9-7 The Crystalens is designed with a flexible hinge in the haptic at the proximal end and a polyamide foot plate at the distal end. The foot plate functions to maximize contact with the capsule and ciliary body, and the hinge transfers the horizontal force into an anteroposterior movement of the optic. *(Courtesy of Eyeonics.)*

vaults the optic forward. A forward movement of the entire ciliary body may also carry the IOL anteriorly. The Crystalens, made of third-generation silicone, is designed with grooved "hinges" within the optic plate and haptics. The use of atropine drops postoperatively facilitates the posterior seating of the IOL in the capsular bag until fibrosis occurs. Oversized polyamide haptics are attached to the ends of the plate lens to prevent rotation of the IOL in the bag and to maintain constant contact with the ciliary body. As the ciliary body contracts, it thickens, causing increased pressure on the polyamide haptics. The compression between the haptics causes the IOL to bow forward. The exaggerated anterior displacement is postulated to result in an effective increase in optical power and near vision. Although this mechanism was not definitively proven in clinical trials, an average of 1.00 D of power was generated at near.

The FDA clinical trials investigated the 4.5-mm Crystalens for primary implantation at the time of cataract surgery. Because the accommodative effect depends on IOL placement posterior to an intact capsulorrhexis, this IOL is not indicated for secondary IOL placement. At 1 year, 100% of patients were reading J3 or better, and 50.4% of patients were reading J1 or better. At 3 years, the number of patients reading J1 increased to 67.7% and the number reading J3 were stable. Most patients had excellent uncorrected distance and intermediate vision at 1 and 3 years. In addition, 98.4% of cataract patients implanted with Crystalens in both eyes could pass a driver's test without glasses, and 98.4% of Crystalens cataract surgery patients could see well enough to read the newspaper and the phone book without glasses.

Questions still remain about the long-term accommodative effect of the Crystalens and whether the movement of this IOL contributes significantly to a patient's reading ability. In laboratory experiments, the Crystalens was flexed 1 million times without mechanical failure. It is not known how many times it flexes in a patient's eye on a yearly basis or whether there is a risk of mechanical failure of the haptics in the patient's lifetime.

An important observation on the preliminary success of accommodating IOLs in restoring accommodative facility in older patients is the apparent maintenance of effective ciliary muscle function despite years without a "normal" accommodative effort. The impact of long-term capsular fibrosis on the dynamic functioning of these IOL designs is not yet known.

Besides holding promise for cataract patients, the accommodating IOL may allow for greater acceptance of clear lens extraction as a refractive procedure for moderate to high hyperopia. Although clear lens extraction for high myopia is associated with a number of serious potential complications, many of these are infrequently seen in hyperopic patients. Nevertheless, the loss of accommodation in a hyperopic patient who normally has a large accommodative amplitude for his or her age is a substantial and often undesirable surgical trade-off in clear lens extraction. The accommodating IOL offers, at least in part, the promise for the pseudophakic patient of emmetropia without presbyopia.

Other IOL Innovations on the Horizon

The Crystalens is thought to work via lens effectivity secondary to a change in the position of the optic in the eye. Thus, its accommodative range is limited. A number of other experimental lenses are undergoing clinical investigation. The Synchrony (Visiogen, Irvine, CA) is a dual-optic accommodating IOL that has already been approved for use in Europe and has entered phase 3 trials in the United States. The SmartLens (Medennium, Irvine, CA) is made from a thermoplastic acrylic gel that can be customized to any size, shape, or power specified by the physician. The Light Adjustable Lens (LAL; Calhoun Vision, Pasadena, CA) is made from a macromer silicone matrix with smaller, embedded photosensitive molecules that will allow for postoperative customization of the power via tunable ultraviolet light treatment. Finally, flexible polymers are being designed for injection into a nearly intact capsular bag, after extraction of the crystalline lens through a tiny, laterally placed capsulorrhexis. Other lenses being developed appear to have much greater accommodative capacity. One such lens is the NuLens Accommodating IOL (NuLens, Herzliya Pituach, Israel). The NuLens changes its power rather than changing its position in the eye. It incorporates a small chamber of silicone gel and a posterior piston with an aperture. The future appears bright, but only time will tell which of these innovations will be successful in clinical practice.

PART III

Refractive Surgery in the Setting of Other Conditions

CHAPTER **10**

Refractive Surgery in Ocular and Systemic Disease

Introduction

Although many ophthalmologists viewed the field of refractive surgery with skepticism only a few decades ago, refractive surgery is now highly accepted and much practiced. As refractive surgery has evolved from the controversial to the routine, the spectrum of indications has enlarged, and an increasing proportion of patients who seek refractive surgery have other known ocular or systemic diseases.

During this period, refractive surgeons have discovered that many of the patients excluded from original FDA clinical trials can be successfully treated with refractive surgery, and some former absolute contraindications have changed to relative contraindications. In other cases, it may not be clear whether refractive surgery poses an unacceptable risk.

The surgeon must always remember that refractive surgery is elective and does involve risks. Refractive surgery is typically contraindicated in the monocular patient; the adverse effect of even small risks is markedly magnified in this patient because any postoperative visual loss may prove devastating.

However, the envelope is constantly being pushed, and refractive surgery is successfully being performed now in patients who were previously considered poor candidates. Some of the categories of patients with relative contraindications to refractive surgery are addressed in the following sections. With increased experience, LASIK and surface ablation have been performed safely and effectively in many patients with ocular or systemic diseases.

As with other surgeries, ophthalmologists should never go beyond their comfort zone when performing refractive surgery. The surgeon may want to obtain a second opinion for a difficult case or refer some patients to more experienced colleagues. In the higher-risk patient, unilateral surgery may offer the advantage of providing assurance that 1 eye is doing well before surgery is performed on the second eye. In addition, when deciding whether a patient with connective tissue disease or immunosuppression is an appropriate candidate for refractive surgery, the surgeon may find that consultation with the patient's primary physician offers important information about the patient's systemic health. The process of consent should be altered not only to inform the patient but also to document the patient's understanding of the additional risks and limitations of postoperative results due to any associated ocular or systemic diseases. The refractive surgeon may want to supplement the standard written consent, highlighting specific concerns, to help ensure and document that the patient understands these additional risks. The ophthalmologist should assiduously avoid the high-risk refractive surgery patient who volunteers to sign any preoperative consent because "I know these complications won't happen to me." This patient has not heard or understood the informed consent.

Preferred Practice Patterns Committee, Refractive Errors Panel. *Refractive Errors and Refractive Surgery*. Preferred Practice Pattern. San Francisco: American Academy of Ophthalmology; 2007.

Ocular Conditions

Dry Eye

Essentially all patients experience at least a transient dry eye following LASIK and surface ablation. Dry eye after LASIK is the most common side effect of refractive surgery. Corneal nerves are severed when the flap is made, and the cornea overlying the flap is significantly anesthetic for 3 to 6 months. As a result, most patients experience a decrease in tear production. Patients who had dry eyes before surgery or whose eyes were marginally compensated before surgery will have the most severe symptoms. In addition, most patients with post-LASIK and surface ablation dry eye will find the tear film and ocular surface disrupted and will often complain of fluctuating visual acuity between blinks and at different times of the day. Fortunately, the symptoms of the great majority of these patients resolve 3 to 6 months following surgery. To optimize outcomes, it is imperative that dry-eye disease be diagnosed and treated before surgery.

Several steps may be taken to reduce the incidence of dry-eye symptoms following refractive surgery. One of the most important is to screen patients more carefully before surgery. Many patients seeking refractive surgery are actually dry-eye patients who are contact lens–intolerant. Because their pre-existing dry-eye syndrome causes these patients to be uncomfortable wearing contact lenses, they often turn to refractive surgery for visual rehabilitation. Any mention of contact lens intolerance during the course of the patient history should strongly suggest the possibility of underlying dry eye.

Refractive surgery may be problematic in dry-eye patients because a normal tear-film layer is important to the healing of the corneal stroma and epithelium. Epidermal growth factor, vitamin A, and IgA in the tears help prevent postoperative infection and help potentiate wound healing. Consequently, severe dry-eye syndrome was previously thought to be a relative contraindication to refractive surgery.

However, in a series of 543 eyes of 290 patients after LASIK, no significant differences were found in uncorrected visual acuity (UCVA) or best-corrected visual acuity (BCVA) among eyes with or without preoperative dry eye. There was no increased incidence of epithelial defects in the patients with preoperative dry eye. The dry-eye group did demonstrate a slower recovery of corneal sensation, more vital staining of the ocular surface, lower tear production, and more severe dry-eye symptoms until 1 year after LASIK. In patients with collagen-vascular disease that was well controlled, LASIK was shown to be an effective treatment option.

Any refractive surgery candidate with signs or symptoms of dry eyes should be thoroughly evaluated. Patient history should include questions about collagen-vascular diseases and conjunctival cicatrizing disorders, because these are relative contraindications to any refractive procedure and would need to be addressed prior to any surgical consideration (see Chapter 3).

External examination should include evaluation of eyelid closure for such conditions as incomplete blink, lagophthalmos, entropion, ectropion, or eyelid notching. On slit-lamp examination, notation should be made of blepharitis, meibomitis, and tear film quantity and quality. Ancillary testing for dry eyes, such as Schirmer testing, tear break-up time, fluorescein corneal staining, and lissamine green or rose bengal conjunctival staining can be performed.

Preferred Practice Patterns Committee, Cornea/External Disease Panel. *Dry Eye Syndrome.* Preferred Practice Pattern. San Francisco: American Academy of Ophthalmology; 2003.

If collagen-vascular diseases or cicatrizing diseases are suspected, appropriate referral or laboratory testing should be performed to rule out these conditions before refractive surgery is considered. Preexisting abnormalities should be treated, and topical tear replacement and/or punctal occlusion can be performed. If appropriate, a preoperative course of topical anti-inflammatories such as topical corticosteroids or cyclosporine may be given. Topical cyclosporine has been shown to improve dry-eye and refractive outcomes in dry-eye patients undergoing LASIK and PRK. Blepharitis and/or meibomitis should be treated. Flaxseed and fish oils work together synergistically to help dry eye in some patients as well.

Although excimer laser ablation may be performed in selected patients with dry eye, these patients must be cautioned about the increased risk of their dry eye becoming worse postoperatively, which may result in additional discomfort and/or visual decrease. The worsening is typically temporary but may be permanent. Proper ocular surface management by means of topical tear replacement therapy, topical medications, and/or punctal occlusion must be provided in the perioperative and postoperative periods.

Salib GM, McDonald MB, Smolek M. Safety and efficacy of cyclosporine 0.05% drops versus unpreserved artificial tears in dry-eye patients having laser in situ keratomileusis. *J Cataract Refract Surg.* 2006;32:772–778.

Smith RJ, Maloney RK. Laser in situ keratomileusis in patients with autoimmune diseases. *J Cataract Refract Surg.* 2006;32:1292–1295.

Toda I, Asano-Kato N, Hori-Komai Y, Tsubota K. Laser-assisted in situ keratomileusis for patients with dry eye. *Arch Ophthalmol.* 2002;120:1024–1028.

Toda I, Yagi Y, Hata S, Itoh S, Tsubota K. Excimer laser photorefractive keratectomy for patients with contact lens intolerance caused by dry eye. *Br J Ophthalmol.* 1996;80:604–609.

Herpesvirus

Many surgeons avoid laser vision correction in patients with a history of herpes simplex virus (HSV) keratitis because of concern that the ultraviolet light exposure from the excimer laser may increase viral shedding and recurrence. Although there is insufficient evidence to determine conclusively whether surface ablation or LASIK increases the risk of recurrence in a patient with prior HSV keratitis, there are many case reports of such in the literature. Because recurrences have taken place months after excimer laser treatment, some authors have concluded that the recurrence simply reflects the natural course of the disease and not reactivation due to excimer laser ablation. Others, however, have postulated that trauma from the lamellar dissection or exposure to the excimer laser reactivates the virus and causes recurrent keratitis. There have also been several published case reports of patients with a history of oral HSV infection and without preexisting corneal disease who developed HSV keratitis after excimer ablation, including one that occurred on the first postoperative day, suggesting that caution should also be exercised in individuals with a history of systemic HSV infection.

The role of excimer laser ablation in inciting recurrence of HSV keratitis has been investigated in the laboratory. Rabbits infected with HSV type 1 had viral reactivation after exposure of the corneal stroma to 193 nm ultraviolet radiation during PRK and after LASIK. Pretreatment with systemic valacyclovir prior to laser treatment decreased the rate of recurrence in the rabbit model.

Reactivation of HSV keratitis has been reported in humans after radial keratotomy (RK), phototherapeutic keratectomy (PTK), PRK, and LASIK. Fagerholm and colleagues reported a 25% incidence of postoperative HSV keratitis in the 17 months after PTK for surface irregularities from prior HSV infections, compared with an 18% recurrence rate in the same time period prior to PTK. They concluded that the procedure does not seem to significantly increase the incidence of recurrences.

A retrospective review of 13,200 PRK-treated eyes with no history of corneal HSV revealed a 0.14% incidence of HSV keratitis. Of these cases, 16.5% occurred within 10 days of the procedure, which the authors postulated could indicate a direct effect of the excimer ultraviolet laser. In 78%, HSV keratitis occurred within 15 weeks, which could be related to the corticosteroid therapy.

Corneal perforation after LASIK has been reported in a patient who had a prior penetrating keratoplasty (PKP) for herpetic disease with resultant high myopia and astigmatism. The HSV keratitis recurred 10 days after the LASIK, with corneal thinning and subsequent perforation.

Reactivation of herpes zoster ophthalmicus (HZO) has also been reported after LASIK, but after topical and oral antiviral treatment, recovery of vision was excellent. Anecdotal reports exist of flap interface inflammation, resembling diffuse lamellar keratitis, after LASIK in the setting of herpes simplex or zoster keratitis. In these cases, topical corticosteroids may also be required.

Because of the potential for visual loss from herpetic recurrence, some refractive surgeons consider prior herpetic keratitis a contraindication to refractive surgery. Caution should be exercised in making the decision to perform surface ablation, PTK, or LASIK in a patient with a history of prior ocular herpetic infection. Patients with pronounced corneal hypoesthesia or anesthesia, vascularization, thinning and scarring, and/or recent herpetic attacks should not be considered candidates for refractive surgery.

Some surgeons will consider LASIK in a patient with a past history of HSV keratitis who has not had any recent recurrences and who has good corneal sensation, minimal to no corneal vascularization or scarring, and normal BCVA. Preoperative and postoperative prophylaxis with systemic and/or topical antivirals should be strongly considered. Any patient with a history of herpes simplex or zoster keratitis must be counseled about the continued risk of recurrence and its concomitant potential for visual loss after excimer laser vision correction.

Asbell PA. Valacyclovir for the prevention of recurrent herpes simplex virus eye disease after excimer laser photokeratectomy. *Trans Am Ophthalmol Soc.* 2000;98:285–303.

Fagerholm P, Ohman L, Orndahl M. Phototherapeutic keratectomy in herpes simplex keratitis: clinical results in 20 patients. *Acta Ophthalmol.* 1994;72:457–460.

Nagy ZZ, Keleman E, Kovacs A. Herpes simplex keratitis after photorefractive keratectomy. *J Cataract Refract Surg.* 2003;29:222–223.

Keratoconus

Keratoconus is a contraindication to LASIK and surface ablation. Performance of LASIK may result in loss of BCVA and may increase the need for corneal transplantation in such cases, as creation of the flap and removal of corneal tissue significantly increase the risk of progressive ectasia, even if the keratoconus was stable prior to treatment. Although different stages of keratoconus can be diagnosed by slit-lamp examination, more sensitive analyses using corneal topography and corneal pachymetry can reveal findings ranging from clearly normal to clearly pathologic. No specific agreed-upon test or measurement is diagnostic of a corneal ectatic disorder, but both of these diagnostic tests should be part of the evaluation because subtle corneal thinning or curvature changes can be overlooked on slit-lamp evaluation.

The existing literature on ectasia and longitudinal studies of the fellow eye of unilateral keratoconus patients indicate that asymmetric inferior corneal steepening or asymmetric bowtie topographic patterns with skewed steep radial axes above and below the horizontal meridian (Fig 10-1) are risk factors for progression to keratoconus and post-LASIK ectasia. LASIK should not be considered in such patients using current technology. Patients with an inferior "crab claw" pattern accompanied by central flattening are at risk to develop pellucid marginal degeneration, even if there are no clinical signs of it (Fig 10-2). This pattern should be designated "pellucid suspect," and LASIK should be avoided in eyes exhibiting this topographic pattern. Global pachymetry measurements may be important

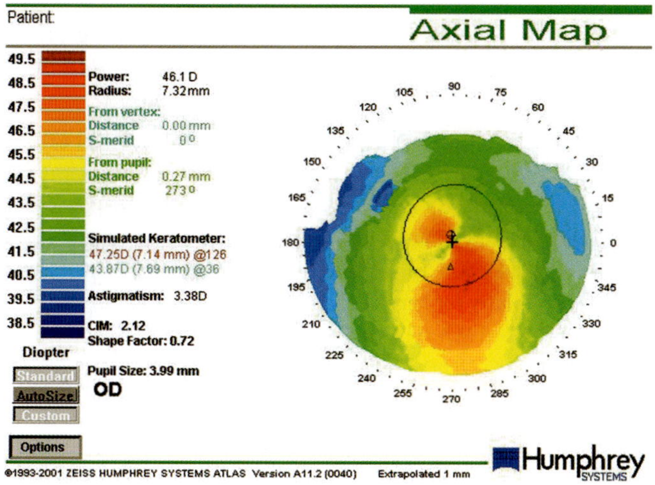

Figure 10-1 Forme fruste keratoconus with skew deviation. *(Courtesy of Eric D. Donnenfeld, MD.)*

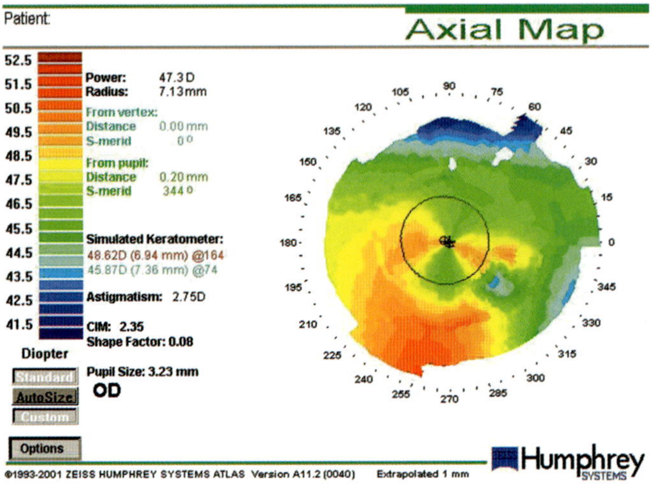

Figure 10-2 Early pellucid marginal degeneration with crab claw appearance. *(Courtesy of Eric D. Donnenfeld, MD.)*

in helping to rule out forme fruste keratoconus. Posterior curvature evaluation with new corneal imaging technology may also prove to be of significant importance.

Often, the refractive surgeon is the first physician to inform a refractive surgery candidate that she or he has forme fruste keratoconus. The patient may have excellent vision with glasses or contact lenses and may be seeking the convenience of a more permanent correction through LASIK. Often the patient is shocked to learn about an eye disease that contraindicates refractive surgery. It is important that the ophthalmologist clearly convey that refractive surgery should not be performed because of the potential for unpredictable results and loss of vision. Otherwise, some patients may be tempted to seek out another refractive surgeon in the hope of having surgery performed.

Intrastromal corneal ring segments (eg, Intacs) have been FDA approved for keratoconus (see Chapter 5). Corneal collagen cross-linking with riboflavin and ultraviolet A light exposure shows promising early results and may prove to be effective in preventing and treating corneal ectasia.

Binder PS, Lindstrom RL, Stulting RD, et al. Keratoconus and corneal ectasia after LASIK. *J Cataract Refract Surg.* 2005;31:2035–2038.

Chan CC, Sharma M, Boxer Wachler BS. Effect of inferior segment Intacs with and without corneal C3-R on keratoconus. *J Cataract Refract Surg.* 2007;33:75–80.

Kirkness CM, Ficker LA, Steele AD, Rice NS. Refractive surgery for graft-induced astigmatism after penetrating keratoplasty for keratoconus. *Ophthalmology.* 1991;98:1786–1792.

Randleman JB, Russell B, Ward MA, Thompson KP, Stulting RD. Risk factors and prognosis for corneal ectasia after LASIK. *Ophthalmology.* 2003;110:267–275.

Post–Penetrating Keratoplasty

Dramatic improvements in microsurgical techniques have resulted in penetrating keratoplasty becoming a more common and successful procedure. Unfortunately, postoperative visual rehabilitation remains challenging. Most patients will not tolerate more than 3.0 D of anisometropia, due to image size disparity or astigmatism of greater than 1.5–3.0 D. Refractive unpredictability following PKP is extremely common due to the inherent imprecision of the operation, with most series documenting mean cylinders of 4.0–5.0 D and significant anisometropia. Irregular astigmatism can be corrected only with gas-permeable contact lenses. Between 10% and 30% of patients require contact lens correction after PKP. However, contact lens fitting may not be possible because of the abnormal corneal curvature.

Surgical alternatives for the correction of post-PKP astigmatism include corneal relaxing incisions, compression sutures, and wedge resections. In a series of 201 corneal transplants for keratoconus, 18% of patients required refractive surgery for the correction of astigmatism. These procedures can significantly decrease corneal cylinder and are highly effective. However, they have minimal effect on spherical equivalent. In addition, they can be unpredictable and may destabilize the graft–host wound.

Pseudophakic patients with significant anisometropia can consider an intraocular lens (IOL) exchange or a piggyback IOL; new options include toric IOLs. Unfortunately, these patients have already often undergone a significant number of intraocular procedures. This alternative requires another such procedure, which increases the risk of endothelial decompensation, glaucoma, and cystoid macular edema and may incite a graft rejection.

Given the success of the excimer laser in treating myopia and astigmatism, photorefractive keratectomy (PRK) has been studied and used to treat post-PKP refractive errors. However, the use of PRK in post-PKP patients is less predictable and less effective than it is for naturally occurring astigmatism and myopia. PRK has the disadvantages associated with epithelial removal in a corneal transplant and the potential for corneal haze when high refractive errors are treated. With increased use of prophylactic mitomycin C, PRK may become a more common treatment option for refractive errors following PKP.

LASIK following PKP is subject to the same constraints as conventional LASIK (Fig 10-3). Monocular patients or patients with limited visual potential in the fellow eye are not good candidates. In addition, patients with wound-healing disorders, significant

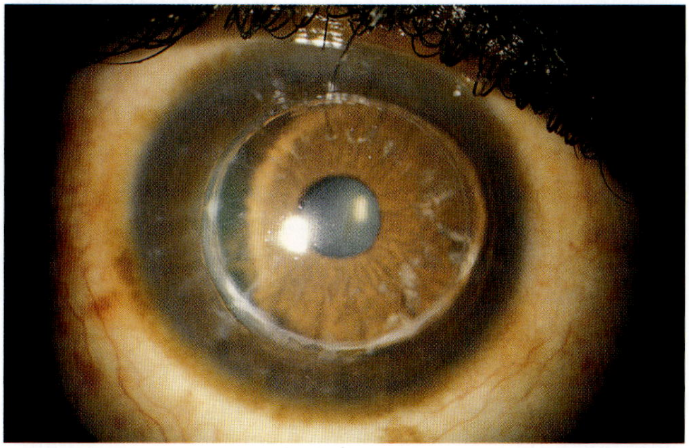

Figure 10-3 A LASIK flap in a patient who had previously undergone PKP for keratoconus. Pre-LASIK manifest refraction −9.00 +6.00 × 85 20/25; pre-LASIK UCVA 20/400; post-LASIK manifest refraction −2.50 +1.25 × 25 20/20^{-2}; post-LASIK UCVA 20/25. *(Courtesy of Jayne S. Weiss, MD.)*

dry-eye syndrome, or a collagen-vascular disease should be offered other options. Finally, patients should have realistic expectations for their rehabilitation following LASIK for PKP. The accuracy of the procedure is not as refined as with conventional LASIK, and patients should expect to require spectacles for residual refractive error. The goal of LASIK following PKP is to return the patient to spectacle-corrected binocularity or enable the patient to wear contact lenses successfully.

It is important to remember that there are no FDA-approved procedures to treat irregular astigmatism. Patients with irregular astigmatism whose corneal curvature prevents contact lens fitting need to be clearly told that the postoperative goal of the laser refractive surgery is solely to allow a comfortable fit with a gas-permeable contact lens.

Preoperative examination of the post-PKP patient who is considering refractive surgery should include investigation of the reasons for the PKP. Herpetic keratitis is a relative contraindication for refractive surgery, as is connective tissue disease. Patients with low endothelial cell counts may be at an increased risk of flap dislocation due to the impairment of the endothelial cell pump function.

Gas-permeable contact lenses should be discontinued for at least 1 month prior to performing refraction. Refraction and corneal topography should be stable, as documented by 2 consecutive readings on separate visits at least 1 month apart. LASIK should not be performed if there are signs of corneal decompensation. Areas of neovascularization should be noted and areas of suspected ectasia should be confirmed with pachymetry to avoid perforation. The surgeon should confirm that there is sufficient scarring/healing in the graft–host interface. Refractive surgery should be avoided if the corneal graft shows evidence of inflammation, diffuse vascularization, ectasia, inadequate healing of the graft–host interface, refractive instability, or signs of rejection or decompensation.

The timing of surgical intervention post-PKP is controversial. All sutures should be removed and refraction should be stable. To avoid wound dehiscence, many surgeons wait at least 1 year after PKP and an additional 4 months after all sutures are removed. An interval of at least 18–24 months after PKP provides sufficient wound healing in most cases.

Because eye alignment under the laser is critical to accurately treating astigmatism, some surgeons mark the vertical or horizontal axis of the cornea at the slit lamp prior to placing the patient under the laser. Suction time should be minimized to decrease stress on the corneal wound and to lessen the potentially devastating complication of wound dehiscence. If the corneal curvature is very steep, cutting a thicker flap during the microkeratome pass may decrease the possibility of buttonhole formation. PRK should also be considered in steep corneas to avoid flap complications, although late-developing corneal haze has been reported.

The creation of a lamellar flap may itself cause a change in the amount and axis of the astigmatism, so some surgeons perform LASIK in 2 stages. First, the flap is cut and then laid back down. Second, one or more weeks later, after the refractive error has stabilized, the flap is lifted and laser ablation is performed. Other surgeons prefer to perform LASIK in 1 step to avoid increasing the potential complications associated with performing 2 separate procedures, including infection, graft rejection, and epithelial ingrowth.

The mean percentage reduction of astigmatism after LASIK following PKP ranges from 54% to 87.9%. Although most series report an improvement in UCVA, up to 42.9% of patients require enhancement due to cylindrical undercorrection. In addition, up to 35%

of patients are reported to lose 1 line of BCVA. Corneal graft rejection has been described after PRK. Higher and more prolonged dosing with topical corticosteroids should be prescribed in the post-PKP refractive surgery patient to decrease the risk of graft rejection.

Busin MB, Arffa RC, Zambianchi L, Lamberti G, Sebastiani A. Effect of hinged lamellar keratotomy on postkeratoplasty eyes. *Ophthalmology.* 2001;108:1845–1850.

Donnenfeld ED, Kornstein HS, Amin A, et al. Laser in situ keratomileusis for correction of myopia and astigmatism after penetrating keratoplasty. *Ophthalmology.* 1999;106:1966–1974.

Lam DS, Leung AT, Wu JT, Tham CC, Fan DS. How long should one wait to perform LASIK after PKP? *J Cataract Refract Surg.* 1998;24:6–7.

Rashad KM. Laser in situ keratomileusis for correction of high astigmatism after penetrating keratoplasty. *J Refract Surg.* 2000;16:701–710.

Tuunanen TH, Ruusuvaara PJ, Uusitalo RJ, Tervo TM. Photoastigmatic keratectomy for correction of astigmatism in corneal grafts. *Cornea.* 1997;16:48–53.

Ocular Hypertension and Glaucoma

Between 9% and 28% of myopic patients have primary open-angle glaucoma (POAG). The frequency of myopia in the glaucomatous population has been reported at between 6.6% and 37.8%, as compared with 3% to 25% in the nonglaucomatous population. Consequently, it is likely that some patients with glaucoma will request refractive surgery.

Of particular concern in patients with ocular hypertension or POAG is the effect of the acute intraocular pressure (IOP) rise to more than 65 mm Hg when suction is applied to cut the stromal flap for LASIK or the epithelial flap for epi-LASIK. Although the normal optic nerve seems to tolerate this level of IOP elevation, we do not yet fully know the resultant effect on the compromised optic nerve. There have been a few reports of new visual field defects immediately after LASIK attributed to mechanical compression or ischemia of the optic nerve head from the temporary increase in IOP.

Evaluation of the patient with ocular hypertension or POAG includes a complete history and ocular examination with peripheral visual field testing and corneal pachymetry. A history of poor IOP control, noncompliance with treatment, maximal medical therapy, or prior surgical interventions may suggest progressive disease, which may contraindicate refractive surgery. As part of the complete examination, the surgeon should note the status of the angle, the presence and amount of optic nerve cupping, and the degree of visual field loss.

Central corneal thickness must be considered in evaluating IOP as measured by the Goldmann applanation tonometer (see Chapter 11). The principle of applanation tonometry assumes a corneal thickness of 520 μm. Studies have demonstrated that thinner than normal corneas give falsely lower IOP readings, whereas thicker corneas give falsely higher readings. For example, the IOP is underestimated by approximately 5.2 mm Hg in a cornea with a central thickness of 450 μm.

LASIK and surface ablation procedures, which remove tissue in the process of sculpting the cornea, invariably create thinner corneas, which may influence IOP measurements obtained postoperatively. There are publications that document the inaccuracy of IOP measurements after PRK or LASIK. These inaccurately low central applanation tonometry measurements have been reported to obscure the diagnosis of corticosteroid-induced glaucoma after these procedures, resulting in optic nerve cupping, visual field loss, and decreased visual acuity (Fig 10-4). Because of difficulty interpreting IOP measurements after PRK or LASIK, these procedures should not be considered when IOP is poorly controlled. Furthermore, patients should be advised of the effect of refractive surgery on their IOP measurements and urged to inform future ophthalmologists about their surgery. Patients should be referred to a glaucoma specialist when indicated.

Retinal nerve fiber layer (RNFL) analysis has developed into a useful tool to diagnose glaucoma and monitor for glaucomatous progression. Although there are case reports of glaucomatous damage or progression following refractive surgery, several well-designed studies have been published that demonstrate no significant change in the RNFL after either LASIK or LASEK.

Choplin NT, Schallhorn SC, Sinai M, Tanzer D, Tidwell JL, Zhou Q. Retinal nerve fiber layer measurements do not change after LASIK for high myopia as measured by scanning laser polarimetry with custom compensation. *Ophthalmology.* 2005;112:92–97.

Sharma N, Sony P, Gupta A, Vajpayee RB. Effect of laser in situ keratomileusis and laser-assisted subepithelial keratectomy on retinal nerve fiber layer thickness. *J Cataract Refract Surg.* 2006;32:446–450.

A

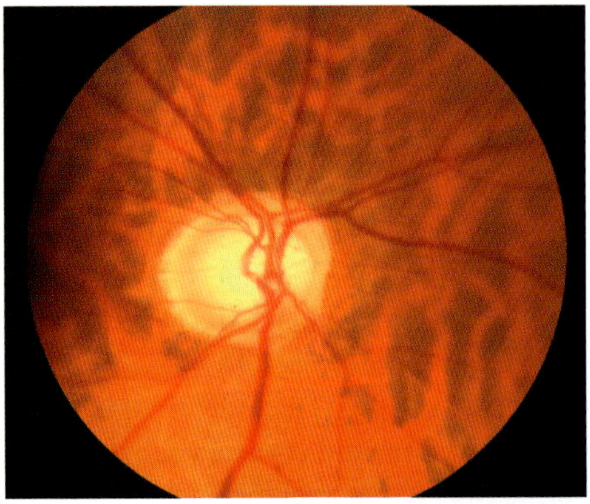

B

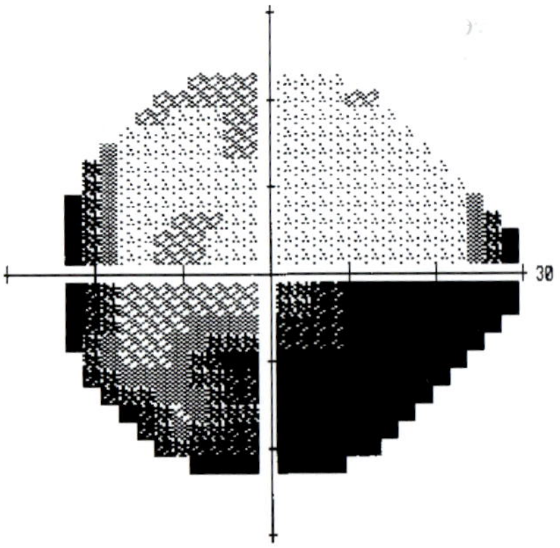

C

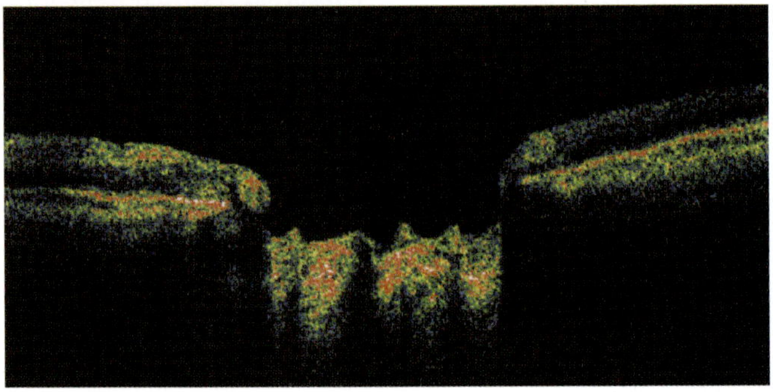

Figure 10-4 Glaucomatous optic nerve atrophy in a patient with "normal IOP" after LASIK. **A,** Increased cup–disc ratio in a patient diagnosed with glaucoma 1 year after LASIK. Patient had decreased vision with BCVA of 20/40 and IOP of 21 mm Hg. **B,** Humphrey 24-2 visual field with extensive inferior arcuate visual field loss corresponding to thinning of the superior optic nerve rim. **C,** Ocular coherence tomography demonstrates marked optic nerve cupping. *(Courtesy of Jayne S. Weiss, MD.)*

Patients with ocular hypertension can often safely undergo refractive surgery. Such a patient must be counseled preoperatively that the refractive surgery treats only the refractive error and not the natural history of the ocular hypertension, which can sometimes progress to glaucoma, with optic nerve cupping and visual field loss. Particular attention should be paid to the risk factors for progression to glaucoma, including age, corneal thickness, cup–disc ratio, and IOP. The patient needs to understand that after excimer laser ablation it is more difficult to accurately assess IOP.

The decision about whether to perform refractive surgery in a patient with glaucoma is controversial. There are no long-term studies on refractive surgery in this population. LASIK is contraindicated in any patient with marked optic nerve cupping, visual field loss, or visual acuity loss. The refractive surgeon may want the patient to sign an ancillary consent form that documents the patient's understanding that POAG may result in progressive visual loss independent of any refractive surgery and that IOP elevation during a LASIK or an epi-LASIK procedure or following LASIK or surface ablation (often due to a corticosteroid response) can cause glaucoma progression.

The surgeon should be aware that placement of a suction ring may not be possible if there is a functioning filtering bleb. Typically, glaucoma should be well controlled before refractive surgery is even considered. In the rare case in which filtering surgery and LASIK are both being planned, it is preferable that LASIK be performed before the filter is placed. Suction time should be minimized to decrease the chance of optic nerve damage from the transient increase in IOP. Alternatively, PRK or LASEK may be preferable because each eliminates the IOP rise associated with use of the microkeratome. The surgeon must be careful in using postoperative corticosteroids because of the potential for IOP elevation. The patient should be informed as to when he or she can resume postoperative topical medications for glaucoma.

To avoid trauma to the flap, IOP should generally not be checked for at least 72 hours. The patient should be told to inform a subsequent ophthalmologist of the prior LASIK, as well as of the preoperative refractive error, so that post-LASIK IOP may be assessed more accurately.

Bushley DM, Parmley VC, Paglen P. Visual field defect associated with laser in situ keratomileusis. *Am J Ophthalmol.* 2000;129:668–671.

Hamilton DR, Manche EE, Rich LF, Maloney RK. Steroid-induced glaucoma after laser in situ keratomileusis associated with interface fluid. *Ophthalmology.* 2002;109:659–665.

Kass MA, Heuer DK, Higginbotham EJ, et al. The Ocular Hypertension Treatment Study: a randomized trial determines that topical ocular hypotensive medication delays or prevents the onset of primary open-angle glaucoma. *Arch Ophthalmol.* 2002;120:701–713.

Lewis RA. Refractive surgery and the glaucoma patient: customized corneas under pressure. *Ophthalmology.* 2000;107:1621–1622.

Morales J, Good D. Permanent glaucomatous visual loss after photorefractive keratectomy. *J Cataract Refract Surg.* 1998;24:715–718.

Shaikh NM, Ahsikh S, Singh K, Manche E. Progression to end-stage glaucoma after laser in situ keratomileusis. *J Cataract Refract Surg.* 2002;28:356–359.

Wilson MR, Martone JF. Epidemiology of chronic open angle glaucoma. In Ritch R, Shields MB, Krupin T, eds. *The Glaucomas.* 2nd ed. St. Louis: Mosby; 1996:chap 35, pp 753–768.

Wong TY, Klein BE, Klein R, Knudtson M, Lee KE. Refractive errors, intraocular pressure, and glaucoma in a white population. *Ophthalmology.* 2003;110:211–217.

Retinal Disease

All patients undergoing refractive surgery should have a preoperative dilated retinal examination. The patient should be informed of the significance, treatment, and prognosis of any vitreoretinal pathology.

High myopia

A highly myopic patient is at increased risk for retinal tears and detachment. The yearly incidence of retinal detachments has been estimated at 0.015% in patients with less than 4.75 D of myopia, increasing to 0.07% in patients with ≥5.00 D of myopia. A study of 1000 patients with myopia greater than −6.00 D revealed a 3.2% incidence of retinal detachment. Scleral depression examination should be performed and referral to a retina specialist should be made, if indicated, in the highly myopic refractive surgery candidate. Symptomatic retinal tears or subclinical retinal detachments should be treated. In the absence of other risk factors, asymptomatic lattice degeneration with or without atrophic holes generally does not require prophylactic treatment. Asymptomatic retinal flap tears or holes usually also do not require treatment (see BCSC Section 12, *Retina and Vitreous*); however, tears or holes associated with high myopia and other risk factors should be considered for treatment. In a study of 29,916 myopic and hyperopic eyes undergoing LASIK, 1.5% required preoperative treatment of retinal pathology.

Patients with high myopia should be counseled that refractive surgery corrects only the refractive aspect of the myopia and not the natural history of the highly myopic eye with its known complications. Highly myopic patients remain at risk for retinal tears and detachment throughout their lives, despite refractive surgery.

Although no causal link has been established between retinal detachment and excimer laser refractive surgery, the potential adverse effects should be considered. The rapid increase and then decrease in IOP could theoretically stretch the vitreous base, and the acoustic shock waves from the laser could play a role in the development of a posterior vitreous detachment. Although the actual risk to eyes with high myopia or preexisting retinal pathology has not been determined through well-controlled, long-term studies, current data suggest that RK, surface ablation, and LASIK do not appear to increase the incidence of retinal detachment. The occurrence of retinal detachment after LASIK has been reported to range from 0.034% to 0.250%. In a series of 1554 eyes that were undergoing LASIK for myopia with a mean refractive error of −13.52 ± 3.38 D, 4 eyes (0.25%) developed retinal detachments at 11.25 ± 8.53 months after the procedure. Three of the eyes had retinal flap tears and 1 eye had an atrophic hole. There was no statistically significant difference in BCVA before and after conventional retinal reattachment surgery. A myopic shift did result from the scleral buckle, however.

Another study of 38,823 eyes with a mean myopia of −6.00 D had a 0.8% frequency of rhegmatogenous retinal detachments at a mean of 16.3 months after LASIK. The eyes that developed retinal detachments had a mean preoperative myopia of −8.75 D. Final BCVA after conventional scleral buckling procedures in such patients is usually good.

Using retrospective review, Blumenkranz reported that the frequency of retinal detachment after excimer laser was similar to the frequency in the general population, averaging 0.034% over 2 years. The operating retinal surgeon must be informed that LASIK has previously been performed because of the potential for flap dehiscence during retinal detachment surgery, especially during corneal epithelial scraping.

Arevalo JF, Ramirez E, Suarez E, et al. Incidence of vitreoretinal pathologic conditions within 24 months after laser in situ keratomileusis. *Ophthalmology.* 2000;107:258–262.

Arevalo JF, Ramirez E, Suarez E, Cortez R, Ramirez G, Yepez JB. Retinal detachment in myopic eyes after laser in situ keratomileusis. *J Refract Surg.* 2002;18:708–714.

Blumenkranz MS. LASIK and retinal detachment: should we be concerned? [editorial]. *Retina.* 2000;5:578–581.

Loewenstein A, Goldstein M, Lazar M. Retinal pathology occurring after excimer laser surgery or phakic intraocular lens implantation: evaluation of possible relationship. *Surv Ophthalmol.* 2002;47:125–135.

Ruiz-Moreno JM, Perez-Santonja JJ, Alió JL. Retinal detachment in myopic eyes after laser in situ keratomileusis. *Am J Ophthalmol.* 1999;128:588–594.

Sakurai E, Okuda M, Nozaki M, Ogura Y. Late-onset laser in situ keratomileusis (LASIK) flap dehiscence during retinal detachment surgery. *Am J Ophthalmol.* 2002;134:265–266.

The risk of retinal detachment after cataract surgery is well described (see BCSC Section 11, *Lens and Cataract*). Cataract surgery is the intraocular surgical procedure most commonly complicated subsequently by retinal detachment. Highly myopic eyes undergoing phakic IOL procedures are at risk for retinal detachment from the underlying high myopia as well as from the intraocular surgery. A retinal detachment rate of 4.8% was reported in a study of phakic IOLs to correct high myopia.

Ruiz-Moreno JM, Alió JL, Perez-Santonja JJ, de la Hoz F. Retinal detachment in phakic eyes with anterior chamber intraocular lenses to correct severe myopia. *Am J Ophthalmol.* 1999;127:270–275.

Clear lens extraction has also been associated with retinal detachment. Colin reported an incidence of postoperative retinal detachment following clear lens extraction of 2.0% after 4 years and 8.1% at 7 years despite prophylactic laser photocoagulation of lattice degeneration, retinal tears, and holes. This study emphasized the need for prolonged surveillance, as the 4-year retinal detachment rate was similar to the rate seen in patients with myopia of greater than –10.00 D who don't undergo surgery but double the predicted rate at 7 years. In other studies, serious vitreoretinal complications also occurred despite preoperative prophylactic treatment of retinal lesions. In some cases, the postoperative retinal tears occurred at the edge of the treated zones. Longer-term follow-up is needed to determine whether these surgeries increase morbidity in the highly myopic eye.

Colin J, Robinet A, Cochener B. Retinal detachment after clear lens extraction for high myopia: seven-year follow-up. *Ophthalmology.* 1999;106:2281–2284.

Ripandelli G, Billi B, Fedeli R, Stirpe M. Retinal detachment after clear lens extraction in 41 eyes with high axial myopia. *Retina.* 1996;16:3–6.

Retinal detachment surgery

Patients who have had prior scleral buckle surgery or vitrectomy may want refractive surgery because of resultant myopia. Prior retinal detachment surgery can result in a myopic shift because of axial elongation of the eye from indentation of the scleral buckle. Refractive surgery can be considered in selected cases if there is symptomatic anisometropia with good BCVA.

The retina should be extensively evaluated preoperatively. Referral to a retinal specialist should be made when indicated. The surgeon should determine whether the scleral buckle or conjunctival scarring will interfere with placement of the suction ring during the microkeratome pass. If so, PRK or LASEK may be considered instead of LASIK.

The patient must be informed that the role of the surgery is solely to treat the refractive error to correct anisometropia or to make her or him less dependent on corrective eye wear. Preoperative pathology, including preexisting macular pathology, will continue to limit UCVA and BCVA after refractive surgery. There are no published long-term series of the results of excimer laser vision correction in patients who have had prior retinal detachment surgery. Both the patient and the doctor should realize that the final visual results may not be as predictable as after other refractive surgeries. Patients should also be aware that if the scleral buckle needs to be removed, the refractive error could change dramatically. Unexpected corneal steepening has been reported in patients undergoing LASIK with previously placed scleral buckles.

Barequet IS, Levy J, Klemperer I, et al. Laser in situ keratomileusis for correction of myopia in eyes after retinal detachment surgery. *J Refract Surg.* 2005;21:191–193.

Panozzo G, Parolini B. Relationships between vitreoretinal and refractive surgery. *Ophthalmology.* 2001;108:1663–1668.

Amblyopia and Strabismus in the Adult and Child

Amblyopia and anisometropic amblyopia

Amblyopia is defined as a decrease in visual acuity without evidence of organic eye disease, typically resulting from unequal visual stimulation during the period of visual development. The prevalence of amblyopia is 2%–4% of the US population, with up to half of these cases representing anisometropic amblyopia. In addition, a percentage of patients also have both anisometropia and strabismus. Anisometropia of more than 3.00 D between the 2 eyes is likely to induce amblyopia. Anisometropic amblyopia may be more resistant to traditional amblyopia therapy, such as glasses, contact lenses, patching, or atropine penalization therapy, partly because of the large aniseikonia induced.

Assessment of the amblyopic patient should include a thorough medical history to identify any known cause of amblyopia, a history of ocular disease or surgery, assessment of ocular alignment and motility, and a comprehensive anterior segment and retinal examination. Referral to a strabismologist should be made when indicated. Preoperative counseling of an amblyopic patient must emphasize that, even after refractive surgery, the vision in the amblyopic eye will not be as good as vision in the nonamblyopic eye. The patient should also understand that BCVA will be the same, or nearly so, with or without refractive surgery.

Typically, refractive surgery is performed in this group of patients to treat high anisometropia or astigmatism (1 eye) or high refractive error (both eyes). Laser vision correction and phakic IOL implantation have been successfully performed in the higher-myopic amblyopic eye in adult patients with anisometropic amblyopia. Some studies suggest that postoperative best spectacle-corrected visual acuities may even improve modestly compared with preoperative levels in a subset of adults who undergo refractive surgery. For example, one study examined phakic IOL implantation in 59 eyes of 48 patients with 3.00 D or more of anisometropia. An average of 3 lines of vision was gained, with 91% of eyes gaining at least 1 line of vision and no eyes losing best-corrected vision. This increase in vision was attributed to an increase in magnification and a decrease in optical aberrations, but, based on a theoretical eye model, no evidence was found of an improvement in the amblyopia.

Alió JL, Ortiz D, Abdelrahman A, de Luca A. Optical analysis of visual improvement after correction of anisometropic amblyopia with a phakic intraocular lens in adult patients. *Ophthalmology.* 2007;114:643–647.

Sakatani K, Jabbur NS, O'Brien TP. Improvement in best-corrected visual acuity in amblyopic adult eyes after laser in situ keratomileusis. *J Cataract Refract Surg.* 2004;30:2517–2521.

Performing refractive surgery in the normal eye of the adult amblyopic patient, however, is controversial. The decision to do so depends on many factors, including the level of BCVA in the amblyopic eye and the normal eye and the ocular alignment. To increase safety, unilateral surgery in the amblyopic eye followed by surgery in the nonamblyopic eye can be considered. However, ocular deviation has been reported after unilateral LASIK for high myopia because of focus disparity resulting in esodeviation and impairment of fusion. A preoperative contact lens trial may be helpful in some cases to assess this potential risk.

Kim SK, Lee JB, Han SH, Kim EK. Ocular deviation after unilateral laser in situ keratomileusis. *Yonsei Med J.* 2000;41:404–406.

In many US states, 20/40 visual acuity is needed in at least 1 eye to obtain an unrestricted driver's license. Once BCVA is worse than 20/40 in the amblyopic eye, the patient is dependent on the normal eye for driving vision. In suburban or rural areas where driving is a necessary daily function, the loss of 20/40 vision in both eyes can be devastating. Consequently, some ophthalmologists may choose to perform refractive surgery only in the normal eye if the BCVA in the fellow, amblyopic eye is 20/40 or better.

A patient with anisometropic amblyopia, for example, who is corrected to 20/40 with –7.00 D in the right eye and to 20/20 with –1.00 D in the left eye may be an excellent candidate for refractive surgery in the amblyopic right eye. This patient likely cannot tolerate glasses to correct the anisometropic amblyopia and may not want or tolerate contact lenses. Even if the post-LASIK UCVA were less than 20/40 in the amblyopic eye, it would be better than the pre-LASIK UCVA of counting fingers.

If the postoperative UCVA in the amblyopic right eye improved to 20/40, the patient could request laser vision correction in the left eye for –1.00 D. However, if the patient were presbyopic, some surgeons would discourage further intervention and discuss potential advantages of the low myopia. In a younger patient with accommodation, some surgeons would inform the patient of the potential risks associated with treating the better eye but would perform the excimer laser vision correction.

If BCVA in the amblyopic eye were 20/200 or worse, however, the patient would be considered legally blind if he were to lose significant vision in the normal fellow eye. In such cases, refractive surgery in the amblyopic eye may or may not offer much benefit, and refractive surgery in the nonamblyopic eye should be regarded as contraindicated in most cases. In the extenuating circumstances where such surgery might be considered, the physician and patient should have an extensive discussion of the potential risks.

Persistent diplopia has been reported after bilateral LASIK in a patient with anisometropic amblyopia and a history of intermittent diplopia in childhood. Preoperatively, this type of patient can adjust to the disparity of the retinal image sizes with spectacle correction. Refractive surgery, however, can result in a dissimilar retinal image size that the patient cannot fuse, resulting in diplopia. This type of diplopia cannot be treated by prisms or muscle surgery.

Holland D, Amm M, de Decker W. Persisting diplopia after bilateral laser in situ keratomileusis. *J Cataract Refract Surg.* 2000;26:1555–1557.

Nemet P, Levenger S, Nemet A. Refractive surgery for refractive errors which cause strabismus: a report of 8 cases. *Binocul Vis Strabismus Q.* 2002;17:187–190.

In children, refractive surgery is controversial because their eyes and refractive state continue to change. More studies on the growing eye and the effect of excimer laser and phakic IOLs on the pediatric corneal endothelium and lens are needed before the effect of refractive surgery in the pediatric age group can be fully understood. Consequently, these procedures are typically contraindicated in children and should be regarded as investigational.

In the literature, however, there are multiple reports of the successful performance of PRK, LASEK, LASIK, and phakic IOL implantation in children, mostly age 8 years and older, when conventional therapies have failed. Most of these children underwent treatment in the more myopic eye to treat anisometropic amblyopia. In these studies, refractive error was decreased and visual acuity was maintained or improved in moderately amblyopic eyes. Refractive surgery did not improve BCVA in older children with densely amblyopic eyes, and stereopsis did not improve in this group. The limited effect on visual acuity was frequently attributable to the fact that the children were beyond amblyogenic age. Many authors have also reported a myopic shift and haze after PRK and LASIK, possibly related to the more vigorous wound-healing response that occurs in children. Thus, although these studies demonstrate the feasibility of performing corneal refractive surgery in this age group, its effectiveness in treating amblyopia cannot be adequately assessed, as amblyopia must typically be treated by the age of 8.

In one study involving a younger population, general anesthesia was used to perform PRK in 40 children, ages 1 to 6 years, who were unable to wear glasses or contact lenses for high myopia or anisometropic amblyopia from myopia. Patients were treated for existing amblyopia, and mean BCVA improved from 20/70 to 20/40. The study found that 60% of eyes developed posttreatment corneal haze, with most patients demonstrating "increasing corneal clarity" within 1 year, although 2 of 27 patients required PTK for the corneal haze. Regression of effect was attributed to a vigorous healing response and the axial myopic shift associated with growth.

There are also several reports of successful implantation of phakic IOLs in children with high anisometropia and amblyopia. This technique eliminates the aforementioned corneal wound-healing problems associated with corneal refractive procedures and may be considered when the refractive error is high and other traditional methods of amblyopia therapy have failed. Depending on the type of phakic IOL, though, other potentially serious complications may ensue, including progressive corneal endothelial cell loss, cataract formation, and persistent inflammation, as well as the usual risks associated with intraocular surgery. Thus, phakic IOLs should also be approached as investigational in children, and larger clinical trials are necessary to adequately evaluate the safety and efficacy of this technique in this age group.

Agarwal A, Agarwal A, Agarwal T, Siraj AA, Narang P, Narang S. Results of pediatric laser in situ keratomileusis. *J Cataract Refract Surg.* 2000;26:684–689.

Astle WF, Huang PT, Ells AL, Cox RG, Deschenes MC, Vibert HM. Photorefractive keratectomy in children. *J Cataract Refract Surg.* 2002;28:932–941.

Lesueur LC, Arne JL. Phakic intraocular lens to correct high myopic amblyopia in children. *J Refract Surg.* 2002;18:519–523.

Nassaralla BR, Nassaralla JJ Jr. Laser in situ keratomileusis in children 8–15 years old. *J Refract Surg.* 2001;17:519–524.

Nucci P, Drack AV. Refractive surgery for unilateral high myopia in children. *J AAPOS.* 2001;5:348–351.

Phillips CB, Prager TC, McClellan G, Mintz-Hittner HA. Laser in situ keratomileusis for treated anisometropic amblyopia in awake, autofixating pediatric and adolescent patients. *J Cataract Refract Surg.* 2004;30:2522–2528.

Accommodative esotropia

Uncorrected hyperopia causes an increase in accommodation leading to accommodative convergence. In accommodative esotropia, esotropia results because of insufficient fusional divergence. Traditional optical treatment includes correction of hyperopia with glasses or contact lenses and muscle surgery for any residual esotropia (see BCSC Section 6, *Pediatric Ophthalmology and Strabismus*). While glasses or contact lenses are being worn, the esotropia is usually kept in check. Hyperopia typically decreases in adolescence, so emmetropia and resolution of the accommodative esotropia may occur with age. If significant hyperopia persists, however, glasses or contact lenses continue to be needed to control the esotropia.

Before refractive surgery, it is important to perform an adequate cycloplegic refraction on patients younger than 35 years of age who have intermittent strabismus or phoria. The surgeon must determine the accurate refraction to avoid inducing postoperative hyperopia. Otherwise, the postoperative hyperopia may result in new onset of an esotropia with an accommodative element.

There have been reports outside the United States of PRK and LASIK for adults with accommodative esotropia. In one study, orthophoria or microesotropia was achieved after LASIK for hyperopia in accommodative esotropia in a series of 9 patients over 18 years of age. However, another study of LASIK in accommodative esotropia in patients from 10 to 52 years of age found that 42% of patients had no reduction in their esotropia and that these patients could not have been predicted on the basis of preoperative sensorimotor testing.

Hoyos JE, Cigales M, Hoyos-Chacon J, Ferrer J, Maldonado-Bas A. Hyperopic laser in situ keratomileusis for refractive accommodative esotropia. *J Cataract Refract Surg.* 2002;28: 1522–1529.

Stidham DB, Borissova O, Borissov V, Prager TC. Effect of hyperopic laser in situ keratomileusis on ocular alignment and stereopsis in patients with accommodative esotropia. *Ophthalmology.* 2002;109:1148–1153.

Systemic Conditions

Human Immunodeficiency Virus

Little has been written on the performance of refractive surgery in patients with known human immunodeficiency virus (HIV) infection. Some surgeons counsel these patients against refractive surgery because of concerns about postoperative complications, including the increased risk of infection associated with their immunosuppression. For example, bilateral keratitis after LASIK has been reported in an HIV-positive patient. If a patient has progressed to acquired immunodeficiency syndrome (AIDS), the underlying severe immunosuppression must be the paramount consideration. More importantly, these patients should be monitored for vision-threatening diseases such as cytomegalovirus retinitis (see BCSC Section 12, *Retina and Vitreous*). Most ophthalmologists consider AIDS a contraindication to refractive surgery.

As HIV-infected patients have begun to live longer productive lives before the onset of AIDS, the question of the appropriateness of refractive surgery in this "healthier" population has become relevant. One concern is the vaporization of the corneal tissue and the potential for aerosolizing live virus during laser ablation, which could pose a risk to laser suite personnel. Because the refractive surgeon may operate on patients who do not know they have been infected with viruses such as HIV or hepatitis, uniform precautions must be applied with all patients.

In one study, excimer ablation of pseudorabies virus, a porcine-enveloped herpesvirus similar to HIV and HSV, did not appear capable of causing infection by transmission through the air. The authors concluded that excimer laser ablation of the cornea in a patient infected with HIV is unlikely to pose a health hazard to the surgeon or the assistants. In another study, after excimer laser ablation of infected corneal stroma, polymerase chain reaction did not detect viable varicella virus (200 nm) but did detect viable polio particles (70 nm).

Inhaled particles ≥5 μm are deposited in the bronchial, tracheal, nasopharyngeal, and nasal walls, and particles smaller than 2 μm are deposited in the bronchioles and alveoli. Even if viral particles are not viable, the excimer laser plume produces particles with a mean diameter of 0.22 μm that can be inhaled. Although the health effects of inhaled particles from the plume have not yet been determined, there have been anecdotal reports of respiratory ailments such as chronic bronchitis in busy excimer laser refractive surgeons. Canister filter masks can filter particles down to 0.1 μm and may be more protective than conventional surgical masks. In addition, evacuation of the laser plume may potentially decrease the amount of breathable debris. Because of the many unknowns involved, some surgeons consider patients with known HIV to be poor candidates for refractive surgery.

If a surgeon is considering performing excimer laser ablation in a "healthy" HIV-infected patient with a normal eye examination and excellent best-corrected vision, extra precautions should be exercised. The refractive surgeon should consider consulting and communicating with the physicians, including infectious disease specialists, who are responsible for caring for the patient's underlying disease. The patient should be extensively counseled preoperatively concerning the visual risks of HIV and the lack of long-term follow-up of refractive surgery in this population. The surgeon may want to treat 1 eye at a time on separate days and should consider additional precautions for the operating room staff, such as wearing filter masks during the procedure and evacuating the laser plume.

Hagen KB, Kettering JD, Aprecio RM, Beltran F, Maloney RK. Lack of virus transmission by the excimer laser plume. *Am J Ophthalmol.* 1997;124:206–211.

Hovanesian JA, Faktorovich EG, Hoffbauer JD, Shah SS, Maloney RK. Bilateral bacterial keratitis after laser in situ keratomileusis in a patient with human immunodeficiency virus infection. *Arch Ophthalmol.* 1999;117:968–970.

Taravella MJ, Viega J, Luiszer F, et al. Respirable particles in the excimer laser plume. *J Cataract Refract Surg*. 2001;27:604–607.

Diabetes Mellitus

The National Diabetes Information Clearinghouse of the National Institutes of Health reported a prevalence of 7% for diabetes mellitus in the United States in 2005. Diabetic patients who are considering refractive surgery should have a thorough preoperative history and examination. The blood sugar of diabetic patients must be under good control at the time of examination to ensure an accurate refraction. A history of laser treatment for proliferative diabetic retinopathy or cystoid macular edema indicates visually significant diabetic complications that typically contraindicate refractive surgery. Any patient who has preexisting, visually significant diabetic ocular complications is not a good refractive surgery candidate. Ocular examination should include inspection of the corneal epithelium to check the health of the ocular surface, detection of cataract formation, and detailed retinal examination. Preoperative corneal sensation should be assessed because corneal anesthesia can impede epithelial healing.

The most common problems associated with LASIK in the diabetic patient appear to be related to the corneal epithelium, with an increased incidence of epithelial defect and epithelial ingrowth. One retrospective review of 30 eyes of diabetic patients who had had LASIK 6 months earlier revealed a complication rate of 47% compared with a complication rate in the control group of 6.9%. The most common problems were related to epithelial healing and included epithelial loosening and defects. A loss of 2 or more lines of best-corrected visual acuity (BCVA) was reported in less than 1% of both the diabetic group and the control group. However, 6 diabetic eyes (6/30) required a mean time of 4.3 months to heal because of persistent epithelial defects. The authors concluded that the high complication rate in diabetic patients was explained by unmasking subclinical diabetic keratopathy. Another retrospective review of 24 diabetic patients who underwent LASIK demonstrated that 63% achieved uncorrected visual acuity (UCVA) of 20/25 or better. Three eyes (6.5%) had an epithelial defect after surgery, with epithelial ingrowth developing in 2 of these eyes. No eye lost BCVA. A different study, which reviewed 22 patients who developed epithelial ingrowth after LASIK, suggested that type 1 diabetes might increase the risk of epithelial ingrowth.

Refractive surgeons should exercise caution in the selection of diabetic patients for refractive surgery. Intraoperative technique should be adjusted to ensure maximal epithelial health. To minimize corneal toxicity, the surgeon should use the minimal amount of topical anesthetic immediately before performing the procedure. Artificial tears, not anesthetic, are used during the microkeratome pass.

Diabetic patients should be counseled preoperatively about the increased risk of postoperative complications and the possibility of a prolonged healing time after LASIK. In addition, the patient needs to be told that the procedure treats only the refractive error and not the natural history of the diabetes, which can lead to future diabetic ocular complications and associated visual loss.

Fraunfelder FW, Rich LF. Laser-assisted in situ keratomileusis complications in diabetes mellitus. *Cornea*. 2002;21:246–248.

Halkiadakis I, Belfair N, Gimbel HV. Laser in situ keratomileusis in patients with diabetes. *J Cataract Refract Surg.* 2005;31:1895–1898.

Jabbur NS, Chicani CF, Kuo IC, O'Brien TP. Risk factors in interface epithelialization after laser in situ keratomileusis. *J Refract Surg.* 2004;20:343–348.

Connective Tissue and Autoimmune Diseases

Most surgeons consider active, uncontrolled connective tissue diseases such as systemic rheumatoid arthritis, lupus erythematosus, and polyarteritis nodosa to be contraindications to refractive surgery because of reports of postoperative corneal melt and perforation. Late corneal scarring has been reported after PRK in a patient with systemic lupus erythematosus.

However, 2 retrospective series suggest that refractive surgery may be considered in patients with well-controlled connective tissue or autoimmune disease. One retrospective study of 49 eyes of 26 patients with inactive or stable autoimmune disease that underwent LASIK revealed no postoperative corneal melts or persistent epithelial defects after LASIK. Another retrospective study of 62 eyes with autoimmune connective tissue disorders that had undergone LASIK revealed that these patients had a somewhat worse refractive outcome when compared with controls but otherwise no severe complications such as corneal melts or laceration or interface alterations.

Alió JL, Artola A, Belda JI, et al. LASIK in patients with rheumatic diseases: a pilot study. *Ophthalmology.* 2005;112:1948–1954.

Cobo-Soriano R, Beltran J, Baviera J. LASIK outcomes in patients with underlying systemic contraindications: a preliminary study. *Ophthalmology.* 2006;113:1118–1124.

Cua IY, Pepose JS. Late corneal scarring after photorefractive keratectomy concurrent with development of systemic lupus erythematosus. *J Refract Surg.* 2002;18:750–752.

Smith RJ, Maloney RK. Laser in situ keratomileusis in patients with autoimmune diseases. *J Cataract Refract Surg.* 2006;32:1292–1295.

Patients with poorly controlled connective tissue disease or autoimmune diseases should not have refractive surgery because they may be at higher risk for corneal melts. Because the amount of risk from an underlying disease cannot be quantified, increased cautions should be exercised if refractive surgery is considered in patients with well-controlled connective tissue disease or autoimmune diseases. Consultation with the treating physician, unilateral surgery, and ancillary informed consent should be considered.

CHAPTER 11

Considerations After Refractive Surgery

The number of patients who have had refractive surgery continues to increase yearly, and ophthalmologists are beginning to be confronted with the management of other conditions, such as glaucoma and contact lens fitting, in patients who have had refractive surgery. Calculating intraocular lens (IOL) power and performing retinal detachment surgery are additional challenges in this population. Finally, corneal transplantation may occasionally be needed. The following discussion considers all of these post–refractive surgery challenges.

IOL Calculations After Refractive Surgery

The difficulties inherent in obtaining accurate IOL calculations after refractive surgery become more important as the population of patients who have undergone refractive surgery ages. Numerous formulas are available to calculate IOL power prior to cataract surgery; these rely primarily on axial length, keratometric measurements, and desired postoperative refraction. Although measurement of axial length after refractive surgery should still be accurate, determining the actual keratometric power of the post–refractive surgery cornea is problematic. The difficulty arises from several factors. Small, effective central optical zones after refractive surgery (especially after radial keratotomy [RK]) can lead to inaccurate measurements because keratometers and Placido disk–based corneal topography units measure the corneal curvature several millimeters away from the center of the cornea. Also, the anterior and posterior corneal curvatures can be very different from each other after refractive surgery (especially after excimer laser surface ablation or LASIK), leading to inaccurate results. Generally, if standard keratometry readings are used to calculate IOL power in a previously myopic patient, the postoperative refraction will be hyperopic because the keratometry readings are higher than the real corneal power. It is not uncommon for IOL exchanges to be necessary in these cases due to refractive surprises.

A variety of methods have been developed to better estimate the central corneal power after refractive surgery. None of these methods is perfectly accurate, and different methods can lead to rather disparate values. The techniques are classified by whether they require information about refraction prior to or after refractive surgery or whether they require keratometry prior to refractive surgery. As many methods as possible should be used to calculate corneal power, and these estimates should be compared with each other and with standard keratometric readings and corneal topographic central power and simulated K readings.

Newer, non–Placido disk-based corneal topography systems claim to directly measure the central corneal curvature. Such technology should make direct calculation of IOL power after refractive surgery as accurate as it is in patients without previous refractive surgery. In the meantime, several methods for determining IOL power are available.

With Pre–Refractive Surgery Refraction and Keratometry and Post–Refractive Surgery Refraction

The most accurate IOL power calculation method is probably the "clinical history method," where pre–refractive surgery information is available, and the precise calculation depends on exactly what clinical information is available. If preoperative refraction and keratometry readings are available, the change in spherical equivalent can be calculated at the spectacle plane or, better yet, at the corneal plane. The postoperative refraction used must be a stable refraction obtained several months after the refractive surgery but before any potential onset of induced myopia from a nuclear sclerotic cataract. For example:

Preoperative average keratometry: 44.00 D
Preoperative spherical equivalent refraction (vertex distance 12 mm): –8.00 D
Preoperative refraction at the corneal plane:
  –8.00 D/(1 – [0.012 × –8.00 D]) = –7.30 D
Postoperative spherical equivalent refraction (vertex distance 12 mm): –1.00 D
Postoperative refraction at the corneal plane:
  –1.00 D/(1 – [0.012 × –1.00 D]) = –0.98 D
Change in manifest refraction at the corneal plane:
  –7.30 D – (–0.98 D) = –6.32 D
Postoperative estimated keratometry: 44.00 – 6.32 D = 37.68 D

With Pre–Refractive Surgery Refraction and Keratometry

Another method, used when preoperative keratometry and refraction information is known, is to perform the IOL power calculation based on the pre–refractive surgery numbers, using the preoperative refraction (assuming the patient was plano after refractive surgery) as the desired refraction after cataract surgery. For example:

Preoperative average keratometry: 44.00 D
Preoperative axial length: 25 mm
Preoperative spherical equivalent refraction: –8.00 D
IOL power using IOL calculation formula (A-constant 118.4): 25.00 D

With Pre–Refractive Surgery Refraction and Post–Refractive Surgery Refraction

When preoperative and postoperative refraction information is available after PRK or LASIK, but not preoperative keratometry information, one method is to simply subtract

20% of the spherical equivalent refractive change from the measured postoperative keratometry reading. For example:

Preoperative spherical equivalent refraction: –8.00 D
Postoperative spherical equivalent refraction: –1.00 D
20% of change in spherical refraction: 0.2 × (–8.00 D – [–1.00 D]) = –1.4 D
Postoperative keratometry reading: 40.00 D
"New" postoperative keratometry reading: 40.00 D – 1.40 D = 38.60 D

With Pre–Refractive Surgery Refraction Only

Feiz and associates describe a theoretical nomogram for adjusting IOL power after LASIK when the only preoperative datum available is the refraction. The IOL calculation is performed with current manual keratometric measurements. The IOL power is then adjusted per their nomogram (Table 11-1).

With No Preoperative Information

When no preoperative information is available, the "hard contact lens method" can be used to calculate corneal power. This method is quite accurate in theory but, unfortunately, not very useful in clinical practice. The BCVA needs to be at least 20/80 for this approach to work. First, a manifest refraction is performed. Then a plano hard contact lens of known base curve (power) is placed on the eye and another manifest refraction

Table 11-1 Nomogram of IOL Power Adjustment for Emmetropia

AFTER MYOPIC LASIK:

When the change in spherical equivalent induced by LASIK (D) is	Increase the IOL power (D) by
1.0	0.36
2.0	0.96
3.0	1.55
4.0	2.15
5.0	2.74
6.0	3.34
7.0	3.93
8.0	4.53
9.0	5.12
10.0	5.72

AFTER HYPEROPIC LASIK:

When the change in spherical equivalent induced by LASIK (D) is	Decrease the IOL power (D) by
1.0	0.00
2.0	0.97
3.0	1.84
4.0	2.70
5.0	3.56
6.0	4.42

From Feiz V, Mannis MJ, Garcia-Ferrer F, et al. Intraocular lens power calculation after laser in situ keratomileusis for myopia and hyperopia. *Cornea.* 2001;20:792–797.

is performed. If the manifest refraction does not change, then the cornea has the same power as the contact lens. If the refraction is more myopic, the contact lens is steeper (more powerful) than the cornea by the amount of change in the refraction; the reverse holds true if the refraction is more hyperopic. For example:

Current spherical equivalent manifest refraction: −1.00 D
A hard contact lens of known base curve (8.7 mm) and power (37.00 D) is placed.
Overrefraction: +2.00 D
Change in refraction: +2.00 D − (−1.00 D) = +3.00 D
Calculation of corneal power: 37.00 D + 3.00 D = 40.00 D

Conclusion

Randleman and associates found that either the refractive history or the hard contact lens overrefraction, or an average of these 2 methods, is the most accurate. The Feiz nomogram, they found, was not as accurate as these.

In general, after calculations by several different methods are compared, the lowest corneal power obtained should be used. Whenever the postoperative refractive error is used to calculate IOL power, it should represent a stable refraction done several months after the refractive surgery so as not to be influenced by a myopic shift brought on by nuclear sclerosis.

The modern third-generation theoretical optical formulas (eg, Holladay 2, Hoffer Q, SRK/T, Haigis) tend to be better for post–refractive surgery IOL calculations than the empirical regression formulas (eg, SRK I, SRK II). The results of more than one IOL power formula should be compared and the highest IOL power selected.

Cataract surgery that is done after RK often induces the cornea to swell somewhat, causing excess flattening and a hyperopic shift. In this case, an IOL exchange should not be performed until the cornea and refraction stabilize, which may take several weeks. As corneal curvature does not tend to change much when cataract surgery is done after PRK or LASIK, it may be possible to examine a patient by retinoscopy or refraction immediately after the cataract surgery, and if the IOL power is not correct, to perform an IOL exchange right away. Patients need to be informed prior to cataract surgery that IOL power calculations are not as accurate if performed after refractive surgery—occasionally such calculations lead to "refractive surprises"—and that additional surgery, such as surface ablation, LASIK, IOL exchange, or a piggyback IOL, may be required to attain a better refractive result.

Feiz V, Mannis MJ. Intraocular lens power calculation after corneal refractive surgery. *Curr Opin Ophthalmol.* 2004;15:342–349.

Feiz V, Mannis MJ, Garcia-Ferrer F, et al. Intraocular lens power calculation after laser in situ keratomileusis for myopia and hyperopia: a standardized approach. *Cornea.* 2001;20:792–797.

Feiz V, Moshirfar M, Mannis MJ, et al. Nomogram-based intraocular lens power adjustment after myopic photorefractive keratectomy and LASIK: a new approach. *Ophthalmology.* 2005;112:1381–1387.

Hill WE, Byrne SF. Complex axial length measurements and unusual IOL power calculations. *Focal Points: Clinical Modules for Ophthalmologists.* San Francisco: American Academy of Ophthalmology; 2004, module 9.

Kim JH, Lee DH, Joo CK. Measuring corneal power for intraocular lens power calculation after refractive surgery: comparison of methods. *J Cataract Refract Surg.* 2002;28:1932–1938.

Latkany RA, Chokshi AR, Speaker MG, Abramson J, Soloway BD, Yu G. Intraocular lens calculations after refractive surgery. *J Cataract Refract Surg.* 2005;31:562–570.

Masket S, Masket SE. Simple regression formula for intraocular lens power adjustment in eyes requiring cataract surgery after excimer laser photoablation. *J Cataract Refract Surg.* 2006;32:430–434.

Odenthal MT, Eggink CA, Melles G, Pameyer JH, Geerards AJ, Beekhuis WH. Clinical and theoretical results of intraocular lens power calculation for cataract surgery after photorefractive keratectomy for myopia. *Arch Ophthalmol.* 2002;120:431–438.

Randleman JB, Loupe DN, Song CD, Waring GO III, Stulting RD. Intraocular lens power calculations after laser in situ keratomileusis. *Cornea.* 2002;22:751–755.

Retinal Detachment Repair After LASIK

Even if patients with highly myopic eyes are made emmetropic after refractive surgery, they need to be informed that their eyes remain at increased risk of retinal detachment. For this reason, the vitreoretinal surgeon should ask about prior refractive surgery. Eyes undergoing retinal detachment repair after LASIK are prone to flap problems, including flap dehiscence and micro- and macrostriae (see Table 6-2). The surgeon may want to mark the edge of the flap prior to surgery to aid in flap replacement should it become dehisced. The risk of flap problems increases dramatically if the epithelium is debrided during the retinal detachment repair. Should a flap dehiscence occur, the flap needs to be carefully repositioned and the interface irrigated. A bandage soft contact lens may be placed at the end of surgery. Postoperatively, the patient should be followed closely for flap problems such as epithelial ingrowth and diffuse lamellar keratitis, especially if an epithelial defect was present in the flap. Although the intraocular pressure (IOP) needs to be monitored carefully in all patients after retinal detachment repair, especially when an intraocular gas bubble is used, several issues about IOP need to be kept in mind in post-LASIK patients. First, IOP measurements may be falsely low due to corneal thinning. Second, elevated IOP can cause a diffuse lamellar keratitis–like picture or even a fluid cleft between the flap and the stroma (resulting in an extremely low IOP measurement).

Corneal Transplantation After Refractive Surgery

Corneal transplantation is occasionally required after refractive surgery. Reasons for needing a corneal graft after refractive surgery include significant corneal scarring, irregular astigmatism, corneal ectasia, and corneal edema. Issues unrelated to refractive surgery, such as trauma or corneal edema after cataract surgery, can also necessitate corneal transplant surgery. The reasons why a graft may be required and ways to avoid problems with the corneal transplant are unique to each refractive surgical procedure.

After RK, a graft may be required secondary to an incision into the visual axis or due to central scarring not responsive to phototherapeutic keratectomy (PTK), with or without mitomycin C; irregular astigmatism; contact lens intolerance; or progressive hyperopia. The RK incisions can gape or dehisce during penetrating keratoplasty trephination, preventing an even, uniform, and deep trephination. One method for avoiding RK wound gape/dehiscence is to mark the cornea with the trephine and then to reinforce the RK incisions outside the trephine mark with interrupted sutures, prior to trephination. The RK incisions may also gape peripheral to the graft–host margin, causing difficulty in obtaining a watertight seal at the end of surgery. X, mattress, or lasso sutures may be required to close these "stellate" wounds.

After excimer laser surface ablation, a corneal graft may be necessary due to central haze or an irregularity not responsive to PTK, with or without mitomycin C; irregular astigmatism; or, in rare instances, corneal ectasia. With the 6- to 8-mm ablation zones typically used, the corneal periphery is generally not thinned, so corneal transplantation after surface ablation, whether partial thickness or full thickness, is usually routine.

After LASIK, corneal transplantation may be required due to central scarring (eg, after infection, buttonhole) not responsive to PTK, with or without mitomycin C; irregular astigmatism; or corneal ectasia. The main problem is that most LASIK flaps are larger than a typical trephine size (8 mm). Trephination through the LASIK flap increases the risk that the flap peripheral to the corneal transplant wound will dehisce. This complication may be avoidable by careful trephination and a gentle suture technique that incorporates the LASIK flap under the corneal transplant suture.

A few cases of inadvertent use of donor tissue that had undergone prior LASIK have been reported. The risk of this untoward event will increase as the donor pool undergoes more LASIK. Eye banks need to develop better techniques to screen out such donor corneas. Should a post-LASIK eye inadvertently be used for corneal transplantation, the patient should be informed. A regraft may be required to address significant anisometropia.

Corneal transplantation is rarely required after placement of intrastromal corneal ring segments. The polymethylmethacrylate (PMMA) ring segments are typically placed near the edge of a standard corneal transplant, so the ring segments should be removed prior to grafting, ideally well before the corneal transplant, to allow the cornea to heal.

Corneal transplantation is also rarely required after laser thermokeratoplasty or conductive keratoplasty. Trephination should be routine in such cases, and the thermal scars should generally be incorporated in the corneal button. Even if they are not, they should not significantly affect wound architecture, graft healing, or corneal curvature.

Prior phakic IOL implants should generally not affect corneal transplant surgery either. However, with phakic IOLs, it is important to monitor for progressive endothelial cell loss, especially with anterior chamber phakic IOLs. The IOL should probably be removed prior to development of corneal edema if progressive cell loss is noted.

Contact Lens Use After Refractive Surgery

Indications

Contact lenses can be used adjunctively to treat a refractive surgery patient before, during, and after the procedure. For example, hydrophilic soft contact lenses can allow a presbyopic patient to experience monovision prior to refractive surgery, thus reducing the risk of postoperative dissatisfaction. Years after refractive surgery, a presbyopic patient with excellent distance acuity may also find a contact lens helpful for near vision. Contact lenses can also be used preoperatively in a patient with a motility abnormality to simulate what vision might be like after refractive surgery and to ensure that diplopia does not develop.

In the perioperative period, hydrophilic soft contact lenses help promote epithelialization, provide patient comfort, and perhaps reduce the risk of epithelial ingrowth and flap dehiscence in the case of a free cap. A soft contact lens can be used following a flap relift that was done for enhancement, interface debridement, or removal of striae if the epithelial edge is irregular. These lenses can also relieve problems related to unexpected myopia or hyperopia after refractive surgery.

Rigid gas-permeable (RGP) contact lenses may help improve vision that is reduced because of irregular astigmatism. In this case, RGP lenses are more effective than soft lenses. Night vision symptoms caused by uncorrected refractive error or irregular astigmatism may also be reduced by using contact lenses. However, if the symptoms are associated with a scotopic pupil diameter that is larger than the treatment zone or related to higher-order aberrations, the symptoms may persist despite contact lens use.

General Principles

Obtaining the past ocular history, including any previous history of contact lens intolerance, can be helpful in predicting the likely postoperative success of a patient with contact lenses. A history of conditions such as dry eye, blepharitis, atopic keratoconjunctivitis, giant papillary conjunctivitis, or infectious or sterile keratitis may adversely affect a patient's ability to tolerate these lenses.

Contact lenses for refractive purposes should not be fitted until surgical wounds and serial refractions are stable. The most practical approach to fitting an RGP lens after refractive surgery is to do a trial fitting with overrefraction.

The clinician needs to discuss with the patient in lay terms the challenges of contact lens fitting after refractive surgery and, if possible, needs to align the patient's expectations with reality. A patient who successfully wore contact lenses prior to refractive surgery is more likely to be a successful contact lens wearer postoperatively than a patient who never wore contact lenses.

Contact Lenses After Radial Keratotomy

Contact lens fitting is a practical solution after RK when further refractive surgery is contraindicated—for example, when there is irregular astigmatism, fluctuating vision, corneal contour instability, progressive hyperopia, or abnormalities of incisions or incision pattern.

Centration is a challenge in fitting contact lenses following RK because the corneal apex is displaced to the midperiphery (Fig 11-1). Popular fitting techniques involve referring to the preoperative keratometry readings and basing the initial lens trial on the flatter curvature. Contact lens stability is achieved by adjusting the lens diameter. In general, larger-diameter lenses take advantage of the eyelid to achieve stability. However, they also increase the effective steepness of the lens due to increased sagittal depth. If preoperative

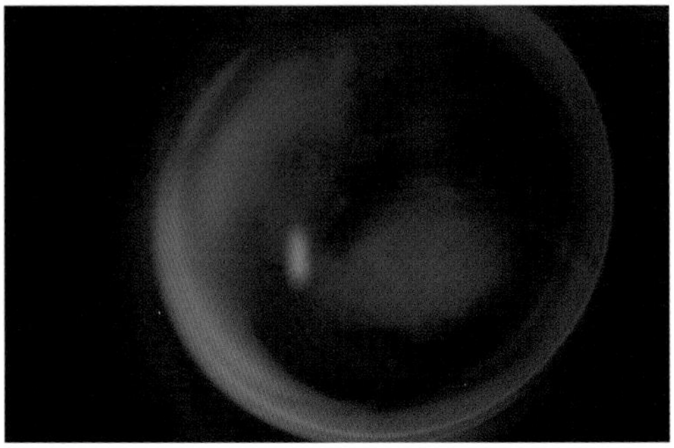

Figure 11-1 Fluorescein staining pattern in a contact lens patient following both RK and LASIK shows pooling centrally and touch in the midperiphery. This pattern is due to central corneal flattening and steepening in the midperiphery. *(Courtesy of Robert S. Feder, MD.)*

keratometry is not available, the ophthalmologist can use a paracentral or midperipheral curve, as measured with postoperative corneal topography, as a starting place.

When a successful fit cannot be obtained with a standard RGP lens, a reverse-geometry lens can be used. In contrast to the standard RGP lens, the reverse-geometry lens is flatter in the center and steeper in the periphery. The secondary curves can be designed as steep as necessary to achieve a stable fit. The larger the optical zone, the flatter the fit.

Once a stable lens fit is obtained, overrefraction is performed to identify the optimal refractive correction. The tear film will fill the gap between the lens and the central cornea and result in a dramatic increase in refractive ametropia in the direction of the preoperative refraction.

Hydrophilic soft lenses can also be used after RK. Toric soft lenses can be helpful when regular astigmatism is present. Soft lenses are less helpful in cases of irregular astigmatism, because they are less able to mask an irregular surface. In addition, soft lenses that typically drape the limbus may stimulate corneal neovascularization, especially when the lens is fitted more tightly. Neovascular proliferation may progress centrally, tracking along the corneal incisions.

Microbial keratitis is always a risk in the contact lens user. A corneal infection near a deep RK scar may progress posteriorly more rapidly. Because of the diurnal variation that occurs after RK, an adequate lens correction in the early morning may be inadequate later in the day, so a patient may require lenses of different powers for different times.

Contact Lenses After Surface Ablation

Immediately following surface ablation, a soft contact lens is placed on the cornea as a bandage to help promote epithelialization and reduce discomfort. The lens is worn until the corneal epithelium has healed. Healing time depends on the size of the epithelial defect created, which is related to the diameter of the treatment zone. The epithelial defect usually closes within 3 to 7 days. A tight-fitting lens should be removed if there is evidence of corneal hypoxia (such as edema, folds in Descemet's membrane, or iritis). In some cases, if an epithelial defect is still present, the lens will need to be exchanged for a properly fitting one.

A surface ablation patient should not be fitted in a contact lens for refractive purposes until the surface is well healed and the refractive correction and corneal contour have stabilized. The corneal contour after hyperopic correction may not stabilize for up to 6 months following surgery. Topical corticosteroids are often used for months following surface ablation. To reduce the risk of infectious keratitis, a patient should, ideally, be off topical corticosteroids prior to lens fitting.

Contact lens fitting after surface ablation may be less challenging than after RK because the disparity between the central and peripheral curves is generally not as dramatic. The risks related to deep incisions in RK are not present in surface ablation. Also, long-term stability may never be achieved in some RK patients; in contrast, once the refractive error stabilizes after surface ablation, it tends to remain stable.

In the absence of irregular astigmatism and significant haze after surface ablation, a soft contact lens can usually provide a comfortable, stable fit resulting in good visual function. Toric soft lenses can be used to treat regular astigmatism, and bifocal lenses are available for the presbyopic post–surface ablation patient with inadequate, unaided distance acuity.

An RGP lens is a better option when irregular astigmatism is present. When the contour disparity between the central and midperipheral cornea is great, a reverse-geometry fitting may be helpful. The goal for fitting an RGP lens is slight clearance of the central cornea, good alignment over the midperipheral cornea, and minimal peripheral liftoff. Aspheric RGP lenses may be better than standard RGP lenses at distributing lens contact in the midperiphery.

Contact Lenses After LASIK

The indications for contact lens fitting after LASIK are similar to those following other types of refractive surgery. The corneal contour following LASIK for myopia is usually stable by 3 months postoperatively; however, following LASIK for hyperopia, the cornea may take up to 6 months to stabilize. Re-treatment is relatively easy to perform for at least 1 year following LASIK surgery because the flap can easily be relifted. In many cases in which a blade microkeratome was used, the flap can be relatively easy to lift even several years following the initial procedure. After initial surgery, contact lens fitting is generally not considered until a decision has been made regarding re-treatment. If a large over- or undercorrection has occurred, a contact lens can be used to provide adequate visual function. However, most surgeons prefer not to have a patient inserting a contact lens into an eye with a newly created LASIK flap.

After LASIK surgery, topical corticosteroids are usually used for at least 1 week, unlike with PRK, where anti-inflammatory medication may be used for months. Thus, the use of corticosteroids after LASIK usually does not restrict contact lens use for refractive purposes. A soft contact lens may be used immediately after LASIK surgery to promote epithelialization and to prevent epithelial ingrowth. It is generally used for 1 or 2 days on an extended-wear basis and then removed by the surgeon. Daily-wear contact lenses for refractive purposes should not be considered until the surgeon feels the risk of flap displacement is low. Just as with surface ablation, the patient can be fitted with hydrophilic soft lenses, soft toric lenses, standard or aspheric RGP lenses, bifocal lenses, or reverse-geometry lenses.

Hybrid contact lenses comprising a central RGP portion surrounded by a soft lens skirt are helpful in certain patients following keratorefractive surgery. The SynergEyes

(Carlsbad, CA) hybrid lens has an extended power range and a higher degree of oxygen permeability than former hybrid lenses.

Contact Lens–Assisted, Pharmacologically Induced Keratosteepening

Contact lens–assisted, pharmacologically induced keratosteepening (CLAPIKS) is a method for treating consecutive hyperopia (ie, hyperopia occurring after PRK or LASIK for myopia). Overcorrected myopia and undercorrected hyperopia have both been treated. The patient is given a tight-fitting soft contact lens to use on an extended-wear basis, as well as ketorolac tromethamine 0.5% (eg, Acular) to administer 4 times per day, and followed weekly until the desired refractive error is obtained. Treatment is continued for an additional 2 weeks to reduce the tendency for regression. The ketorolac is increased to 6 times per day if no effect is noted.

Behind this treatment is the theory that contact lens wear increases drug penetration into the cornea by inducing hypoxia, which reduces epithelial metabolism, decreases cell mitosis, and reduces tight junctions between cells. Upon penetration, the medication should, theoretically, induce corneal steepening by causing anterior stromal thickening and basal epithelial pleomorphism. It is also possible that the contact hypoxia alone may induce increased corneal steepening.

The potential risks of using a tight-fitting lens on an extended-wear basis are corneal edema, iritis, sterile or infectious keratitis, and corneal neovascularization. Although the ketorolac may reduce inflammation associated with the contact lens, the patient should be watched closely for signs of contact lens intolerance. Long-term use of any preserved topical medication can be associated with toxicity. Further study of large series of patients with adequate follow-up will evaluate the long-term benefit of this procedure and determine whether it becomes a well-accepted technique for managing postoperative hyperopia.

Augustine JM, Gonzalez K. Manage overcorrected LASIK with CLAPIKS. *Prim Care Optom News.* 2001;10:21.

McDonald JE II, Mertins A. Contact lens assisted, pharmacologically induced keratosteepening (CLAPIKS). In: Durrie DS, O'Brien TP, eds. Refractive surgery: back to the future. *Subspecialty Day Program 2002.* San Francisco: American Academy of Ophthalmology; 2002.

Scheid TR. Contact lens fitting and management after refractive surgery. In: Scheid TR, ed. *Clinical Manual of Specialized Contact Lens Prescribing.* Boston: Butterworth-Heinemann; 2002:127.

Glaucoma After Refractive Surgery

The force required for applanation of a Goldmann tonometer is proportional to the central corneal thickness. As a result, an eye that has a thin central cornea may have an artifactually low IOP as measured by Goldmann tonometry. Patients with normal-tension glaucoma have significantly thinner corneas than patients with primary open-angle glaucoma. When a correction factor based on corneal thickness is applied, over 30% of these patients demonstrate abnormally high IOP. The correction factor may be less with both the Tono-Pen (Medtronic, Jacksonville, FL) and the pneumotonometer.

An artifactual IOP reduction occurs following surface ablation and LASIK for myopia, both of which reduce central corneal thickness. Similar inaccuracies of IOP measurement can occur with surface ablation and LASIK for hyperopia. The mean reduction in IOP measurement following excimer laser refractive surgery is 0.63 mm Hg per diopter of correction, with fairly wide variation. Postoperatively, some patients may experience no change in IOP measurement, whereas others may experience an increase. In general, the reduction of measured IOP is greater for LASIK than for surface ablation. Surface ablation patients with a preoperative refractive error ≤5.00 D may have a negligible decrease in IOP measurements.

Measuring IOP from the nasal side following LASIK surgery has been shown to reduce the artifactual IOP reduction by half (3.9 to 2.0 mm Hg). These data support the use of the Tono-Pen or pneumotonometer from the side (ie, over the uninvolved cornea) to minimize artifactual IOP reduction after excimer laser refractive surgery. The PASCAL Dynamic Contour Tonometer (Ziemer, Port, Switzerland) is capable of accurately measuring IOP independent of corneal thickness. Although some refractive surgeons cautiously measure IOP as soon as a week after LASIK, others wait a month or more because of concerns about disrupting the flap.

Topical corticosteroids used after refractive surgery pose a serious risk of corticosteroid-induced IOP elevation, particularly because accurate IOP measurement is difficult to obtain. By 3 months postoperatively, up to 15% of surface ablation patients may develop IOP above 22 mm Hg. Men appear to be more vulnerable than women to the corticosteroid effect. If the actual elevation of IOP is not detected, optic nerve damage and visual field loss can occur.

In patients with diffuse lamellar keratitis following LASIK, aqueous fluid may accumulate in the flap interface and falsely lower IOP measurement. Glaucomatous optic nerve damage and visual field loss have been reported in this setting. A syndrome of a diffuse lamellar keratitis pattern (with onset after the first postoperative week) associated with elevated IOP has been described. The syndrome does not respond to increased corticosteroids but rather resolves when the IOP is lowered.

If topical corticosteroids are used postoperatively over a long time, periodic, careful disc evaluation is essential. Optic nerve and nerve fiber layer imaging may facilitate the evaluation. Periodic visual fields may be more effective than IOP measurement for identifying at-risk patients before severe visual field loss occurs (see Fig 10-4).

Refractive surgery patients who develop glaucoma are initially treated with IOP-lowering medications and their IOP is carefully measured. If medications or laser is insufficient to lower IOP, glaucoma surgery may be recommended. Patients who have had refractive surgery should be warned prior to glaucoma surgery of the potential for transient vision loss from inflammation, hypotony, or change in refractive error. The glaucoma surgeon should be made aware of the patient's previous LASIK in order to avoid trauma to the corneal flap.

Belin MW, Hannush SB, Yau CW, Schultze RL. Elevated intraocular pressure-induced interlamellar stromal keratitis. *Ophthalmology.* 2002;109:1929–1933.

Brandt JD, Beiser JA, Kass MA. Central corneal thickness in the Ocular Hypertension Treatment Study (OHTS). *Ophthalmology.* 2001;108:1779–1788.

Dohadwala AA, Damji KF. Positive correlation between Tono-Pen intraocular pressure and central corneal thickness. *Ophthalmology.* 1998;105:1849–1854.

Ehlers N, Bramsen T, Sperling S. Applanation tonometry and central corneal thickness. *Acta Ophthalmol (Copenh).* 1975;53:34–43.

Hamilton DR, Manche EE, Rich LF, Maloney RK. Steroid-induced glaucoma after laser in situ keratomileusis associated with interface fluid. *Ophthalmology.* 2002;109:659–665.

Kass MA, Heuer DK, Higginbotham EJ, et al. The Ocular Hypertension Treatment Study: a randomized trial determines that topical ocular hypotensive medication delays or prevents the onset of primary open-angle glaucoma. *Arch Ophthalmol.* 2002;120:701–713.

Kaufmann C, Bachmann LM, Thiel MA. Comparison of dynamic contour tonometry with Goldman applanation tonometry. *Invest Ophthalmol Vis Sci.* 2004;45:3118–3121.

Lee GA, Khaw PT, Ficker LA, Shah P. The corneal thickness and intraocular pressure story: where are we now? *Clin Experiment Ophthalmol.* 2002;30:334–337.

Park HJ, Uhm KB, Hong C. Reduction in intraocular pressure after laser in situ keratomileusis. *J Cataract Refract Surg.* 2001;27:303–309.

CHAPTER 12

International Perspectives in Refractive Surgery

Introduction

Refractive surgery is the fastest growing ophthalmic subspecialty in the United States, and similar, if not greater, growth rates are seen internationally. Most refractive surgical procedures are performed outside of the United States and outside of US practice patterns. Across western Europe and the Asia-Pacific region, trends vary according to ethnic variance in the frequency of refractive errors, socioeconomic factors, and differences in regulatory issues. This chapter presents information on the variety and prevalence of refractive errors globally and on international trends in refractive surgery, and it summarizes the regulations for refractive surgery devices in different countries. In addition, the chapter reviews new clinical studies and refractive surgery therapies currently performed outside the United States.

Global Estimates of Refractive Surgery

It is estimated that 3.4 million refractive surgery procedures were performed worldwide in 2004, 2 million of them outside the United States. In 2005, global demand for refractive surgery grew by approximately 13% to 3.8 million procedures. Much of the growth came from the Asia-Pacific region, largely as a result of a burgeoning middle class in China and India. In addition, refractive surgery, specifically laser in situ keratomileusis (LASIK), has recently gained acceptance on a large scale in Japan. The total estimated number of refractive procedures in Asia grew from 674,000 in 2003 to 940,000 in 2006 (Fig 12-1).

Worldwide market projections for refractive surgery clearly show that the United States and Asia are the 2 dominant markets for refractive surgery, with approximately 1.57 million refractive procedures performed in the United States and 1.29 million procedures performed in Asia in 2006. It is estimated that Asia will be the site of fastest growth in the future, with 1.83 million procedures expected to be performed in 2010 (Fig 12-2).

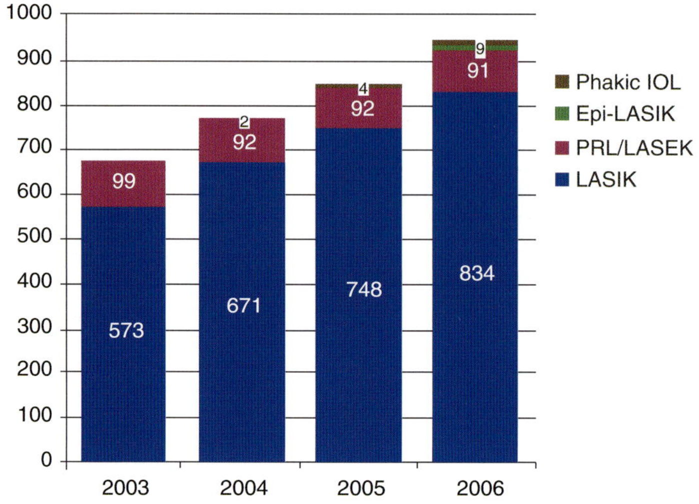

Figure 12-1 Growth of refractive procedures in Asia. *(Reproduced from A review of the 2005 ophthalmic surgery industry.* Ophthalmic Market Perspectives. *Vol 11:1. Market Scope. Accessed 6 January 2006.)*

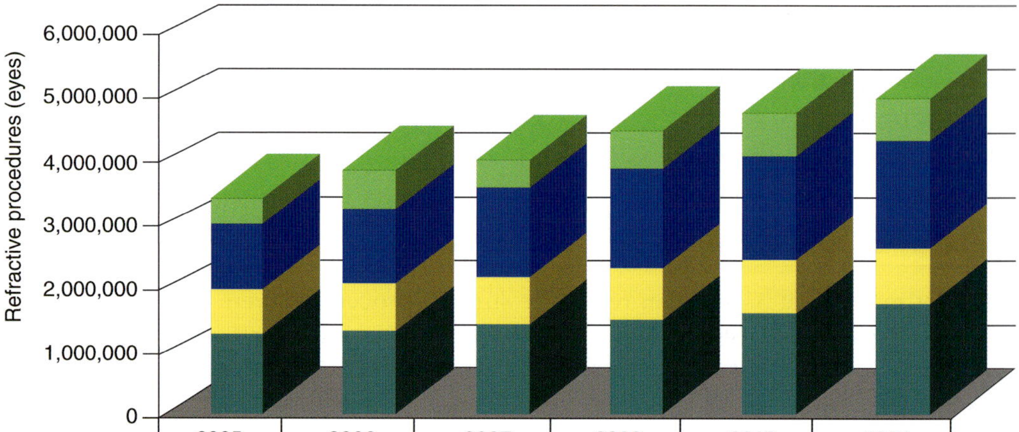

	2005	2006	2007	2008	2009	2010
All Other	375,000	425,000	450,000	475,000	500,000	525,000
Asia	1,072,000	1,285,000	1,485,000	1,685,000	1,750,000	1,825,000
Western Europe	771,000	790,000	815,000	848,000	870,000	890,000
North America	1,497,000	1,565,500	1,651,500	1,746,500	1,847,000	1,957,500

Figure 12-2 Worldwide market projections for refractive surgery. *(Reproduced from Market Scope LLC. Comprehensive Report of the Refractive Market, 2005.)*

Variation in Global Prevalence of Refractive Errors

Although the prevalence of refractive errors and myopia varies among geographic regions and different ethnic groups, it is highest in East Asian countries. The etiology of myopia and other refractive errors is not known but is thought to result from genetic and/or environmental influences.

A genetically supported basis is suggested by familial pathologic myopia and twin studies, as well as by the link between high myopia and certain ocular syndromes. However, these forms of myopia account for only a very small percentage of total myopia, and studies show that support for a genetic basis for normal or school myopia is weak. Most researchers today point toward problems of the emmetropization process in school, or juvenile-onset, myopia. *Emmetropization* is essentially an active process by which the refractive state of the anterior segment and the axial length of the eye are balanced toward an emmetropic state by positive feedback mechanisms (still to be fully elucidated) during ocular development in childhood.

The prevalence rates of myopia in East Asian countries are currently the highest in the world. In Taiwan, Singapore, China, Hong Kong, and Japan, the prevalence of myopia among young adults 15–24 years of age is 50%–80%. In countries with a primarily Caucasian population, prevalence in this same age group is much lower: United States, 27%–33%; Australia, 37%; India (generally considered Caucasian in genetic origin), 5%–10%. The accompanying trend toward higher rates of myopia progression and higher dioptric powers in East Asian populations is a general indication that the upper range of refractive error treated is also higher in these countries compared with the United States or Europe.

For the past 4 decades, while the prevalence of myopia has been increasing in East Asia, it has also been increasing in North America and Europe. Numerous studies show a predilection for myopia to develop in urban and highly economically developed populations—that is, those with greater environmental pressures. Risk factors in such a "myopigenic" environment include educational programs and the impact of increasing near work activities, such as reading, writing, and computer use. Studies of these risk factors now suggest that all human populations, under appropriate conditions, are likely to develop high prevalences of myopia.

Predictably, the growth in refractive surgery reflects the increasing prevalence of myopia in urbanized and developed societies. This increase mirrors somewhat the rising status of refractive surgery in these same populations.

Morgan I, Rose K. How genetic is school myopia? *Prog Retin Eye Res.* 2005;24:1–38.

Saw SM. A synopsis of the prevalence rates and environmental risk factors for myopia. *Clin Exp Optom.* 2003;86:289–294.

Saw SM, Chua WH, Wu HM, Yap E, Chia KS, Stone RA. Myopia: a gene-environment interaction. *Ann Acad Med Singapore.* 2000;29:290–297.

International Trends in Refractive Surgery

International trends in refractive surgery reflect developments in the United States and developed European and Asian nations, but new trends have been emerging. For example, refractive surgery market statistics show that laser refractive procedures (mainly LASIK) represented approximately 50% of all refractive surgery in 2004, but procedures using new lens refractive technologies are expected to exceed 30% of the refractive market by 2008.

Kalomara Information. Advances in ophthalmology: markets in the treatment of eye disorders and corrective vision. Market Research. http://www.marketresearch.com/. Accessed 29 June 2006.

Preferences as to which excimer lasers are used for LASIK vary internationally. In the United States, of a total of 1400 excimer lasers that were in use in 2005, the 3 major laser systems were VISX (Santa Clara, CA) lasers (675 units, 48% of market), Alcon (Ft Worth, TX) LADARVision lasers (300 units, 21%), and Bausch & Lomb (Rochester, NY) Technolas lasers (140 units, 10%). In contrast, of the 3300 excimer lasers in use outside the United States, the majority were Bausch & Lomb lasers (850 units, 26%), followed by VISX (600 units, 18%), Nidek (Fremont, CA) (550 units, 17%), and the ALLEGRETTO WAVE (WaveLight, Sterling, VA) (450 units, 14%). Unlike in the United States, where wavefront-guided custom ablations continue to prevail, customized LASIK is less popular internationally. Exactly twice as many lasers were sold internationally (320 units) in 2006 than were sold in the United States (160 units). The estimated US rate of adoption of wavefront-guided treatment in 2005 was approximately 50% and rising; internationally, this rate in 2007 is closer to 25%–30%. One possible cause for this difference in the popularity of wavefront-guided treatment may be its higher cost.

The choice of microkeratomes for LASIK is similar internationally (Bausch & Lomb: 46.1% market share in the United States, 48.4% internationally; Moria [Antony Cedex, France]: 25.9% in the United States, 24.2% internationally). The introduction of the IntraLase (Irvine, CA) femtosecond laser for LASIK flap creation has led to its increasing use in both the United States and internationally. In 2005, a total of 215 IntraLase units were in use in the United States compared to 112 lasers in use in other countries.

With regard to surface ablation procedures, photorefractive keratectomy (PRK) remains popular for the treatment of low myopia. The use of mitomycin C for higher degrees of correction is increasing in Asia, which may also explain the resurgence in the interest in surface ablation globally. In Asia and other countries with relatively high rates of high myopia, PRK was used extensively in the mid to late 1990s, until the significant risks of corneal haze in high-degree ablation were recognized, and it was largely replaced by LASIK for such treatments. Laser subepithelial keratomileusis (LASEK) and epi-LASIK procedures are becoming increasingly popular in some European countries (eg, Italy).

Phakic intraocular lenses (PIOLs) are widely used throughout Europe and Asia, mainly for the treatment of high or extreme myopia. Intracorneal stromal ring segment (ICRS) surgery remains generally limited to an emerging indication for keratoconus and post–refractive surgery keratectasia. As in the United States, Intacs (Addition Technology, Des Plaines, IL) is the most commonly used ICRS in Europe and Asia; Ferrara ring (Ferrara Ophthalmics, Belo Horizonte, Brazil) use is limited to South America. Ferrara rings are not approved by the US Food and Drug Administration (FDA). The main differences between this device and the Intacs device is that Ferrara rings are triangular in cross section, have a smaller optical zone (5 mm), and are implanted freehand at a corneal stromal depth of 80%. Intacs rings are 6-sided, with an optical zone of 7 mm, and they are implanted at a depth of 68% (see Chapter 5).

In Europe, as in the United States, there is a general focus on the convergence of refractive and cataract surgeries, with PIOLs and presbyopia-correcting IOLs bridging the gap between cataract and refractive technologies. A gradual shift is taking place toward lens-related refractive surgery as an alternative to the traditional forms of corneal surgery—namely, PRK, LASIK, LASEK, and epi-LASIK. In the United States, the Verisyse (AMO, Santa Ana, CA) and the Visian ICL (STAAR, Monrovia, CA) are the only FDA-approved PIOLs (see Chapter 8).

In Europe, numerous PIOLs are available, including 3 posterior chamber IOLs (ICL and Toric ICL [STAAR] and PRL [Zeiss, Dublin, CA]), 3 anterior chamber iris-fixated IOLs (Artisan/Verisyse and toric versions [Ophtec, Groningen, Netherlands/AMO], Artiflex [Ophtec]), and 6 anterior chamber angle-supported IOLs (Phakic 6 [O.I.I., Ontario, CA], Icare [Corneal, Pringy, France], Vivarte Presbyopic [Zeiss], Newlife [Zeiss], Kelman Duet [Tekia, Irvine, CA], and Vivarte/GBR [Zeiss]). PIOLs were introduced fairly early in Europe, starting with the ICL, which received CE marking approval from the European Union (see the discussion in the following section) in 1997. The PRL, Toric ICL, and Artiflex devices received CE marking approvals in 2001, 2003, and 2005, respectively. Use of the PRL lens has dropped significantly since lens subluxation into the vitreous cavity was reported in Spain and Italy. The Vivarte/GBR angle-supported PIOL was withdrawn in France in 2005 and the Vivarte Presbyopic, Newlife, and Icare angle-supported PIOLs were withdrawn from France in 2006 due to concerns regarding significant endothelial cell loss. This earlier use of PIOLs in Europe probably explains the more mature state of the technology in this part of the world.

In Norway, Sweden, and Spain, posterior chamber IOLs (ICL and Toric ICL) are the most commonly used PIOLs. In Germany and France, anterior chamber PIOLs are the most used; in Italy, anterior chamber and posterior chamber PIOLs are used about equally. In the United Kingdom, PIOLs are generally used only as piggyback implants to correct postcataract refractive surprises.

In Asia, the most common refractive procedure is LASIK, which can often be performed even in cases of high myopia because of both newer microkeratomes that can cut thinner flaps and improved tissue-efficient algorithms. In Korea, arguably the Asian country with the highest penetration of refractive surgery, a 2004 survey (unpublished data from Kyung Hwan Shin) conducted by the Korean Society of Cataract and Refractive Surgery (KSCRS) revealed that for myopia less than –12 D, LASIK surgery accounted for 82% of all forms of refractive surgery, followed by LASEK (11%) and PRK (7%). For myopia exceeding –12 D, PIOLs were the preferred option. Wavefront-guided procedures were performed in only half (51%) of cases. (In contrast, surveys conducted at the 2006 American Society of Cataract and Refractive Surgery [ASCRS] meeting suggested that 75% of US surgeons routinely used customized ablation in their practice.) In Japan, the prevalence of refractive surgery is lower because of lingering concerns based on the rash of corneal decompensation cases that occurred over the years among patients who had had posterior radial keratotomy surgery, which was developed by Tsutomu Sato in Japan in the 1930s. In addition, similar to the situation in the United States, there are stringent medical device regulations and regulations on medical advertising. Alcon, Bausch & Lomb, and WaveLight, for example, have yet to attain excimer laser regulatory approvals in Japan; Nidek lasers predominate, as Nidek is based in Japan. Although it is estimated that only 250–300 surgeons currently perform refractive surgery in Japan, despite the country's having the world's tenth largest population (almost 128 million), the situation may be changing. In 2000, only about 20,000 refractive procedures were performed in the country, but the number of procedures more than doubled in 2003, to an estimated 48,000.

International Regulation of Refractive Surgery Practices and Devices

Standards and levels of regulation vary from country to country, but many developing nations accept or conform to regulatory standards from established administrations such as the US FDA and the regulatory framework of the European Union (EU).

International regulation of medical devices was established by the Global Harmonization Task Force (GHTF) in 1992, with the development of the International Harmonized System for medical device control. The 5 founding members were the European Union, United States, Canada, Australia, and Japan. Membership remains restricted to these 5 countries, although other countries may participate as observers. Chairmanship of the GHTF is rotated among representatives of the 5 founding countries.

In Europe, the European Union has adopted a risk-based classification, comparable to that of the US FDA, consisting of 4 classes (I, II, III, and IV). The European Union began medical regulation in 1990, with 3 directives for medical devices; these have led to a harmonized conformity of standards among European countries and to the CE marking system. Regulatory controls focus primarily on safety, with less emphasis on efficacy, unlike those of the US FDA.

In Australia, the Therapeutic Goods Administration (TGA) is the governing body regulating medical devices; this agency looks toward the European Union (CE marking directives) and the US FDA for regulatory guidance on refractive technologies.

In Asia, the fastest growing region for refractive surgery, the status of regulatory control of medical devices varies by nation, ranging from legally enforceable legislation to voluntary guidelines. Some countries use existing drug and food control legislation to control a limited range of medical devices. Many countries (eg, China, Korea), however, recognize or have adopted regulatory standards set by the European Union or the US FDA within their respective internal regulatory frameworks. In India, medical device regulation is still undergoing regulatory reorganization. In Japan, strict internal regulatory controls have limited the importation of refractive surgical devices and surgical procedures. Phototherapeutic keratectomy (PTK) and PRK were approved in Japan in 1998 and 2000, respectively, whereas LASIK has not been formally approved as a refractive procedure.

Some Asian countries have adopted, or are in the process of adopting, a harmonized approach to device regulation, through the Asian Harmonization Working Party (AHWP), a nongovernmental agency formed in 1996, with direct links to the GHTF. Representatives to the AHWP come from both regulatory authorities and industry in the member nations of Brunei, China, Hong Kong, Indonesia, Korea, Malaysia, the Philippines, Saudi Arabia, Singapore, Taiwan, Thailand, and Vietnam. These member nations are currently at various stages of voluntary adoption of the international harmonization system proposed by the GHTF.

Summary

The field of refractive surgery continues to expand and develop, both in the United States and internationally. Clinical trials on new refractive technologies are often initiated outside the United States, in Europe and Asia, before clinical studies are carried out in the United States. Differences in practice patterns among refractive surgeons worldwide, coupled with differences in medical device regulation, result in a varied approach to the treatment and management of refractive conditions around the world. The collective experience of refractive surgeons worldwide with these new technologies has major implications for ongoing development in the field of refractive surgery today.

Basic Texts

Refractive Surgery

Azar DT, Gatinel D, Thanh Hoang-Xuan II, eds. *Refractive Surgery.* 2nd ed. Philadelphia: Elsevier Mosby; 2007.

Boyd BF, Agarwal S, Agarwal A, Agarwal A, eds. *LASIK and Beyond LASIK: Wavefront Analysis and Customized Ablations.* El Dorado, Panama: Highlights of Ophthalmology; 2001.

Feder R, Rapuano CJ. *The LASIK Handbook: A Case-based Approach.* Philadelphia: Lippincott, Williams & Wilkins; 2007.

Garg A. *Mastering the Techniques of Customized LASIK.* New Delhi: Jaypee Brothers; 2007.

Hardten DR, Lindstrom RL, Davis EA, eds. *Phakic Intraocular Lenses: Principles and Practice.* Thorofare, NJ: Slack; 2004.

Probst LE, ed. *LASIK: Advances, Controversies, and Custom.* Thorofare, NJ: Slack; 2003.

Troutman RC, Buzard KA. *Corneal Astigmatism: Etiology, Prevention, and Management.* St Louis: Mosby; 1992.

Related Academy Materials

Focal Points: Clinical Modules for Ophthalmologists

Individual modules are available in PDF format at aao.org/focalpointsarchive. Print modules are available only through an annual subscription.

Klyce SD. Wavefront analysis (Module 10, 2005).
Koch DD. Cataract surgery after refractive surgery (Module 5, 2001).
Lawless MA. Surgical correction of hyperopia (Module 4, 2004).
Majmudar PJ. LASIK complications (Module 13, 2004).
Packer M, Fine IH, Hoffman RS. Refractive lens exchange (Module 6, 2007).
Price FW Jr. Lasik (Module 3, 2000).
Schallhorn SC. Wavefront-guided LASIK (Module 1, 2008).
Wallace RB III. Multifocal lens implementation (Module 11, 2004).

Print Publications

Arnold AC, ed. *Basic Principles of Ophthalmic Surgery* (2006).
Rockwood EJ, ed. *ProVision: Preferred Responses in Ophthalmology.* Series 4. Self-Assessment Program. 2-vol set (2007).

Online

American Academy of Ophthalmology. Ophthalmic News and Education Network: Clinical Education Case Web site; http://www.aao.org/education/products/cases/index.cfm
American Academy of Ophthalmology. Ophthalmic News and Education Network: Clinical Education Course Web site; http://www.aao.org/education/products/courses/index.cfm
Basic and Clinical Science Course (Sections 1–13); http://www.aao.org/education/bcsc_online.cfm
Maintenance of Certification Exam Study Kit, Refractive Management/Intervention, version 2.0 (2007); http://www.aao.org/moc
Rockwood EJ, ed. *ProVision:Preferred Responses in Ophthalmology.* Series 4. Self-Assessment Program. 2-vol set (2007); http://one.aao.org/CE/EducationalContent/Provision.aspx
Specialty Clinical Updates: Refractive Management/Intervention. *Cataract.* Vol 1 (2004); http://www.aao.org/education/products/scu/index.cfm

CDs/DVDs

Basic and Clinical Science Course (Sections 1–13) (CD-ROM; 2008).
Front Row View: Video Collections of Eye Surgery. Series 1 (DVD; 2006).
Front Row View: Video Collections of Eye Surgery. Series 2 (DVD; 2007).

Preferred Practice Patterns

Preferred Practice Patterns are available at http://one.aao.org/CE/PracticeGuidelines/PPP.aspx.

Preferred Practice Patterns Committee, Refractive Management/Intervention Panel. *Refractive Errors and Refractive Surgery* (2007).

Ophthalmic Technology Assessments

Ophthalmic Technology Assessments are available at http://one.aao.org/CE/PracticeGuidelines/Ophthalmic.aspx. Assessments are published in the Academy's journal, *Ophthalmology*. Individual reprints may be ordered at http://www.aao.org/store.

Ophthalmic Technology Assessment Committee. *Excimer Laser Photorefractive Keratectomy (PRK) for Myopia and Astigmatism* (1994).
Ophthalmic Technology Assessment Committee. *Intrastromal Corneal Ring Segments for Low Myopia* (2001).
Ophthalmic Technology Assessment Committee. *Laser In Situ Keratomileusis for Myopia and Astigmatism: Safety and Efficacy* (2002).
Ophthalmic Technology Assessment Committee. *Laser In Situ Keratomileusis for Hyperopia, Hyperopic Astigmatism, and Mixed Astigmatism* (2004).
Ophthalmic Technology Assessment Committee. *Wavefront-Guided LASIK for the Correction of Primary Myopia and Astigmatism* (2008).

Complementary Therapy Assessments

Complementary Therapy Assessments are available at http://one.aao.org/CE/PracticeGuidelines/Therapy.aspx.

Complementary Therapy Task Force. *Visual Training for Refractive Errors* (2004).

To order any of these materials, please order online at www.aao.org/store or call the Academy's Customer Service toll-free number 866-561-8558 in the U.S. If outside the U.S., call 415-561-8540 between 8:00 AM and 5:00 PM PST.

Credit Reporting Form

Basic and Clinical Science Course, 2008–2009
Section 13

The American Academy of Ophthalmology is accredited by the Accreditation Council for Continuing Medical Education to provide continuing medical education for physicians.

The American Academy of Ophthalmology designates this educational activity for a maximum of 30 *AMA PRA Category 1 Credits*™. Physicians should only claim credit commensurate with the extent of their participation in the activity.

If you wish to claim continuing medical education credit for your study of this Section, you may claim your credit online or fill in the required forms and mail or fax them to the Academy.

To use the forms:

1. Complete the study questions and mark your answers on the Section Completion Form.
2. Complete the Section Evaluation.
3. Fill in and sign the statement below.
4. Return this page and the required forms by mail or fax to the CME Registrar (see below).

To claim credit online:

1. Log on to the Academy website (www.aao.org/cme).
2. Select Review/Claim CME.
3. Follow the instructions.

Important: These completed forms or the online claim must be received at the Academy by June 2011.

I hereby certify that I have spent _____ (up to 30) hours of study on the curriculum of this Section and that I have completed the study questions.

Signature: ____
Date

Name: ____

Address: ____

City and State: ______________________ Zip: ______________________

Telephone: (_______) ______________________ Academy Member ID# ______________
area code

Please return completed forms to:
American Academy of Ophthalmology
P.O. Box 7424
San Francisco, CA 94120-7424
Attn: CME Registrar, Customer Service

Or you may fax them to: 415-561-8575

2008–2009
Section Completion Form

Basic and Clinical Science Course

Answer Sheet for Section 13

Question	Answer	Question	Answer	Question	Answer
1	a b c d e	18	a b c d	34	a b c d e
2	a b c d e	19	a b c d	35	a b c d e
3	a b c d e	20	a b c d e	36	a b c d
4	a b c d	21	a b c d	37	a b c d
5	a b c d	22	a b c d	38	a b c d
6	a b c d	23	a b c d	39	a b c d e
7	a b c d	24	a b c d	40	a b c d
8	a b c d	25	a b c d	41	a b c d
9	a b c d	26	a b c d e	42	a b c d e
10	a b c d e	27	a b c d	43	a b c d e
11	a b c d e	28	a b c d e	44	a b c d
12	a b c d e	29	a b c d e	45	a b c d
13	a b c d	30	a b c d e	46	a b c d
14	a b c d e	31	a b c d e	47	a b c d e
15	a b c d	32	a b c d e	48	a b c d e
16	a b c d e	33	a b c d e	49	a b c d e
17	a b c d				

Section Evaluation

Please complete this CME questionnaire.

1. To what degree will you use knowledge from BCSC Section 13 in your practice?

   ☐ Regularly

   ☐ Sometimes

   ☐ Rarely

2. Please review the stated objectives for BCSC Section 13. How effective was the material at meeting those objectives?

   ☐ All objectives were met.

   ☐ Most objectives were met.

   ☐ Some objectives were met.

   ☐ Few or no objectives were met.

3. To what degree is BCSC Section 13 likely to have a positive impact on health outcomes of your patients?

   ☐ Extremely likely

   ☐ Highly likely

   ☐ Somewhat likely

   ☐ Not at all likely

4. After you review the stated objectives for BCSC Section 13, please let us know of any additional knowledge, skills, or information useful to your practice that were acquired but were not included in the objectives. [Optional]

5. Was BCSC Section 13 free of commercial bias?

   ☐ Yes

   ☐ No

6. If you selected "No" in the previous question, please comment. [Optional]

7. Please tell us what might improve the applicability of BCSC to your practice. [Optional]

Study Questions

Although a concerted effort has been made to avoid ambiguity and redundancy in these questions, the authors recognize that differences of opinion may occur regarding the "best" answer. The discussions are provided to demonstrate the rationale used to derive the answer. They may also be helpful in confirming that your approach to the problem was correct or, if necessary, in fixing the principle in your memory.

1. Which of the following is true regarding keratoconus?
   a. Patients with keratoconus have corneal thinning in the paracentral region.
   b. LASIK should be avoided in keratoconus.
   c. In the absence of clinical findings, topography is helpful in diagnosing keratoconus.
   d. All of the above are true.
   e. None of the above are true.

2. Which of the following is true after conventional laser ablations for myopia (LASIK, surface ablations)?
   a. Lower-order (second-order) aberrations are generally reduced.
   b. Higher-order aberrations often increase.
   c. The central corneal curvature is flattened and the corneal apical radius of curvature is increased.
   d. Corneal asphericity changes often accompany myopic laser ablations.
   e. All of the above are true.

3. Which of the following is correct based on Munnerlyn's approximation of the depth of ablation after PRK for myopia?
   a. The ablation depth is proportional to the treatment circumference.
   b. For the same amount of intended dioptric correction, increasing the size of the ablation zone results in deeper treatment.
   c. The ablation depth is proportional to the square of the intended dioptric correction.
   d. All of the above are true.
   e. None of the above are true.

4. Contact lenses should not be worn for at least what period of time before the refraction and treatment?
   a. soft contact lenses, 3 days; rigid gas-permeable contact lenses, 7 days
   b. soft contact lenses, 3 days; rigid gas-permeable contact lenses, 10 days
   c. soft contact lenses, 7 days; rigid gas-permeable contact lenses, 10 days
   d. soft contact lenses, 3–14 days; rigid gas-permeable contact lenses, 14–21 days

5. Important aspects of the preoperative refractive surgery evaluation include all the following *except:*
   a. social history
   b. past ocular history
   c. past and current medical history
   d. none of the above

6. Required parts of the preoperative refractive surgery examination include all of the following *except:*
   a. slit-lamp examination
   b. measurement of corneal curvature
   c. specular microscopy
   d. corneal thickness measurement

7. Important issues when considering monovision include all of the following *except:*
   a. patient age
   b. degree of myopia
   c. success with monovision in the past
   d. ocular dominance

8. LASIK and PRK are both commonly used to treat which refractive range?
   a. −14 to +8 D
   b. −8 to +4 D
   c. −5 to +2 D
   d. −5 to +5 D

9. Thermokeratoplasty (laser thermal keratoplasty and/or conductive keratoplasty)
   a. is best for patients over 40 years of age
   b. is not associated with significant refractive regression
   c. creates a multifocal cornea, giving most patients good uncorrected distance and near vision
   d. is effective at treating astigmatism

10. The risk associated with clear lens extraction may be greater in a patient with high myopia than in a patient with hyperopia because
    a. biometry is less accurate
    b. accommodation will be lost
    c. retinal detachment risk is greater
    d. the risk of infection is greater
    e. a phakic IOL will be more difficult to insert

11. Which of the following is potentially the best candidate for a phakic IOL (PIOL)?
    a. a 60-year-old with a clear lens and an anterior chamber depth of 2.8 mm
    b. a 35-year-old patient with −9.00 myopia with a central corneal thickness of 498 μm
    c. a highly motivated 17-year-old college student with a deep anterior chamber and −10.00 refraction OU
    d. a 40-year-old corticosteroid-dependent asthmatic with a correction of −7.00 OU
    e. a 30-year-old man with a deep anterior chamber and a refraction of −9.00 +3.50 × 035 OS

12. In a previously normal cornea, all of the following are complications of incisional keratotomy (radial and astigmatic) *except:*
    a. corneal ectasia
    b. corneal perforation
    c. traumatic rupture of the globe through the keratotomy incision
    d. bacterial keratitis
    e. loss of best spectacle-corrected visual acuity

13. The mechanism for necrosis of the stroma overlying a corneal inlay made of an impermeable substance such as glass can best be described as
    a. reflection of ultraviolet light from the inlay, causing keratocyte death
    b. hypoxia of the overlying stroma
    c. lack of nutrients from the underlying cornea
    d. trauma at the time of surgery

14. Which of the following is the most common complication of LASIK?
    a. infectious keratitis
    b. ectasia
    c. dry eye
    d. buttonholes
    e. free caps

15. All of the following are relative advantages of intrastromal corneal ring segments (Intacs) *except:*
    a. The refractive result is potentially reversible.
    b. The central clear zone is not violated.
    c. Astigmatism is easily corrected.
    d. The ring segments can be replaced with segments of a different size.

16. Which of the following are effective treatments for dry eye following LASIK?
    a. oral fish oils and flaxseed oil
    b. topical cyclosporine
    c. punctal occlusion
    d. all of the above
    e. none of the above

17. Which of the following has been shown to reduce the risk of haze following PRK?
    a. topical mitomycin C
    b. fourth-generation fluoroquinolones
    c. oral nonsteroidal anti-inflammatory drugs
    d. tetracycline family antibiotics

18. The laser–tissue interaction by which the excimer laser reshapes the cornea is termed
    a. photocoagulation
    b. photodisruption
    c. photoablation
    d. photodynamics

19. Based on our current knowledge of corneal ectatic disorders and ectasia after LASIK, which of the following is true?
    a. Ectatic corneal disorders are the most common indication for keratoplasty in the United States.
    b. Ectasia develops only in eyes with clearly identifiable risk factors.
    c. A computer-generated diagnosis of "keratoconus suspect" is always a contraindication to LASIK surgery.
    d. There is no specific test or measurement that is diagnostic of a corneal ectatic disorder.

20. Possible risk factors for the development of ectasia following laser vision correction include
    a. high myopia
    b. low preoperative corneal thickness
    c. low residual stromal thickness (RST) after ablation
    d. asymmetric corneal steepening
    e. all of the above

21. Larger-diameter microkeratome flaps are associated with which of the following?
    a. steep corneal curvature
    b. low microkeratome suction
    c. thicker corneas
    d. reused blades

22. The LASIK flap adheres to the cornea on the first postoperative day because of which of the following?
    a. the endothelial pump
    b. re-epithelialization of the gutter
    c. sutures
    d. a bandage soft contact lens

23. LASIK enhancements are most commonly performed by which of the following methods?
    a. performing PRK on the flap surface
    b. cutting a new flap
    c. lifting the original flap
    d. reducing the remaining stromal bed to less than 250 μm

24. Dry eye after LASIK is primarily attributed to which of the following?
    a. deinnervation of the flap
    b. phototoxicity to the conjunctival goblet cells
    c. lacrimal gland insufficiency
    d. medicamentosa

25. Which of the following is a characteristic of diffuse lamellar keratitis (DLK)?
    a. It is infectious.
    b. It occurs only in primary LASIK procedures.
    c. It is usually treated with topical NSAIDs.
    d. It can cause corneal melting if undertreated.

26. In LASIK patients, infectious keratitis must be differentiated from diffuse lamellar keratitis (DLK); DLK typically involves all of the following *except:*
    a. It is usually visible within the first 24 hours.
    b. It usually begins at the flap periphery.
    c. The inflammatory cells are confined to the area of the flap interface.
    d. The inflammatory cells typically surround a more intense central infiltrate.
    e. There is minimal pain or photophobia.

27. Which of the following is true regarding conductive keratoplasty (CK)?
    a. In CK, a probe is used to directly heat only the corneal stroma.
    b. Conductive keratoplasty is approved for the temporary treatment of 0.75 to 3.00 D of hyperopia with astigmatism of 0.75 D or less.
    c. Conductive keratoplasty is contraindicated for patients with a decentered corneal apex.
    d. After CK, the refractive error gradually drifts toward increasing myopia.

28. How is heat applied to the cornea during CK?
    a. A probe delivers localized laser pulses to surrounding tissue.
    b. The tip of the probe applies heat directly to the corneal stroma.
    c. The tip of the probe applies heat directly to both the corneal epithelium and the stroma.
    d. Radiofrequency energy flows through the conducting tip to the eyelid speculum.
    e. None of the above are true.

29. LASIK surgery has been reported to
    a. cause glaucomatous damage or progression in isolated cases
    b. not cause retinal nerve fiber layer (NFL) loss in normal patients in controlled prospective studies
    c. affect the Goldmann applanation IOP reading after surgery
    d. all of the above
    e. none of the above

30. Which of the following is(are) an absolute contraindication(s) to LASIK?
    a. rheumatoid arthritis
    b. amblyopia
    c. prior penetrating keratoplasty
    d. keratoconus
    e. all of the above

31. Which of the following statements about phakic intraocular lenses (PIOLs) is true?
    a. The PIOL is inserted after the cataract has been removed.
    b. PIOLs are used in conjunction with clear lens extraction.
    c. PIOLs can correct myopia and hyperopia.
    d. A PIOL cannot be used if the cornea is thin.
    e. A PIOL should not be used if the cornea is flat.

32. Which of the following is not an advantage of bioptics?
    a. Bioptics extends the range of refractive error that can be treated.
    b. Bioptics has the benefit of being adjustable.
    c. Bioptics has the benefit of being less limited by corneal thickness than LASIK.
    d. Bioptics can be performed with a PCPIOL or an iris claw lens.
    e. Bioptics corrects the need for reading glasses in the presbyopic patient by virtue of its dual lens capability.

33. Which of the following statements about PIOLs is false?
    a. Because the optics of all PIOLs are foldable, astigmatism is not a significant problem.
    b. Endophthalmitis is a risk of this procedure.
    c. If the patient develops a cataract at a later time, the PIOL will need to be removed.
    d. No matter which model of PIOL is used, a stable cycloplegic refraction obtained after discontinuing contact lens wear is necessary.
    e. A healthy corneal endothelium is a requirement for PIOL use.

34. The ideal candidate for a multifocal IOL has which of the following characteristics?
    a. The patient has >1.50 D of astigmatism upon cycloplegic refraction.
    b. The pupil is <4.0 mm in diameter.
    c. The patient has good potential vision.
    d. The patient seeks to minimize glare.
    e. The patient requests unilateral surgery.

35. Which of the following about the use of ophthalmic devices is true?
    a. It is considered medical malpractice to use a device off-label.
    b. All ophthalmic medical devices are reviewed by the Ophthalmic Devices Panel of the FDA.
    c. The Ophthalmic Devices Panel recommends approval if a device demonstrates reasonable safety and efficacy.
    d. If FDA approval is delayed, both the FDA and the company must keep the reasons confidential.
    e. All of the above are true.

36. Recent findings contradicting the Schachar theory of accommodation include all of the following *except:*
    a. Scanning electron microscopy in human eye tissues reveals no zonular insertions at the anterior ciliary muscle.
    b. Improved near vision in some patients after scleral expansion surgery is due to small changes in accommodative amplitude shown on infrared optometry.
    c. Crystalline lens diameter decreases with accommodation on various imaging techniques.
    d. Scanning laser imaging shows that the focal length of the crystalline lens remains unchanged with the application of equatorial radial stretching forces.

37. Which person would be the least appropriate candidate for conductive keratoplasty treatment for presbyopia?
    a. a 47-year-old long-haul truck driver with a distance manifest refraction of +1.25 sphere OU
    b. a 56-year-old emmetropic nurse supervisor
    c. a 44-year-old lawyer with a manifest refraction of +1.75 OU
    d. a 36-year-old librarian with a manifest refraction of +0.50 OU

38. Presbyopia progression theories are associated with all of the following physiologic findings *except:*
    a. a decreased response of the anterior lens curvature to a posterior vitreous pressure gradient generated by ciliary body contraction
    b. a decrease in ciliary muscle strength of approximately one third by age 85
    c. a decrease in lens capsule elasticity
    d. an increase in lens volume and anteroposterior (axial) lens thickness

39. The most important finding of the Prospective Evaluation of Radial Keratotomy (PERK) study was
    a. RK is effective for treating hyperopia
    b. PRK is more predictable than RK
    c. RK results in long-term unstable refraction
    d. the greater the number of incisions, the greater the effect on the cornea
    e. All the above were important findings.

40. Which of the following statements regarding the catenary theory of accommodation is true?
    a. Zonular fibers are under tension during the accommodated state.
    b. In this model, presbyopia involves age-related increasing lens volume with reduced curvature response of the anterior lens surface to posterior pressure on the lens.
    c. This theory helps explain the reduced accommodative amplitude typically seen after posterior vitrectomy.
    d. Ciliary body contraction during accommodation generates an increased anterior chamber pressure relative to that of the vitreous cavity.

41. "Coupling" with incisional correction of astigmatism is
    a. the concept of induced corneal steepening in the axis 90° from the axis of the astigmatic incision
    b. the same for arcuate and transverse incisional keratotomy
    c. not important when considering incisional surgery
    d. a ratio describing the amount of steepening in the axis of the incision compared to the amount of flattening 90° away

42. Intrastromal ring segments, or Intacs,
    a. were originally FDA approved to correct low myopia
    b. are placed in the peripheral cornea and cause indirect central corneal flattening
    c. are similar to Ferrara rings, which have a smaller optical zone
    d. may be helpful in improving vision in patients with keratoconus
    e. All the above are correct.

43. Which of the following is false concerning LASIK and glaucoma?
    a. IOP increases to more than 65 mm Hg when suction is applied.
    b. Central corneal thickness must be considered in evaluating applanation IOP.
    c. Ocular hypertension is not a contraindication to LASIK.
    d. The medical regimen should always be determined after LASIK is performed so that the post-LASIK IOP can be measured before instituting therapy.
    e. LASIK is contraindicated in any patient with marked optic nerve cupping, visual field loss, or loss of visual acuity.

44. Important pieces of information when attempting to calculate IOL power after refractive surgery include all the following *except:*
    a. preoperative axial length
    b. preoperative keratometry readings
    c. preoperative manifest refraction
    d. degree of attempted and achieved corrections

45. What is the most important reason that IOL calculation is less accurate after refractive surgery?
    a. inability to obtain accurate central corneal power measurements
    b. myopic shift due to nuclear sclerotic cataract
    c. diurnal variation in corneal curvature
    d. none of the above

46. Retinal detachments after LASIK are
    a. much more common than after PRK
    b. much less common than after PRK
    c. much harder to repair than after PRK
    d. none of the above

47. Contact lenses can be used after refractive surgery to do which of the following?
    a. prevent regression
    b. prevent astigmatism
    c. improve visual acuity in cases of irregular astigmatism
    d. reduce the chance of ectasia
    e. test a patient's candidacy for monovision

48. Excimer laser keratorefractive surgery does which of the following?
    a. induces a form of glaucoma
    b. falsely elevates IOP
    c. can damage the optic nerve without elevating IOP
    d. falsely lowers Goldmann applanation IOP measurements
    e. leads to corticosteroid-induced glaucoma

49. Potential complications of Intacs include all the following *except:*
    a. cataract
    b. epithelial defect
    c. neovascularization of the incision
    d. photophobia
    e. All the above are potential complications.

Answers

1. **d.** Patients with keratoconus have corneal thinning in the paracentral area. This can be diagnosed using slit-lamp biomicroscopy and optical or ultrasonic pachymetry. Topographic changes in keratoconus include central and inferior corneal steepening, hemimeridional asymmetry, and a high inferior–superior (I–S) number. LASIK should be avoided in keratoconus to prevent progressive ectasia of the cornea.
2. **e.** In conventional non–wavefront-guided laser treatment of myopia, the central cornea is flattened. Defocus (a second-order aberration) is corrected at the expense of induced spherical (high-order) aberrations.
3. **b.** Munnerlyn's approximation of the ablation depth per diopter of correction = $\text{diameter}^2/3$, where the diameter is in millimeters and the depth is in micrometers. Thus, the ablation depth is proportional to the square of the diameter. The depth of tissue ablation per diopter of correction is greater for wider ablation zones.
4. **d.** Contact lens wear can change the shape of the cornea and affect refractive error. In extreme cases, it can significantly distort the corneal curvature (a condition called *corneal warpage*). Removal of contact lenses prior to the refractive surgery evaluation and surgery is important to allow the corneal curvature to return to normal. Although recommendations vary, soft contact lenses are generally discontinued for at least 3–14 days and rigid gas-permeable contact lenses for 14–21 days. A stable refraction and a normal-appearing corneal curvature are important prior to any refractive surgery. Repeat examinations after discontinuation of contact lenses should be performed in patients who do not have stable refractions and normal corneal curvatures.
5. **d.** Social history, past ocular history, and past and current medical history are all important in the preoperative refractive surgery evaluation. Social history includes important information about visual requirements and the likelihood of ocular trauma. Past ocular history might alert the surgeon to recurrent erosion syndrome. Medical history is important to determine whether there are conditions that might affect ocular healing, such as diabetes or a connective tissue disorder.
6. **c.** The slit-lamp examination, including looking carefully for evidence of epithelial basement membrane dystrophy, is important in verifying that the cornea is healthy. Measurement of corneal curvature with corneal topography is important to ensure the cornea is regular and without evidence of ectasia (such as with keratoconus or pellucid marginal degeneration). Also, excessively steep or flat corneas increase the risk of flap complications from the microkeratome. Corneal thickness measurements are necessary to determine whether there is adequate corneal thickness to perform certain keratorefractive procedures, especially LASIK. Specular microscopy is not routinely performed prior to refractive surgery. If an endothelial abnormality is suspected, then specular microscopy can be performed.
7. **b.** Patients under age 35 are generally not interested in monovision. Success with monovision in the past indicates that the patient is likely to have success in the future. Ocular dominance is tested, because most patients are happiest with the nondominant eye corrected for near. However, monovision should be demonstrated in trial spectacles and/or contact lenses to assess the patient's preoperative satisfaction with this approach. Patients with both low and high myopia can enjoy successful monovision.

8. **b.** LASIK is generally used to correct from –10 to +4 D and PRK from –8 to +4 D. Unlike LASIK, PRK for higher levels of myopia is associated with a greater incidence of postoperative corneal haze. Consequently, most surgeons prefer LASIK to PRK for higher levels of myopia (above –6 D). If LASIK is contraindicated for reasons such as insufficient corneal thickness, some surgeons will perform PRK with "prophylactic" mitomycin C to attempt to decrease the possibility of corneal haze postoperatively.
9. **a.** Thermokeratoplasty is associated with refractive regression, does not correct astigmatism, and does not reliably create a multifocal cornea that results in good uncorrected distance and near vision. The best answer is a.
10. **c.** Clear lens extraction in high myopia is associated with a higher risk of retinal detachment. The risk increases over time. When postoperative years 1 and 7 were compared, a fourfold increase in risk was documented.
11. **b.** This patient may be appropriate for PIOL insertion. Acceptable criteria include age 21 or older, internal anterior chamber depth of at least 3.0 mm, a clear lens with a low risk of cataract formation, a stable refraction, and no more than 2.00 D of astigmatic correction.
12. **a.** Unlike with LASIK, there is no removal of corneal tissue in incisional keratotomy. In LASIK, if excessive tissue is removed, it may result in corneal ectasia; corneal ectasia should not result after radial or astigmatic keratotomy. However, corneal incisions may cause corneal instability, with diurnal fluctuation of vision and/or continued effect of surgery over time. Any type of refractive surgery performed on a cornea with abnormal preoperative topography, such as forme fruste keratoconus or pellucid marginal degeneration, may be associated with unpredictable postoperative results.
13. **c.** The inlay impedes the flow of nutrients to the overlying stroma and can result in necrosis. Reflection of ultraviolet light from the inlay is not a recognized cause of necrosis. The epithelium and superficial stroma rely on diffusion from the tear film for oxygen. Trauma at the time of surgery can damage the stroma but is not generally responsible for the necrosis seen after inlay implantation.
14. **c.** Infectious keratitis, ectasia, buttonholes, and free caps are all complications of LASIK and all are fortunately very rare. However, dry eye disease occurs in almost every patient who undergoes LASIK. Dry eye is caused in part by corneal anesthesia due to transection of the corneal nerves by creation of the flap and ablation of the neural plexus with the excimer laser. Dry eye usually lasts 3–6 months before resolving and is most commonly manifested by fluctuating visual acuity.
15. **c.** The PMMA corneal ring segments can be removed, making the refractive results potentially reversible. Unlike most other forms of keratorefractive surgery, surgery is not performed on the cornea overlying the pupil. The ring segments can be replaced to alter the refractive result. Intacs are not approved to treat astigmatism.
16. **d.** Treatment of dry eye disease following LASIK is often multifactorial and involves management of meibomian gland disease, immunomodulation of the lacrimal gland, and conservation of existing tears. For this reason, omega-3 fatty acids such as flaxseed oil and fish oils and cyclosporine improve the quality of the tear film; and punctal occlusion preserves the existing tear film. These therapies may be given together or sequentially to manage dry eye following LASIK.

17. **a.** Mitomycin C has been shown to reduce corneal scarring—and thus haze—by preventing the activation of fibroblasts following excimer laser ablation. The concentration of mitomycin C is usually 0.02% or 0.2 mg/mL. The mitomycin C is placed on the ablated surface for approximately 12 seconds to 2 minutes at the end of the laser exposure. The duration of mitomycin C application varies by diagnosis and surgeon preference.
18. **c.** Photoablation. The high-energy photons emitted by the 193-nm excimer laser rupture the collagen peptide backbone of the cornea and eject the protein fragments into the air, ablating the desired cornea.
19. **d.** Ectatic corneal disorders are the second most common indication for keratoplasty, accounting for about 15% of corneal transplants performed in the United States. Although several possible risk factors for post-LASIK ectasia have been identified in the literature, ectasia can develop in eyes with no currently identifiable risk factors. A computer-generated diagnosis of "keratoconus suspect" is not necessarily a contraindication to LASIK, as this decision should be based on the entire clinical picture. No specific test or measurement is diagnostic of a corneal ectatic disorder.
20. **e.** All of the factors listed are presumed risk factors for ectasia.
21. **a.** A steep cornea protrudes higher above the suction ring and therefore more corneal surface area is exposed to the mechanical microkeratome.
22. **a.** The endothelial pump creates a negative suction pressure in the corneal stroma.
23. **c.** In most cases, the surgeon can lift the original flap for at least several years after the original procedure. A residual stromal bed of at least 250 μm is recommended to avoid postoperative ectasia.
24. **a.** The transection of the corneal nerves in the creation of the flap leads to a neurotrophic epitheliopathy.
25. **d.** Diffuse lamellar keratitis (DLK) is a nonspecific inflammatory response to a variety of toxic insults and is usually noninfectious. Although DLK may be associated with primary or enhancement LASIK procedures, it may also occur in other settings, such as after corneal epithelial erosion. DLK is treated primarily with topical corticosteroids. Severe cases of DLK (stage 4) are at risk for collagenase release and corneal melting.
26. **d.** DLK typically is visible within the first 24 hours after surgery, begins at the flap periphery, is usually confined to the area of the flap interface, involves a diffuse distribution of inflammatory cells without a focal infiltrate, and is associated with minimal pain or photophobia.
27. **b.** The probe heats the corneal epithelium as well as the stroma. Although a decentered corneal apex may have less than optimal results, it is not a contraindication to CK. After CK, there is regression toward increasing hyperopia.
28. **d.** Radiofrequency energy is used during CK, and the resistance to the current creates localized heat.
29. **d.** Although there are isolated case reports of glaucomatous damage or progression following LASIK surgery, several controlled prospective studies in normal patients have not demonstrated NFL loss or glaucomatous damage following LASIK. LASIK surgery can cause glaucoma progression in patients with preexisting glaucoma, due to the period of elevated IOP during attachment of the suction ring used in flap creation. Postoperative Goldmann applanation IOP readings are usually lower than preoperative values due to the thinner corneal thickness after ablation.

30. **d.** LASIK should not be performed in keratoconus because this may lead to progression of the corneal ectasia, with worsening of uncorrected and best-corrected visual acuity, which may necessitate earlier corneal transplantation. LASIK can be performed in well-controlled rheumatoid arthritis and in amblyopia when the amblyopic eye retains functional vision. LASIK has also been performed successfully after suture removal in eyes with well-healed penetrating keratoplasty wounds.

31. **c.** PIOLs can correct a wide range of refractive error, from high myopia to high hyperopia. PIOLs are inserted over the clear lens. They have the advantage of not being dependent on corneal thickness or steepness.

32. **e.** Patients who have bioptics will still require reading glasses unless the treatment is adjusted for monovision. The other statements are all true.

33. **a.** The optics of PCPIOLs, such as the Visian ICL (STAAR), are foldable, but some iris-fixated IOL optics and ACPIOLs are made of PMMA and cannot fold. This increases the risk of surgically induced astigmatism. The other statements are true.

34. **c.** The ideal candidate for a multifocal IOL has <1.00 D of astigmatism, has a pupil >4.0 mm in diameter in order to fully benefit from the multifocal effect, has less concern about glare, requires bilateral surgery, and has good potential vision.

35. **c.** The Ophthalmic Devices Panel of the FDA recommends approval if a device demonstrates reasonable safety and efficacy. If a treating clinician does not follow labeling recommendations for a device, it is being used "off-label." Although this is not malpractice if it follows the standard of care for treatment in that community, the clinician should consider discussing the off-label usage with the patient. The Ophthalmic Devices Panel is an advisory panel that most typically reviews first-of-a-kind medical devices and premarket approval (PMA) applications that raise new issues of safety and efficacy. The FDA and its agents are bound by rules of confidentiality, but the company is not and, if it wishes, can release information.

36. **b.** Subjective improvement in near vision is experienced by some patients after they undergo any of the various methods of scleral expansion surgery. These improvements have not been completely explained, are usually transient, and are possibly the result of depth of focus changes, patient effort, test learning, and nonlenticular optical shifts. Dynamic testing with infrared optometers has revealed no increase in the amplitude of accommodation after scleral expansion surgery.

37. **d.** All of these patients may benefit somewhat from the induction of mild myopia (modified monovision) in the nondominant eye. The truck driver could regain the ability to see the dashboard clearly while having a 95% chance of maintaining better than 20/25 binocular distance vision. The nurse and the lawyer could both gain uncorrected near vision in their nondominant eye. The librarian, whose day is spent in constant close-in work, would probably not tolerate the induced myopia—even in her nondominant eye—due to her young age and her intact ability for full accommodation.

38. **b.** A reduction in the overall mobility of the ciliary muscle fibers is seen with advancing presbyopia, a reduction believed to be due to an increase in connective tissue between the fibers. In cross section, the ciliary body changes with age from a lenticular-shaped structure to a more triangular one. A number of recent studies, however, reveal that little if any contractile strength of the ciliary muscle fibers is lost in the normal aging process of the eye. (Without the preserved strength/function of the muscle, the recent success seen with the new accommodating IOLs would not be possible.)

39. **c.** The PERK study evaluated 8-incision RK for myopia. It did not evaluate different numbers of incisions or compare RK results to PRK results. The 5- and 10-year PERK results demonstrated progressive flattening and induced hyperopia in a significant number of patients.

40. **b.** The catenary, or hydraulic support, theory of accommodation proposes that the lens, zonules, and anterior vitreous act as a functional diaphragm between the vitreous cavity and the anterior chamber. Contraction of the ciliary body generates an elevated posterior pressure in the vitreous cavity, causing anterior movement of the lens–zonule diaphragm. As with the Helmholtz theory, this contraction also results in a relaxation of the zonular fibers during accommodation. Presbyopic changes are believed to be due to a reduced response of anterior lens curvature to the vitreous pressure generated by ciliary body contraction in accommodation.

41. **a.** Correcting astigmatism with incisional surgery can be performed with arcuate (curved) incisions or transverse (straight) incisions. Both cause flattening in the axis of the incision and steepening 90° away. The amount of flattening and steepening depends on the type and length of the incision. The ratio of flattening to steepening is the "coupling ratio." When it is 1, there is no change in spherical equivalent.

42. **e.** Intacs were originally FDA approved in 1999 to treat −1.00 to −3.00 D of myopia; in 2004, Intacs received a humanitarian device exemption (HDE) for the treatment of keratoconus. The ring segments are polymethylmethacrylate (PMMA) arcs that are placed in the deep midperipheral cornea, causing central flattening. Intacs are placed at an optical zone of approximately 7 mm; Ferrara rings are slightly thicker than Intacs and are placed at an optical zone of about 5 mm.

43. **d.** Optimal topical IOP-lowering therapy should be determined before LASIK is considered in the glaucoma patient. Because of the difficulty in interpreting IOP measurements, PRK and LASIK should not be considered until the IOP is well controlled.

44. **a.** One of the most accurate methods for determining the power of the IOL after refractive surgery is the historical method, which uses the preoperative keratometry readings, preoperative manifest refraction, and attempted and achieved corrections. The preoperative axial length does not change significantly after refractive surgery. New axial length measurements are also accurate after refractive surgery.

45. **a.** Although both myopic shift due to nuclear sclerosis and diurnal variation in corneal curvature do occur, the primary difficulty in obtaining accurate IOL calculations after refractive surgery is the inability to obtain accurate central corneal power measurements from the instruments used, which were developed to measure curvature in "normal" eyes.

46. **d.** There is no convincing evidence that retinal detachments are more or less frequent after LASIK than after PRK (when the degree of preoperative myopia is controlled for). Although the surgeon should avoid trauma to the LASIK flap to decrease the risk of flap dehiscence and epithelial defect, retinal detachment surgery is no more difficult in LASIK than in PRK.

47. **c.** Contact lenses will not prevent anatomical changes or reduce their occurrence in the cornea postoperatively. If monovision is being considered, it should be done before refractive surgery. Contact lenses can improve visual function in cases of irregular astigmatism.

48. **d.** After laser surgery for myopia, the measured Goldmann applanation IOP is lower than the actual IOP. This can result in glaucomatous damage despite normal IOP readings. IOP should be measured from the side of the cornea, and the optic nerve should be carefully evaluated on an ongoing basis to reduce the likelihood of undetected glaucomatous damage. Newer technology may improve the accuracy of IOP measurements after laser refractive surgery by neutralizing the effect of corneal thickness.

49. **a.** Intacs are placed in channels located at approximately two thirds of corneal depth. These channels are made with a mechanical separator or a femtosecond laser. The surgery can cause an epithelial defect; the incision may become vascularized. Intacs cause photophobia in some patients, rarely requiring removal. As the surgery is extraocular, it is not associated with cataract formation.

Index

(*f* = figure; *t* = table)

Aberrations. *See also specific type*
higher-order, 17–18, 18*f*, 19*f*, 20*f*
wavefront-optimized/wavefront-guided ablation and, 17, 30–31, 146–147
after LASIK, 144–145
lower-order, 16, 16*f*, 17*f*
after surface ablation, 105
Accommodating intraocular lenses, 182–184, 198–200, 199*f*
Accommodation, 187–191, 188*f*, 189*f*, 190*f*
catenary (hydraulic support) theory of, 190–191
Helmholtz (capsular) theory of, 187–188, 188*f*
Schachar theory of, 188–190, 189*f*, 190*f*
Accommodative esotropia, refractive surgery and, 219
ACPIOL (anterior chamber phakic intraocular lenses). *See* Phakic intraocular lenses, anterior chamber
Acquired immunodeficiency syndrome, refractive surgery and, 219–221
AcrySof IQ intraocular lens, 184
AcrySof ReSTOR intraocular lens, 180, 181, 181*f*, 193–194, 193*f*
AcrySof toric intraocular lens, 178, 178*f*, 179, 180
ACS. *See* Anterior ciliary sclerotomy
AcuFocus corneal inlay, 74
Adjustable refractive surgery (ARS), 171–172, 173*t*
Age/aging
accommodative response/presbyopia and, 187
refractive surgery and, 44
radial keratotomy and, 63
surface ablation, 92
overcorrection and, 104
wavefront aberrations and, 17
AIDS, refractive surgery and, 219–221
Air–tear film interface, optical power of eye and, 5
ALK. *See* Automated lamellar keratoplasty
Alloplastic intracorneal implants
corneal biomechanics affected by, 24, 24*f*
corneal inlays
in keratophakia, 74
for presbyopia, 74, 195
corneal onlays, in epikeratoplasty (epikeratophakia), 76–77
Amblyopia, refractive surgery and, 216–219
Amiodarone, refractive surgery in patient taking, 92
Anesthesia (anesthetics), for phakic IOL insertion, 162
Angle-supported intraocular lenses, 159*t*, 160*t*, 162–163, 163*f*
Anisometropia
amblyopia caused by (anisometropic amblyopia), refractive surgery and, 216–219
after penetrating keratoplasty, refractive surgery for, 209
Anterior chamber
depth of, in phakic IOL selection, 162
flat or shallow, refractive surgery and, 48
Anterior chamber intraocular lenses. *See* Intraocular lenses
Anterior ciliary sclerotomy, for presbyopia, 197
Anterior segment, examination of before refractive surgery, 48
Antibiotics
after LASIK, 123
prophylactic, for surface ablation, 94
after surface ablation, 99, 100
Antihistamines, refractive surgery in patient taking, 43
Antimicrobial prophylaxis, for surface ablation, 94
Aphakia, epikeratoplasty (epikeratophakia) for, 75–77, 75*f*, 76*f*
Applanation tonometry
corneal thickness affecting, 211
after LASIK, 47
after surface ablation, 108
Aqueous tear deficiency, refractive surgery and, 47, 47*f*
ARC-T trial, 70
Arcuate incisions (tangential/linear incisions), for keratorefractive surgery, corneal biomechanics affected by, 20–23, 23*f*, 68
Arcuate keratotomy (AK), 68–71, 69*t*, 70*f*
complications of, 71
instrumentation for, 69, 70*f*
ocular surgery after, 71
outcomes of, 70
surgical technique for, 70
ArF laser. *See* Argon-fluoride excimer laser
Argon-fluoride excimer laser, for photoablation, 29, 89–92, 90–91*f*. *See also* Photoablation
Array multifocal lens, 180, 193
ARS. *See* Adjustable refractive surgery
Arthritis, rheumatoid, refractive surgery contraindicated in, 222
Artificial tears, for dry eye after LASIK, 136
Astigmatic keratotomy, 21–22*t*, 23*f*
wound healing/repair and, 27
Astigmatic photorefractive keratectomy (toric PRK), 101–102
Astigmatism
after angle-supported anterior chamber phakic IOL insertion, 163
in cataract patient, toric intraocular lenses for, 177–180, 178*f*
after clear lens extraction/refractive lens exchange, 174–175
corneal topography in detection/management of, 8–10, 9*f*
hyperopic
LASIK for, 126
PRK for, 102
irregular
after arcuate keratotomy, 71
corneal topography in detection/management of, 10, 49
keratorefractive surgery and, 14, 49
after limbal relaxing incisions, 71
after penetrating keratoplasty, refractive surgery for, 209, 210
wavefront analysis and, 14

mixed
LASIK for, 126
PRK for, 102
myopic, LASIK for, 125–126
after penetrating keratoplasty
corneal topography in management of, 13–14
refractive surgery for, 209, 210–211
after radial keratotomy, 65
regular
corneal topography in detection/management of, 8, 9*f*
wavefront aberration produced by, 16, 16*f*
secondary, wavefront aberration produced by, 18, 19*f*
surgical correction of. *See also specific procedure*
arcuate keratotomy for, 68–71, 69*t*, 70*f*
conductive keratoplasty for, 154
incisional corneal surgery for, 67–71, 68*f*, 69*f*, 69*t*, 70*f*
LASIK for
hyperopia and, 126
mixed astigmatism and, 126
myopia and, 125–126
light-adjustable IOLs for, 184–185, 185*f*
limbal relaxing incisions for, 68–71, 68*f*, 69*f*, 70*f*
PRK for, 101–102
hyperopic astigmatic, 102
mixed astigmatic, 102
toric (photoastigmatic keratectomy), 101–102
toric intraocular lenses for, 177–180, 178*f*
wavefront-guided laser ablation for, 146–147
Autoimmune diseases, refractive surgery in patient with, 222
Automated lamellar keratoplasty, 110
Axial curvature, 6–7, 7*f*
Axial power, 6–7, 7*f*

Bandage contact lenses
after LASIK
epithelial erosions and, 132
epithelial ingrowth prevention and, 142
striae and, 133, 135
after surface ablation, 97*f*, 99, 230
for overcorrection, 104
sterile infiltrates associated with, 107–108, 107*f*
Bichrome (red-green/duochrome) test, before refractive surgery, 45
Biomechanics of cornea, 19–27
keratorefractive surgery affecting, 20–27, 28–29*t*
alloplastic material addition and, 24, 24*f*
collagen shrinkage and, 27, 27*f*
incisional effect and, 20–23, 23*f*, 67–68, 68*f*
laser effect and, 24–25, 25*f*, 26*f*
tissue addition/subtraction and, 23–24, 23*f*
Biometry/biometrics, in IOL selection, clear lens extraction/refractive lens exchange and, 176
Biomicroscopy, slit-lamp
before refractive surgery, 47, 47*f*, 48*f*, 49*f*
in striae in LASIK flaps, 132, 134*t*
Bioptics, 157, 171–172, 173*t*
Bitoric ablation, 25
Blend zone, 90*f*, 94
Blepharitis, refractive surgery in patients with, 47, 48*f*
Blood, in LASIK interface, 142, 143*f*
Blunt trauma, LASIK flap dislocation and, 136
Breast feeding, refractive surgery contraindicated during, 43
Broad-beam lasers, for photoablation, 29
central island formation and, 104
Bull's-eye optic, for corneal inlay for presbyopia, 196
Buttonhole flap, 130, 130*f*

Capsular opacification, with multifocal IOLs, 194
Capsular theory (Helmholtz hypothesis) of accommodation, 187–188, 188*f*
Cataract
after iris-fixated phakic IOL insertion, 167*t*, 169
after posterior chamber phakic IOL insertion, 167*t*, 169–170, 170
refractive surgery in patient with, 48
Cataract surgery
after arcuate keratotomy, 71
astigmatism and, toric IOL for, 177–180, 178*f*
intraocular lens implantation and, 192–194
after limbal relaxing incisions, 71
after radial keratotomy, 67, 226
with refractive surgery, 192–194
retinal detachment after, 215
Catenary (hydraulic support) theory of accommodation, 190–191
Center-surround optic, for corneal inlay for presbyopia, 196
Centering procedures
for LASIK, 122–123
radial keratotomy outcome affected by, 62
for surface ablation, 98–99, 98*f*
decentered ablation and, 105–106, 106*f*
Central islands
after LASIK, 137
after surface ablation, 104, 105*f*
Central optical clear zone
in radial keratotomy, 62
outcome affected by, 62, 65
in surface ablation, preoperative laser programming and, 94
Children, refractive surgery in, 218
Ciliary muscle, in accommodation, 187–190, 188*f*, 189*f*
CK. *See* Conductive keratoplasty
CLAPIKS (contact lens–assisted, pharmacologically induced keratosteepening), 232
Clear lens extraction (refractive lens exchange), 53*t*, 172–177
advantages of, 177
complications of, 177
disadvantages of, 177
indications for, 172
informed consent for, 172–174
IOL calculations for, 176
patient selection for, 172–174
retinal detachment and, 174, 175, 177, 215
surgical planning/techniques for, 174–176
"Clinical history method," for IOL power calculation after refractive surgery, 224
Clinical studies, for unapproved medical device, 36
Closed-loop trackers, 101
Collagen, stromal, corneal haze after surface ablation and, 106

Collagen shrinkage, 22*t*, 27, 27*f*, 149–155. *See also* *specific procedure*
conductive keratoplasty for, 22*t*, 27, 27*f*, 150–155
corneal biomechanics affected by, 27, 27*f*
history of, 149–150
laser thermokeratoplasty for, 27, 150
Collagen-vascular diseases. *See also* Connective tissue disorders
refractive surgery in patient with, 205
Colvard pupillometer, 46
Coma (wavefront aberration), 17, 18*f*
Compromised host, refractive surgery in, 43
Computerized corneal topography, 6–14, 49–50, 50*f*. *See also* Cornea, topography of
Conductive keratoplasty, 22*t*, 27, 27*f*, 150–155, 151*f*, 152*f*, 152*t*, 153*f*, 154*t*
corneal transplantation after, 228
for presbyopia, 151, 153, 192
Confrontation testing, before refractive surgery, 46
Conjunctiva, examination of, before refractive surgery, 47
Connective tissue disorders, refractive surgery in patient with, 205, 222
surface ablation, 92
Consecutive hyperopia, 104
contact lens–assisted, pharmacologically induced keratosteepening (CLAPIKS) for, 232
Consent, informed, for refractive surgery
clear lens extraction/refractive lens exchange and, 172–174
LASIK and, 54–58
in patient with ocular or systemic disease, 203–204
phakic intraocular lens insertion and, 162
Contact lens–assisted, pharmacologically induced keratosteepening (CLAPIKS), 232
Contact lens method, for IOL power calculation after refractive surgery, 225–226
Contact lenses
bandage
after LASIK, 231
epithelial erosions and, 132
epithelial ingrowth prevention and, 142
striae and, 133, 135
after surface ablation, 97*f*, 99, 230
overcorrection and, 104
sterile infiltrates and, 107–108, 107*f*
discontinuing use of, before refractive surgery, 44
history of use of, before refractive surgery, 43
keratosteepening and (contact lens–assisted, pharmacologically induced keratosteepening/ CLAPIKS), 232
after LASIK, 231–232
monovision and, as trial for surgery, 191
for myopia reduction (orthokeratology), 86–87
after radial keratotomy, 229–230, 230*f*
after refractive/keratorefractive surgery, 228–232
after surface ablation, 230–231
Contrast sensitivity
with multifocal IOLs, 182
with phakic IOLs, 165
Cornea
biomechanics of, 19–27
keratorefractive surgery affecting, 20–27, 28–29*t*
alloplastic material addition and, 24, 24*f*
collagen shrinkage and, 27, 27*f*
incisional effect and, 20–23, 23*f*, 67–68, 68*f*
laser effect and, 24–25, 25*f*, 26*f*
tissue addition/subtraction and, 23–24, 23*f*
curvature of. *See also* Cornea, topography of
axial, 6–7
power and, 5–6, 6–7, 7*f*
radius of, instantaneous (meridional/tangential power), 7, 7*f*
refractive surgery affecting, IOL power calculation and, 223
ectasia of. *See* Ectasia/ectatic disorders
edema of
after incisional surgery, 61
orthokeratology causing, 86–87
after radial keratotomy, 67
refractive surgery contraindicated in, 47
endothelium of
anterior chamber phakic IOLs affecting, 167*t*, 168, 170
iris-fixated phakic IOLs affecting, 167*t*, 169
posterior chamber phakic IOLs affecting, 167*t*, 169
surface ablation and, 108
epithelium of
debridement of for surface ablation, 95, 96*f*
preservation techniques for
in epi-LASIK, 96–97
in LASEK, 95–96, 97*f*
wound healing/repair of, after surface ablation, 27
delayed, 107
erosions of
after LASIK, 131–132
refractive surgery in patient with, 47, 48*f*
examination of, before refractive surgery, 47, 48*f*
flat, flap creation and, 50, 114
melting of (keratolysis), refractive surgery and, 222
oblate shape of, 6, 8
perforation of
LASIK and, 130–131
radial keratotomy and, 63, 65, 65*f*
prolate shape of, 6, 8
intrastromal corneal ring segments and, 77–78
refractive power of, estimation of after refractive surgery, 223–224
shape of, 5–6, 7–8
aspheric, 6, 8
curvature and power and, 5–8, 7*f*
refractive surgery and, 5–6
steep, flap creation and, 50, 114
thickness of
intraocular pressure evaluation and, 211
measurement of. *See also* Pachymetry
minimum requirements for LASIK and, 114–115
corneal perforation and, 131
before refractive surgery, 50–51
refractive surgery affected by, corneal topography and, 12–13
topography of, 5–6, 6–14, 49–50, 50*f*
central islands after surface ablation and, 104, 105*f*
computerized, 6–14, 49–50, 50*f*
elevation-based, 6, 8, 8*f*
before LASIK, 114
limitations of, 12
after penetrating keratoplasty, 13–14
Placido-based, 6
in pellucid marginal degeneration, 13

after radial keratotomy, 64
refractive surgery and, 5–6, 6–14, 49–50, 50*f*, 93
clinical situations illustrating role of, 12–14
indications for, 8–10, 9*f*
postoperative, 10, 11*f*
transplantation of. *See also* Keratoplasty, penetrating
after refractive surgery, 227–228
warpage of
contact lens wear causing, refractive surgery and, 44, 49
topography in identification of, 10, 49
wound healing/repair of, keratorefractive surgery and, 27–28
delays in, 107
Corneal dystrophies, epithelial, basement membrane (map-dot-fingerprint/anterior membrane), refractive surgery in patients with, 47, 49*f*
LASIK, 114
surface ablation, 93
Corneal flap folds, after LASIK, 132–136, 134*t*, 135*f*. *See also* Striae
Corneal grafts. *See* Cornea, transplantation of
Corneal haze. *See* Haze formation
Corneal inlays, 73–87
alloplastic, 74
homoplastic, 73–74
in keratophakia, 73–75
for presbyopia, 74, 195–196
Corneal onlays, 73–87
alloplastic, in epikeratoplasty (epikeratophakia), 76–77
Corneal power maps, 6–7, 49
Corneal refractive therapy (orthokeratology), 86–87
Corneal ring segments, intrastromal, 53*t*, 77–86
advantages of, 77–78
complications of, 83–85, 83*f*, 84*f*, 85*f*
corneal biomechanics affected by, 24, 24*f*, 77–78
corneal transplantation after, 228
disadvantages of, 78
instrumentation for, 79, 79*t*
international trends in use of, 238
for keratoconus, 13, 81–83, 82*f*, 208
after LASIK, 85
for myopia, 77–81, 77*f*, 78*f*, 79*t*, 80*f*
patient selection for, 78–79
outcomes of, 80–81
removal of, 81
technique for, 79–80, 80*f*
Corneal surgery, incisional, 61–71
for astigmatism correction, 67–71, 68*f*, 69*f*, 69*t*, 70*f*
for myopia, 61–67, 63*f*, 64*f*, 65*f*, 66*f*
Corticosteroids (steroids)
corneal wound healing and, 28
after LASIK, 123
after refractive surgery, elevated IOP/glaucoma and, 47, 108, 212, 213, 233
after surface ablation, 99, 100
complications associated with, 108
corneal haze and, 106
for regression in overcorrection, 104
for regression in undercorrection, 104
Coupling, 20, 23*f*, 67–68, 68*f*
Cryolathe, 109
Crystalens, for refractive errors/presbyopia, 182–183, 198–200, 199*f*
Curvature (corneal). *See also* Cornea, topography of
axial, 6–7
power and, 5–6, 6–7, 7*f*
radius of, instantaneous (meridional/tangential power), 7, 7*f*
refractive surgery affecting, IOL power calculation and, 223
Custom ablation. *See also* Wavefront-guided laser ablation
for presbyopia, 194–195, 195*f*
Cutting head, of microkeratome, 110, 111–112*f*
Cycloplegic refraction. *See also* Refraction
before refractive surgery, 45

Debridement, epithelial, for surface ablation, 95, 96*f*
Decentered ablation, 105–106, 106*f*
Decentration, of phakic intraocular lenses, 170, 170*f*
Defibrillator-cardioverters, implantable (ICDs), laser surgery in patient with, 43
Defocus, positive and negative, 16, 16*f*
Deformable intraocular lenses, 183
Dexamethasone, after surface ablation, elevated IOP associated with, 108
Diabetes mellitus, refractive surgery in patient with, 92, 221–222
Diathermy, for conductive thermokeratoplasty, 27, 149
Difference map
after intrastromal corneal ring segment placement, 82, 82*f*
after keratorefractive surgery, 10, 11*f*
Diffractive multifocal intraocular lenses, 180, 193–194
Diffuse lamellar (interface) keratitis (DLK), after LASIK, 137–138, 137*f*, 138*t*, 139*t*, 140*f*
femtosecond laser flap creation and, 119
glaucoma/IOP measurement and, 233
Dilated fundus examination, before refractive surgery, 49
Diplopia, after LASIK, 145
in amblyopia patient, 217–218
Diurnal variation in vision, after radial keratotomy, 64
DLK. *See* Diffuse lamellar (interface) keratitis
Donor cornea, prior LASIK affecting, 228
Dry eye syndrome
after LASIK, 114, 136, 204
microkeratome hinge position and, 112
LASIK in patient with, 136, 204
refractive surgery and, 47, 204–205
after surface ablation, 108, 204
epithelial defect and, 107
Dual-optic intraocular lenses, 183, 200
Duochrome (red-green/bichrome) test, before refractive surgery, 45
Dystrophies, corneal, refractive surgery in patients with, 47, 49*f*
LASIK, 114
surface ablation, 93

Ectasia/ectatic disorders, corneal
after LASIK, 143–144
intrastromal corneal ring segments for, 85, 143
refractive surgery contraindicated in, corneal topography in detection of, 10

Elevated intraocular pressure
after iris-fixated phakic IOL insertion, 167*t*
after LASIK, 211–213, 212*f*
pressure-induced stromal keratitis and, 138–139
after posterior chamber phakic IOL insertion, 167*t*
refractive surgery and, 211–213, 212*f*
after surface ablation, 108
Elevation-based topography, 6, 7*f*, 8
Elevation maps, 8, 8*f*
Emmetropization, myopia and, 237
Endothelium, corneal
anterior chamber phakic IOLs affecting, 167*t*, 168, 169
iris-fixated phakic IOLs affecting, 167*t*, 169
posterior chamber phakic IOLs affecting, 167*t*, 179
surface ablation and, 108
epi-LASIK. *See* Epithelial laser in situ keratomileusis
Epikeratoplasty (epikeratophakia), 21*t*, 24, 75–77, 75*f*, 76*f*
laser-adjustable synthetic, 76–77
Epithelial defects
after LASIK, 131–132
in diabetic patients, 221
refractive surgery in patients with, 47, 48*f*
after surface ablation, 107
Epithelial downgrowth (ingrowth), after LASIK, 140–142, 141*f*, 142*f*
in diabetic patients, 221
haze formation and, 28
Epithelial dystrophies, basement membrane, refractive surgery in patients with, 47, 49*f*
LASIK, 114
surface ablation, 93
Epithelial erosions
after LASIK, 131–132
refractive surgery in patient with, 47, 48*f*
Epithelial laser in situ keratomileusis (epi-LASIK), 28, 92–109. *See also* Surface ablation
calibration of excimer laser for, 93
central islands and, 104, 105*f*
centration and ablation in, 98–99, 98*f*
complications of, 103–108
corneal haze and, 106–107, 106*f*
corneal wound healing and, 28
corticosteroid-induced complications after, 108
decentered ablation and, 105–106, 106*f*
dry eye after, 108
endothelial effects of, 108
enhancements/reoperation and, 103
epithelial debridement for, 95, 96*f*
epithelial defects and, 107
epithelial preservation techniques for, 96–97
glaucoma/ocular hypertension and, 108, 213
global estimates of, 236*f*
infiltrates and, 107–108, 107*f*
international trends in use of, 238
laser ablation technique in, 98–100, 98*f*
optical aberrations and, 105
outcomes of, 100–103
overcorrection and, 103–104
patient selection for, 92–93
postablation measures and
immediate, 99
operative day, 99
subsequent postoperative care, 100
preoperative planning/laser programming for, 93–94
surgical technique for, 93–97
tracking devices for, 101
undercorrection and, 104
Epithelium, corneal
debridement of for surface ablation, 95, 96*f*
healing of after surface ablation, 27
delayed, 107
preservation techniques for
in epi-LASIK, 96–97
in LASEK, 95–96, 97*f*
Erbium:YAG (Er:YAG) laser, for scleral expansion, 198
Erosions, epithelial
after LASIK, 131–132
refractive surgery in patient with, 47, 48*f*
Esotropia, accommodative, refractive surgery and, 219
Examination, ophthalmic, before refractive surgery, 45–49, 47*f*, 48*f*, 49*f*
ancillary tests and, 49–52
Excimer laser, for photoablation, 29, 89–92, 90–91*f*. *See also specific procedure*
herpes simplex virus keratitis and, 205–206
international preferences and, 238
LASIK, 122–123, 123*f*
ablation technique and, 122–123, 123*f*
preoperative inspection of, 113
preoperative programming of, 116–117
for presbyopia, 194–195, 195*f*
surface ablation
ablation technique and, 98–100, 98*f*
calibration of, 93
preoperative programming of, 93–94
wavefront-guided, 147
higher-order aberrations and, 17, 146–147
Eye, examination of, before refractive surgery, 45–49, 47*f*, 48*f*, 49*f*
ancillary tests and, 49–52
Eye banking, screening for prior LASIK and, 228
Eyelids, examination of, before refractive surgery, 47

FDA. *See* Food and Drug Administration
Feiz nomogram, 225, 225*t*, 226
Femtosecond laser
for LASIK flap creation, 113, 118–120, 119*f*, 120*f*, 121*f*, 121*t*
advantages/disadvantages of, 119, 120, 121*t*
ocular aberrations and, 144
steep or flat corneas and, 50, 114
for photodisruption, 29
Ferrara rings, 77. *See also* Intrastromal corneal ring segments
international trends in use of, 238
Filtering procedures, LASIK and, 213
Fitting (contact lens), after refractive surgery, 228–232
510(k) (premarket notification) application, 36–37
Flap folds, after LASIK, 132–136, 134*t*, 135*f*. *See also* Striae
Flaps, LASIK
buttonhole, 130, 130*f*
dislocation/subluxation of, 136
striae and, 133
femtosecond creation of, 113, 118–120, 119*f*, 120*f*, 121*f*, 121*t*
steep or flat corneas and, 50, 114

haze formation and, 28
infected, 139–140, 139*t*, 140*f*, 141*f*
microkeratome creation of, 110–113, 111–112*f*, 117–118, 117*f*, 118*f*
complications associated with, 129–131, 130*f*, 131*f*
ocular aberrations associated with creation of, 144
penetrating keratoplasty and, 210
replacement of, 123
retinal detachment repair and, 227
retreatment and, 127–129, 128*f*
steep or flat corneas and, 50, 114
striae in, 132–136, 134*t*, 135*f*
Flat anterior chamber. *See* Anterior chamber, flat or shallow
Flexible (soft) contact lenses
after LASIK, 231
after radial keratotomy, 230
refractive surgery and, 228–229
after surface ablation, 230–231
Fluorometholone, after surface ablation, elevated IOP associated with, 108
Flying-spot lasers, for photoablation, 29–30
Foldable posterior chamber phakic intraocular lenses, 164–165, 164*f*, 165*f*
Food and Drug Administration, 33–39
adverse event reporting to, 39
delays in device approval by, 38–39
lasers approved by, 34–35*t*
medical device classification by, 33–36
medical device pathways to market and, 36–37
Food, Drug, and Cosmetic Act, 33
Forme fruste. *See also* Keratoconus
ectasia after LASIK and, 143
phakic IOLs for, 161
refractive surgery contraindicated in, 10, 207, 207*f*
topography in detection of, 10
Fourier analysis, of wavefront aberrations, 15–16
Free cap formation, in LASIK, 130, 131*f*
Fundus evaluation, before refractive surgery, 49
clear lens extraction/refractive lens exchange, 175

Ghost images
with multifocal IOLs, 182
after surface ablation, 105
GHTF (Global Harmonization Task Force), 240
Glare
with anterior chamber phakic IOLs, 167*t*, 168, 169
with iris-fixated phakic IOLs, 167*t*, 169
with multifocal IOLs, 182
with posterior chamber phakic IOLs, 167*t*, 170
after radial keratotomy, 65
after surface ablation, 105
Glaucoma. *See also* Elevated intraocular pressure
refractive surgery and, 46–47, 211–213, 212*f*, 232–234
Global Harmonization Task Force (GHTF), 240
Globe, rupture of, after radial keratotomy, 65, 66*f*
Glycosaminoglycans, corneal haze after surface ablation and, 106
Goldmann applanation tonometry
corneal thickness affecting, 211, 232
after refractive surgery, 232–233
LASIK, 47, 233
surface ablation, 108, 233
Grafts, corneal. *See* Cornea, transplantation of

Haigis formula, for IOL power determination, 226
clear lens extraction/refractive lens exchange and, 176
Halos
with anterior chamber phakic IOLs, 167*t*, 168, 169
with iris-fixated phakic IOLs, 167*t*, 169
with multifocal IOLs, 182
with posterior chamber phakic IOLs, 167*t*, 169
after surface ablation, 105
Hanna arcuate trephine, 69
Hard contact lens method, for IOL power calculation after refractive surgery, 225–226
Hartmann-Shack wavefront analysis/aberrometry, 14, 15*f*
Haze formation
after LASIK, diffuse lamellar keratitis and, 137
after surface ablation, 106–107, 106*f*
mitomycin C in reduction of, 98–99
wound healing and, 27–28, 107
HDE. *See* Humanitarian Device Exemption
Helmholtz hypothesis (capsular theory) of accommodation, 187–188, 188*f*
Herpes zoster ophthalmicus, refractive surgery and, 206
Herpesviruses, ocular infection caused by, refractive surgery and, 92, 205–207
High myopia, correction of
bioptics for, 172, 173*t*
clear lens extraction/refractive lens exchange for, 174, 176, 215
LASIK for, 125, 214
phakic IOLs for, 161
retinal detachment and, 174, 214–215, 227
Higher-order aberrations, 17–18, 18*f*, 19*f*, 20*f*
after LASIK, 144
after surface ablation, 105
wavefront-optimized/wavefront-guided ablation and, 17, 30–31, 146–147
Hinge position, dry eye syndrome and, 112
Historical methods, for IOL power calculation after refractive surgery, 224
History, refractive surgery and, 41–45, 42*t*
HIV (human immunodeficiency virus), viability of after excimer laser ablation, 220
HIV infection/AIDS, refractive surgery in patients with, 219–221
Ho:YAG laser. *See* Holmium:YAG (Ho:YAG) laser
Hoffer Q formula, for IOL power selection, 226
clear lens extraction/refractive lens exchange and, 176
Holladay 2 formula, for IOL power determination, 226
clear lens extraction/refractive lens exchange and, 176
Holmium:YAG (Ho:YAG) laser
for collagen shrinkage, 22*t*, 29
photothermal effects of, 29
for thermokeratoplasty, 27, 150
Homoplastic corneal inlays, in keratophakia, 73–74
Hormone replacement therapy, refractive surgery in patient taking, 43
Human immunodeficiency virus (HIV), viability of after excimer laser ablation, 220
Humanitarian Device Exemption (HDE), 37
Hybrid contact lenses, after LASIK, 231–232
Hydraulic support (catenary) theory of accommodation, 190–191
Hydrodissection, in clear lens extraction/refractive lens exchange, 175

Hydrogel polymers, for corneal inlays for presbyopia, 195–196
Hyperopia
assessment of, before refractive surgery, 45
consecutive/myopia overcorrection and, 104
contact lens–assisted, pharmacologically induced keratosteepening (CLAPIKS) for, 232
after radial keratotomy, 64–65, 66
surgical correction of
clear lens extraction/refractive lens exchange for, 174, 175, 176
conductive keratoplasty for, 151–152, 152*f*, 152*t*
keratophakia for, 73–75
LASIK for, 25–26, 25*f*, 26*f*, 126
light-adjustable IOLs for, 184–185, 185*f*
monovision for, 44–45
multifocal IOLs for, 158–161
phakic IOLs for, 161
photothermal therapy for, 29
PRK for, 102
wavefront-guided laser ablation for, 30–31
wavefront aberration produced by (negative defocus), 16
Hyperopic astigmatism
LASIK for, 126
PRK for, 102
Hypertension, ocular. *See also* Elevated intraocular pressure
refractive surgery and, 211–213, 212*f*
Hyphema, iris-fixated phakic IOL insertion and, 169

I–S number, 13
ICRS. *See* Intrastromal corneal ring segments
IDE. *See* Investigational device exemption
Imitrex. *See* Sumatriptan
Immunocompromised host, refractive surgery and, 219–221
Implantable cardioverter-defibrillators (ICDs), laser surgery in patient with, 43
In situ keratomileusis, 109. *See also* Laser in situ keratomileusis (LASIK)
Incisional corneal surgery, 61–71
for astigmatism, 67–71, 68*f*, 69*f*, 69*t*, 70*f*
for myopia, 61–67, 63*f*, 64*f*, 65*f*, 66*f*
Incisions
for keratorefractive surgery, corneal biomechanics affected by, 20–23, 23*f*, 67–68, 68*f*
for radial keratotomy, 62, 63*f*
depth affecting outcome and, 63
Infectious keratitis, after LASIK, 139–140, 139*t*, 140*f*, 141*f*
Informed consent for refractive surgery
clear lens extraction/refractive lens exchange and, 172–174
LASIK and, 54–58
in patient with ocular or systemic disease, 203–204
phakic intraocular lens insertion and, 162
Infrared pupillometer, 46
Inlays, corneal, 73–87
alloplastic, 74
homoplastic, 73–74
in keratophakia, 73–75
for presbyopia, 74, 195–196
Instantaneous radius of curvature (meridional/tangential power), 7, 7*f*
Intacs, 77. *See also* Intrastromal corneal ring segments
international trends in use of, 238
Interface debris, after LASIK, 142, 143*f*
Interface keratitis
diffuse (diffuse lamellar keratitis/sands of the Sahara), after LASIK, 137–138, 137*f*, 138*t*, 139*t*, 140*f*
femtosecond laser flap creation and, 119
glaucoma/IOP measurement and, 233
infectious, 139–140, 139*t*, 140*f*, 141*f*
pressure-induced, 138–139, 138*f*
Interlenticular membranes, piggyback IOLs and, 176
Intracorneal implants, alloplastic
corneal biomechanics affected by, 24, 24*f*
in epikeratoplasty (epikeratophakia), 76–77
in keratophakia, 74
for presbyopia, 74
Intracorneal lens/ring, 21*t*. *See also* Intrastromal corneal ring segments
Intraocular lenses (IOLs), for refractive errors. *See also specific type*
accommodating, 182–184, 198–200, 199*f*
with clear lens extraction, 176. *See also* Clear lens extraction
piggybacking and, 176
deformable, 183
dual-optic, 183, 200
innovations in, 200
light-adjustable, 184–185, 185*f*
multifocal, 180–182, 181*f*
for presbyopia, 181, 192–193
phakic, 157, 157–171. *See also* Phakic intraocular lenses
corneal transplantation and, 228
with LASIK (bioptics), 157, 171–172, 173*t*
retinal detachment and, 169, 171, 215
power determination of
clear lens extraction/refractive lens exchange and, 176
after refractive surgery, 223–227, 225*t*
for presbyopia, 181, 192–194, 193*f*
after radial keratotomy, 67
single-optic, 182–183. *See also* Crystalens
toric, 177–180, 178*f*
wavefront-designed, 184
Intraocular pressure
elevated/increased. *See* Elevated intraocular pressure
flap creation affected by, 117–118
measurement of
before refractive surgery, 46–47
after refractive surgery, 211–212, 212*f*, 232–233
pressure-induced stromal keratitis after LASIK and, 138–139, 233
surface ablation, 108
Intraocular surgery. *See* Ocular (intraocular) surgery
Intrastromal corneal ring segments, 53*t*, 77–86
advantages of, 77–78
complications of, 83–85, 83*f*, 84*f*, 85*f*
corneal biomechanics affected by, 24, 24*f*, 77–78
corneal transplantation after, 228
disadvantages of, 78
instrumentation for, 79, 79*t*
international trends in use of, 238

for keratoconus, 13, 81–83, 82*f*, 208
after LASIK, 85
for myopia, 77–81, 77*f*, 78*f*, 79*t*, 80*f*
patient selection for, 78–79
outcomes of, 80–81
removal of, 81
technique for, 79–80, 80*f*
Investigational device exemption (IDE), 36
IOLs. *See* Intraocular lenses
IOP. *See* Intraocular pressure
Iridotomy, for phakic IOL insertion, 162
Iris-fixated phakic intraocular lenses, 160*t*, 163–164, 164*f*. *See also* Phakic intraocular lenses
complications of, 167*t*, 169
results with, 166*t*
Iritis
after anterior chamber phakic IOL insertion, 169
after iris-fixated phakic IOL insertion, 167*t*, 169
Irregular astigmatism
after arcuate keratotomy, 71
corneal topography in detection/management of, 10, 49
keratorefractive surgery and, 14, 49
after limbal relaxing incisions, 71
after penetrating keratoplasty, refractive surgery for, 209, 210
wavefront analysis and, 14
Isotretinoin, refractive surgery in patient taking, 43, 92

KC. *See* Keratoconus
Keloid scar formation, history of, refractive surgery in patient with, 92, 114
Keratectasia, after LASIK, 143
Keratectomy, 22*t*
laser, 22*t*
multizone, 25, 25*f*
photorefractive. *See* Photorefractive keratectomy
phototherapeutic (PTK)
for corneal haze after surface ablation, 107
for epithelial erosions after LASIK, 132
herpes simplex virus keratitis and, 206
for striae in LASIK flaps, 135
Keratitis
diffuse lamellar/interface (DLK), after LASIK, 137–138, 137*f*, 138*t*, 139*t*, 140*f*
femtosecond laser flap creation and, 119
glaucoma/IOP measurement and, 233
in HIV infection/AIDS, after LASIK, 220
infectious/microbial
after LASIK, 139–140, 139*t*, 140*f*, 141*f*
contact lens wear after radial keratotomy and, 230
herpes simplex, 205–207
stromal, pressure-induced, after LASIK, 138–139, 138*f*
Keratoconjunctivitis sicca. *See* Dry eye syndrome
Keratoconus
ectasia after LASIK and, 143
intrastromal corneal ring segments for, 13, 81–83, 82*f*, 208
phakic IOLs for, 161
refractive surgery contraindicated in, 10, 47, 207–208, 207*f*, 208*f*
corneal topography in detection of, 10, 12–13, 49
thermokeratoplasty for, 149, 154
Keratocytes, stromal, corneal haze after surface ablation and, 106
Keratolysis (corneal melting), refractive surgery and, 222
Keratometry, refractive surgery and, 49
IOL power calculation and, 223, 224
postoperative estimation of, 50, 223
Keratomileusis, 20*t*, 23, 109. *See also* Laser in situ keratomileusis (LASIK); Laser subepithelial keratomileusis (LASEK)
Keratophakia, 24, 73–75
Keratoplasty
conductive, 22*t*, 27, 27*f*, 150–155, 151*f*, 152*f*, 152*t*, 153*f*, 154*t*
corneal transplantation after, 228
for presbyopia, 151, 153, 192
lamellar
automated, 110
wound healing/repair and, 27
penetrating
after arcuate keratotomy, 71
astigmatism after, refractive surgery for, 209, 210–211
corneal topography after, 13–14
after radial keratotomy, 66–67
after refractive surgery, 227–228
refractive surgery after, 208–211, 209*f*
Keratorefractive surgery (KRS). *See also specific procedure and* Refractive surgery
classification of, 20, 21–22*t*
corneal biomechanics affected by, 20–27, 28–29*t*
corneal shape and, 6
corneal topography and, 5–6, 6–14, 49–50, 50*f*. *See also* Cornea, topography of
corneal wound healing and, 27–28
glaucoma/ocular hypertension and, 46–47, 211–213, 212*f*
for irregular astigmatism, 14
laser biophysics and, 29–31
in ocular and systemic disease, 203–222. *See also specific disorder*
patient evaluation for, 41–58, 42*t*, 53*t*. *See also* Keratorefractive surgery (KRS), preoperative evaluation for
patient expectations and, 41–42, 42*t*
postoperative considerations and, 223–234
preoperative evaluation for, 41–58, 42*t*, 53*t*
ancillary tests in, 49–52, 50*f*
corneal topography in, 5–6, 6–14, 49–50, 50*f*. *See also* Cornea, topography of
discussion of findings/informed consent and, 52, 54–58
examination in, 45–49, 47*f*, 48*f*, 49*f*
history in, 41–45, 42*t*
retinal detachment after, 214–215
wavefront aberrations after, 17–18, 18*f*, 19*f*, 20*f*
wavefront-guided, for irregular astigmatism, 14
Keratoscopy, computerized, 6
Keratosteepening, contact lens–assisted, pharmacologically induced (CLAPIKS), 232
Keratotomy, 21–22*t*
arcuate, 68–71, 69*t*, 70*f*
complications of, 71
instrumentation for, 69, 70*f*

ocular surgery after, 71
outcomes of, 70
surgical technique for, 70
astigmatic, 21–22*t*, 23*f*
wound healing/repair and, 27
radial. *See* Radial keratotomy
KRS. *See* Keratorefractive surgery

Lactation, refractive surgery contraindicated during, 43
LAL. *See* Light-adjustable intraocular lenses
Lamellar keratoplasty
automated, 110
wound healing/repair and, 27
Lamellar surgery, 21*t*. *See also* Laser in situ keratomileusis (LASIK)
corneal biomechanics affected by, 23–24, 23*f*
corneal wound healing and, 27
LASEK. *See* Laser subepithelial keratomileusis
Laser-adjustable synthetic epikeratoplasty, 76–77
Laser in situ keratomileusis (LASIK), 21*t*, 23, 23*f*, 53*t*, 109–146
ablation techniques for, 122–123, 123*f*
for accommodative esotropia, 219
for amblyopia/anisometropic amblyopia, 217–218
in astigmatism
hyperopic, 126
mixed, 126
myopic, 125–126
after penetrating keratoplasty, 210–211
central islands and, 137
in children, 218
CLAPIKS after, 232
complications of, 129–145, 145–146
in diabetic patients, 221
in connective tissue/autoimmune diseases, 222
corneal curvatures affected by, 223
corneal sensation affected by, 136
corneal thickness and, 51, 114–115
corneal transplantation after, 228
corneal wound healing and, 28
decentration and, 137
in diabetic patients, 221
diffuse lamellar keratitis (DLK) after, 137–138, 137*f*, 138*t*, 139*t*, 140*f*
femtosecond laser flap creation and, 119
dry eye after, 114, 136, 204
microkeratome hinge position and, 112
ectasia after, 143–144
intrastromal corneal ring segment placement and, 85, 143
epithelial. *See* Epithelial laser in situ keratomileusis
epithelial erosions and, 131–132
epithelial ingrowth after, 140–142, 141*f*, 142*f*
haze formation and, 28
excimer laser ablation in, 122–123, 123*f*
filtering surgery and, 213
flap creation for. *See also* Flaps, LASIK
femtosecond laser, 113, 118–120, 119*f*, 120*f*, 121*f*, 121*t*
steep or flat corneas and, 50, 114
microkeratome, 110–113, 111–112*f*, 117–118, 117*f*, 118*f*
complications associated with, 129–131, 130*f*, 131*f*
ocular aberrations and, 144
flap dislocation and, 136
flap replacement in, 123
glaucoma/ocular hypertension and, 211–213, 212*f*
global estimates of, 235, 235*f*
haze formation and, 28
herpes simplex virus keratitis and, 205–206
history of, 109–110
in HIV infection/AIDS, 220
for hyperopia, 25–26, 25*f*, 26*f*, 126
with astigmatism, 126
infectious keratitis after, 139–140, 139*t*, 140*f*, 141*f*
informed consent for, 54–58
instrumentation for, 110–113, 111–112*f*
interface debris after, 142, 143*f*
international trends in use of, 237–238, 238
intraocular lens power calculation after, 223–227, 225*t*
intraocular pressure measurements after, 211–212, 212*f*, 233
intrastromal corneal ring segment placement and, 85
lasers approved for, 34–35*t*
microkeratome for, 110–113, 111–112*f*, 117–118, 117*f*, 118*f*
complications associated with, 129–131, 130*f*, 131*f*
for mixed astigmatism, 126
for myopia, 25, 124–126
with astigmatism, 125–126
corneal biomechanics affected by, 23, 23*f*, 25
high myopia, 125
low myopia, 124
moderate myopia, 124–125
spherical aberrations after, 17
optical aberrations after, 144–145
outcomes of, 124–129, 145
patient selection for, 114–116
after penetrating keratoplasty, 209–210, 209*f*
with phakic IOL insertion (bioptics), 157, 171–172, 173*t*
preoperative laser inspection and, 113
preoperative laser programming for, 116–117
preoperative patient preparation and, 116, 116*f*
preoperative patient selection and, 114–116
pressure-induced stromal keratitis after, 138–139, 138*f*
after radial keratotomy, 66
re-treatment and, 127–129, 128*f*
residual myopia after, intrastromal corneal ring segments for, 85
residual stromal bed thickness after, 51–52, 114–115
ectasia and, 143–144
retinal detachment/retinal detachment repair and, 214, 227
striae and, 132–136, 134*t*, 135*f*
cornel haze and, 28
surface ablation for enhancement of, 129
surgical suite for, 116
surgical techniques for, 116–123
wavefront aberrations after, 17–18, 18*f*, 19*f*, 20*f*, 144–145
wavefront-guided, 115–116, 127, 146–147
Laser iridotomy, for phakic IOL insertion, 162
Laser keratectomy, 22*t*. *See also* Photorefractive keratectomy
Laser subepithelial keratomileusis (LASEK), 92–109. *See also* Surface ablation
calibration of excimer laser for, 93
central islands and, 104, 105*f*

centration and ablation in, 98–99, 98*f*
in children, 218
complications of, 103–108
corneal haze and, 106–107, 106*f*
corneal wound healing and, 28
corticosteroid-induced complications after, 108
decentered ablation and, 105–106, 106*f*
dry eye after, 108
endothelial effects of, 108
enhancements/reoperation and, 103
epithelial debridement for, 95, 96*f*
epithelial defects and, 107
epithelial preservation techniques for, 95–96, 97*f*
glaucoma/ocular hypertension and, 108, 212, 213
global estimates of, 236*f*
infiltrates and, 107–108, 107*f*
international trends in use of, 238
laser ablation technique in, 98–100, 98*f*
optical aberrations and, 105
outcomes of, 100–103
overcorrection and, 103–104
patient selection for, 92–93
postablation measures and
immediate, 99
operative day, 99
subsequent postoperative care, 100
preoperative planning/laser programming for, 93–94
surgical technique for, 93–97
tracking devices for, 101
undercorrection and, 104
Laser thermokeratoplasty, 27, 150
corneal transplantation after, 228
Lasers
biophysics of, 29–31
corneal biomechanics affected by, 24–26, 25*f*, 26*f*
for refractive surgery
FDA-approved, 34–35*t*
international preferences and, 238
tissue interactions and, 29
wavefront-guided, 147
LASIK. *See* Laser in situ keratomileusis
Lens (crystalline)
evaluation of, before refractive surgery, 48
zonular fibers/zonules of, in accommodation, 187–190, 188*f*, 189*f*, 190*f*
Lens fibers, zonular (zonules of Zinn), in accommodation, 187–190, 188*f*, 189*f*, 190*f*
Lensectomy, refractive (clear lens extraction/refractive lens exchange), 53*t*, 172–177
advantages of, 177
complications of, 177
disadvantages of, 177
indications for, 172
informed consent for, 172–174
IOL calculations for, 176
patient selection for, 172–174
retinal detachment and, 174, 175, 177, 215
surgical planning/techniques for, 174–176
Lenticules, 73
in epikeratoplasty, 75–77, 75*f*
in keratophakia, 73–75
in LASIK, 109
Light-adjustable intraocular lenses (Light Adjustable Lens), 184–185, 185*f*, 200
Limbal relaxing incisions, 68–71, 68*f*, 69*f*, 70*f*
instrumentation for, 69, 70*f*
ocular surgery after, 71
outcomes of, 70
technique for, 60, 69*t*
Linear incisions (tangential/arcuate incisions), for keratorefractive surgery, corneal biomechanics affected by, 20–23, 23*f*, 68
Lower-order aberrations, 16, 16*f*, 17*f*
after LASIK, 144
LTK. *See* Laser thermokeratoplasty
Lupus erythematosus, systemic, refractive surgery contraindicated in, 222

Macrostriae/macrofolds, in LASIK flaps, 133, 134*t*, 135*t*. *See also* Striae
Manifest (noncycloplegic) refraction. *See also* Refraction, clinical
before refractive surgery, 45
Map-dot-fingerprint dystrophy (epithelial basement membrane/anterior membrane dystrophy), refractive surgery in patients with, 47, 49*f*
LASIK, 114
surface ablation, 93
Marginal degeneration, pellucid, 13, 49, 50*f*
refractive surgery contraindicated in, 207–208, 208*f*
Medical Device Amendments, to Food, Drug, and Cosmetic Act, 33
Medical devices
adverse event reporting and, 39
FDA approval of
clinical data required for, 36
delays in, 38–39
FDA classification of, 33–36
labeling, 38
pathways to market for, 36–37
Medical history, refractive surgery and, 42*t*, 43
Meibomian glands, dysfunction of, refractive surgery and, 47
Meridional power (instantaneous radius of curvature), 7, 7*f*
Microfolds/microstriae, in LASIK flaps, 133–136, 134*t*, 135*f*. *See also* Striae
Microkeratomes, for LASIK, 109, 110–113, 111–112*f*, 117–118, 117*f*, 118*f*
complications associated with, 129–131, 130*f*, 131*f*
ocular aberrations and, 144
Microstriae/microfolds, in LASIK flaps, 133–136, 134*t*, 135*f*. *See also* Striae
Mitomycin/mitomycin C
enhancement of LASIK flaps and, 129
in ocular surgery after radial keratotomy, 66
in surface ablation, 98–99
corneal haze prevention/corneal wound healing and, 28, 66, 98–99, 107
international trends in use of, 238
for undercorrection, 104
Mixed astigmatism
LASIK for, 126
PRK for, 102
Modified monovision, 44–45, 191
Monovision, 191–192
modified, 44–45, 191
Motility, ocular. *See* Ocular motility

Multifocal ablation, for presbyopia, 194–195, 195*f*
Multifocal intraocular lenses, 180–182, 181*f*
for presbyopia, 181, 192–194, 193*f*
Multizone keratectomies, 25, 25*f*
Munnerlyn formula, 24–25
Mydriasis/mydriatics, multifocal IOLs and, 182, 194
Myopia
global variation in prevalence of, 237
high. *See* High myopia
hyperopia overcorrection and, 104
orthokeratology for correction of, 86–87
prevalence of, 237
residual
after intrastromal corneal ring segment placement, 81
after LASIK, intrastromal corneal ring segments for, 85
after radial keratotomy, 63
surgical correction of. *See also specific procedure*
bioptics for, 172, 173*t*
clear lens extraction/refractive lens exchange for, 174, 176
hyperopia after (consecutive hyperopia), 104
contact lens–assisted, pharmacologically induced keratosteepening (CLAPIKS) for, 232
incisional corneal surgery for, 61–67, 63*f*, 64*f*, 65*f*, 66*f*
intrastromal corneal ring segments for, 77–81, 77*f*, 78*f*, 79*t*, 80*f*
LASIK for, 25, 124–126. *See also* Laser in situ keratomileusis
with astigmatism, 125–126
high myopia, 125
low myopia, 124
moderate myopia, 124–125
light-adjustable IOLs for, 184–185, 185*f*
monovision for, 191–192
phakic IOLs for, 161
PRK for, 26*f*, 101
spherical aberrations after, 17
radial keratotomy for, 61–67, 63*f*, 64*f*, 65*f*, 66*f*
retinal detachment and, 174, 214–215, 227
wavefront-guided laser ablation for, 30–31
wavefront aberration produced by (positive defocus), 16, 16*f*
Myopic astigmatism, LASIK for, 125–126
Myopic spherical photorefractive keratectomy, 26*f*, 101

Nd:YAG laser. *See also* Femtosecond laser
for LASIK flap creation, 113
Negative defocus, 16
Nerve fiber layer, refractive surgery and, 212
Night vision abnormalities
after posterior chamber phakic IOL insertion, 170
after radial keratotomy, 65
after surface ablation, 105
Noncycloplegic (manifest) refraction. *See also* Refraction, clinical
before refractive surgery, 45
Nonsteroidal anti-inflammatory drugs (NSAIDs), after surface ablation, 99
delayed re-epithelialization and, 107
for overcorrection, 104
NuLens Accommodating IOL, 200
Nursing (breast feeding), refractive surgery contraindicated during, 43

OBL. *See* Opaque bubble layer
Oblate cornea, 6, 8
Occupation, refractive surgery selection and, 42–43
Ocular aberrations. *See* Aberrations
Ocular history, refractive surgery and, 42*t*, 43–44
Ocular hypertension. *See also* Elevated intraocular pressure
refractive surgery and, 211–213, 212*f*
Ocular motility, assessment of, before refractive surgery, 46
Ocular (intraocular) surgery. *See also specific procedure*
after arcuate keratotomy, 71
after limbal relaxing incisions, 71
after radial keratotomy, 65–67
for refractive errors, 157–185. *See also specific procedure*
accommodating intraocular lenses, 182–184, 198–200, 199*f*
clear lens extraction/refractive lens exchange, 53*t*, 172–177
light-adjustable intraocular lenses, 184–185, 185*f*
multifocal intraocular lenses, 180–182, 181*f*
phakic intraocular lens implantation, 157–171, 159–160*t*
toric intraocular lenses, 177–180, 178*f*
wavefront-designed intraocular lenses, 184
Onlays, corneal, 73–87
alloplastic, 76–77
Opaque bubble layer, with femtosecond laser, 120
Open-angle glaucoma, refractive surgery and, 211–212, 212*f*, 232–234
Open-loop trackers, 101
Ophthalmic Devices Panel, 33, 37–38
Optical aberrations. *See* Aberrations
Optical zone
in radial keratotomy, 62
outcome affected by, 62, 65
in surface ablation, preoperative laser programming and, 94
Orbit, anatomy of, assessment of before refractive surgery, 46
surface ablation, 92
Orthokeratology, 86–87
Overcorrection, with surface ablation, 103–104

Pacemakers, laser surgery in patient with, 43
Pachymetry (pachymeter)
for intrastromal corneal ring segment placement, 80
before LASIK, 114–115
corneal perforation and, 131
before phakic intraocular lens insertion, 162
before refractive surgery, 50–51
Pain, postoperative, management of after surface ablation, 99
Patient selection
for clear lens extraction/refractive lens exchange, 172–174
for conductive keratoplasty, 152–153
for intrastromal corneal ring segments for myopia, 78–79

for LASIK, 114–116
for monovision, 191–192
for multifocal IOLs, 180–181
for phakic intraocular lenses, 161–162
for radial keratotomy, 62
for surface ablation, 92–93
for toric IOLs, 178–179
PCPIOL (posterior chamber phakic intraocular lenses). *See* Phakic intraocular lenses, posterior chamber
Pellucid marginal degeneration, 13, 49, 50*f*
refractive surgery contraindicated in, 207–208, 208*f*
Penetrating keratoplasty. *See* Keratoplasty, penetrating
Peribulbar anesthesia, for phakic IOL insertion, 162
PERK (Prospective Evaluation of Radial Keratotomy) study, 62
Persistent corneal epithelial defect
after LASIK, 132
after surface ablation, 107
Phacoemulsification, in clear lens extraction/refractive lens exchange, 175
Phakic intraocular lenses, 53*t*, 157, 157–171, 159–160*t*
advantages of, 158
for amblyopia, 216–217
ancillary preoperative tests for, 162
anterior chamber, 162–163, 163*f*
angle-supported, 159*t*, 162–163, 163*f*
complications of, 167*t*, 168–169
results with, 166*t*
background of, 157–158
in children, 218
complications of, 167*t*, 168–171, 170*f*
contraindications to, 161
corneal transplant surgery and, 228
disadvantages of, 158–161
global estimates of use of, 236*f*
indications for, 161
informed consent for, 162
international trends in use of, 238, 239
iris-fixated, 160*t*, 163–164, 164*f*
complications of, 167*t*, 169
results of, 166*t*
with LASIK (bioptics), 157, 171–172, 173*t*
outcomes of, 165–168, 166*t*, 167*t*
patient selection/evaluation for, 161–162
posterior chamber, 164–165, 164*f*, 165*f*
complications of, 167*t*, 169–171, 170*f*
decentration of, 170–171
with LASIK (bioptics), 171–172, 173*t*
results with, 167*t*
preoperative patient evaluation and, 161–162
retinal detachment and, 169, 171, 215
sulcus-supported, 160*t*
surgical technique for insertion of, 162–165, 163*f*, 164*f*, 165*f*
Phorias, refractive surgery and, 46
Photoablation, 29, 89–147, 90–91*f*. *See also specific procedure*
custom. *See also* Wavefront-guided laser ablation
for presbyopia, 194–195, 195*f*
herpes simplex virus keratitis and, 205–206
LASIK, 21*t*, 23, 23*f*, 53*t*, 109–146
surface ablation, 53*t*, 92–109
types of lasers for, 29–30
wavefront-guided, 146–147. *See also* Wavefront-guided laser ablation
Photoastigmatic keratectomy (toric PRK), 101–102
Photodisruption, 29
Photomydriasis, multifocal IOLs and, 182
Photorefractive keratectomy (PRK), 23, 23*f*, 92–109. *See also* Surface ablation
for accommodative esotropia, 219
calibration of excimer laser for, 93
central islands and, 104, 105*f*
centration and ablation in, 98–99, 98*f*
in children, 218
CLAPIKS after, 232
complications of, 103–108
corneal biomechanics affected by, 24–25, 26*f*
corneal haze and, 106–107, 106*f*
corneal topography after, 10, 11*f*
corneal wound healing/repair and, 27–28
delays in, 107
corticosteroid-induced complications after, 108
decentered ablation and, 105–106, 106*f*
dry eye after, 108
endothelial effects of, 108
enhancements/reoperation and, 103
epithelial debridement for, 95, 96*f*
epithelial defects and, 107
glaucoma/ocular hypertension and, 108, 211–212
global estimates of, 236*f*
herpes simplex virus keratitis and, 206
hyperopic, 102
hyperopic astigmatic, 102
infiltrates and, 107–108, 107*f*
international trends in use of, 238
intraocular lens power calculation after, 223–227
laser ablation technique in, 98–100, 98*f*
lasers approved for, 35*t*
mixed astigmatic, 102
myopic, 26*f*, 101
spherical aberrations after, 17
optical aberrations after, 105
outcomes of, 100–103
overcorrection and, 103–104
patient selection for, 92–93
after penetrating keratoplasty, 209, 210
postablation measures for
immediate, 99
operative day, 99
subsequent postoperative care, 100
preoperative planning/laser programming for, 93–94
surgical technique for, 93–97
toric (photoastigmatic keratectomy), 101–102
tracking devices for, 101
undercorrection and, 104
wavefront aberrations after, 17–18, 18*f*, 19*f*, 20*f*
Photosensitivity, femtosecond laser flap creation and, 120
Phototherapeutic keratectomy (PTK)
for corneal haze after surface ablation, 107
for epithelial erosions after LASIK, 132
herpes simplex virus keratitis and, 206
for striae in LASIK flaps, 135
Photothermal laser therapy, 29

Picosecond laser, for LASIK flap creation, 113
Piggybacking, with intraocular lenses, clear lens extraction/refractive lens exchange and, 176
Pigment dispersion syndrome
after iris-fixated phakic IOL insertion, 167*t*
after posterior chamber phakic IOL insertion, 167*t*
PIOL. *See* Phakic intraocular lenses
PISK. *See* Pressure-induced stromal keratitis
Piston, wavefront aberrations and, 16
PK/PKP (penetrating keratoplasty). *See* Keratoplasty, penetrating
Placido-based topography/Placido disk, 6, 7
for IOL power calculation after refractive surgery, 224
in pellucid marginal degeneration, 13
PMA. *See* Premarket approval
PMMA. *See* Polymethylmethacrylate
Pneumotonometry/pneumotonometer, for IOP measurement after refractive surgery, 108, 232, 233
Polyarteritis nodosa, refractive surgery contraindicated in, 222
Polymethylmethacrylate (PMMA)
intrastromal corneal ring segments made from, 77
phakic IOLs made from, 158
Polysulfone, for corneal inlays, 74, 195
Positive defocus, 16, 16*f*
Posterior chamber intraocular lenses. *See* Intraocular lenses
Posterior segment, assessment of before refractive surgery, 49
Postoperative care of refractive surgery patient, 223–234
LASIK and, 123
surface ablation
immediate postablation measures for, 99
operative day postablation treatment and, 99
subsequent postoperative care and, 100
Power (optical)
intraocular lens, determination of
clear lens extraction/refractive lens exchange and, 176
refractive surgery and, 223–227, 225*t*
refractive, of cornea, 5–6
Power maps, 6–7, 49
Power prediction formulas, for IOLs, 226
clear lens extraction/refractive lens exchange and, 176
Pregnancy, refractive surgery contraindicated during, 43
Premarket approval (PMA), 36, 37
delays in, 38–39
Premarket Notification 510(k) application, 36–37
Preoperative assessment/preparation for refractive surgery, 41–58, 42*t*, 53*t*
LASIK
patient preparation, 116, 116*f*
patient selection, 114–116
phakic intraocular lens insertion, 162–163
surface ablation, 92–93, 94–95
wavefront-guided laser ablation, 147
PresbyLens, 196
Presbyopia, 187–200
catenary (hydraulic support) theory of accommodation and, 190–191
Helmholtz (capsular) theory of accommodation and, 187–188, 188*f*
refractive surgery and, 44–45
Schachar theory of accommodation and, 188–190, 189*f*, 190*f*
surgical correction of, 187–200
accommodative, 196–200, 197*f*, 199*f*
clear lens extraction/refractive lens exchange for, 174
conductive keratoplasty for, 151, 153, 192
corneal inlays for, 74, 195–196
custom/multifocal ablations for, 194–195, 195*f*
intraocular lenses for, 181, 192–194, 193*f*
accommodating IOLs, 198–200, 199*f*
experimental IOLs, 200
multifocal IOLs, 181, 192–194, 193*f*
monovision and, 44–45, 191–192
nonaccommodative, 191–196, 193*f*, 195*f*
scleral surgery for, 196–198, 197*f*
Pressure-induced stromal keratitis, after LASIK, 138–139, 138*f*
PresVIEW scleral expansion bands, 197
Prisms, wavefront aberrations and, 16, 17*f*
PRK. *See* Photorefractive keratectomy
Prolate cornea, 6, 8
intrastromal corneal ring segments and, 77–78
Prospective Evaluation of Radial Keratotomy (PERK) study, 62
PTK. *See* Phototherapeutic keratectomy
Punctate epithelial defects/erosions, corneal, refractive surgery in patient with, 47, 48*f*
Pupillary block, after anterior chamber phakic IOL insertion, 168
Pupils
examination of before refractive surgery, 45–46
surface ablation, 92–93
ovalization of
after anterior chamber phakic IOL insertion, 167*t*, 168, 169
after iris-fixated phakic IOL insertion, 167*t*
size of
measurement of before refractive surgery, 45–46
surface ablation, 92–93
wavefront aberrations and, 17
"Pushing plus," before refractive surgery, 45

Q formula, Hoffer, for IOL power selection, 226
clear lens extraction/refractive lens exchange and, 176
Q value, 8
Quadrafoil, 18, 20*f*

Radial incisions
for keratorefractive surgery, corneal biomechanics affected by, 20–23
for radial keratotomy, 62, 63*f*
depth affecting outcome and, 63
Radial keratotomy (RK), 21*t*, 61–67, 63*f*, 64*f*, 65*f*, 66*f*
cataract surgery after, 67, 226
complications of, 65, 65*f*, 66*f*
contact lens use after, 229–230, 230*f*
corneal topography after, 64
corneal transplantation after, 66–67, 227–228
difference map in, 10, 11*f*

herpes simplex virus keratitis and, 206
hyperopic shift and, 64–65, 66
intraocular lens power calculation after, 67, 223–227
keratometric power measurements affected by, 223
ocular surgery after, 65–67
outcomes of, 62–65
patient selection for, 62
penetrating keratoplasty after, 66–67, 227–228
refraction after, 64
stability of, 64–65
surgical technique for, 62, 63*f*, 64*f*
visual acuity after, 64
Radial thermokeratoplasty, 150
Radiofrequency, for conductive keratoplasty, 150–155, 151*f*, 152*f*, 152*t*, 153*f*, 154*t*
Radius of curvature, instantaneous (meridional/tangential power), 7, 7*f*
Red-green test, duochrome/bichrome, before refractive surgery, 45
Refraction
after radial keratotomy, 64
stability of, 64–65
refractive surgery and, 45
IOL power calculation and, 224–225, 225*t*
Refractive errors. *See also specific type*
global variation in prevalence of, 237
Refractive lens exchange (clear lens extraction), 53*t*, 172–177
advantages of, 177
complications of, 177
disadvantages of, 177
indications for, 172
informed consent for, 172–174
IOL calculations for, 176
patient selection for, 172–174
retinal detachment and, 174, 175, 177, 215
surgical planning/techniques for, 174–176
Refractive power of cornea, 5
keratometry in measurement of, 5–6
Refractive surgery. *See also specific procedure*
adjustable (ARS), 171–172, 173*t*
amblyopia and strabismus and, 216–219
in autoimmune disease, 222
cataract/cataract surgery and, 192–194
CLAPIKS after, 232
classification of, 20, 21–22*t*
in connective tissue diseases, 205, 222
contact lens use after, 228–232
corneal biomechanics and, 20–27, 28–29*t*
corneal topography and, 5–6, 6–14, 49–50, 50*f*. *See also* Cornea, topography of
indications for, 8–10, 9*f*
postoperative evaluation and, 10, 11*f*
corneal transplant after, 227–228
corneal wound healing and, 27–28
in diabetes mellitus, 221–222
glaucoma/ocular hypertension and, 46–47, 211–213, 212*f*, 232–234
global estimates of, 235, 236*f*
in HIV infection/AIDS, 219–221
indications for, 203–204
international perspectives in, 235–241
global estimates of surgery procedures and, 235, 236*f*
regulation of practices and devices and, 240
trends in surgery and, 237–240
variation in refractive error prevalence and, 237
intraocular lens power calculations after, 223–227, 225*t*
for irregular astigmatism, 14
after penetrating keratoplasty, 209, 210
keratorefractive procedures, 5. *See also* Keratorefractive surgery
laser biophysics and, 29–31
lenticular procedures, 5. *See also specific procedure*
in ocular and systemic disease, 203–222. *See also specific disorder*
patient evaluation for, 41–58, 42*t*, 53*t*. *See also* Refractive surgery, preoperative evaluation for
patient expectations and, 41–42, 42*t*
after penetrating keratoplasty, 208–211, 209*f*
penetrating keratoplasty after, 227–228
postoperative considerations and, 223–234
preoperative evaluation for, 41–58, 42*t*, 53*t*
ancillary tests in, 49–52, 50*f*
corneal topography in, 5–6, 6–14, 49–50, 50*f*. *See also* Cornea, topography of
discussion of findings/informed consent and, 52, 54–58
examination in, 45–49, 47*f*, 48*f*, 49*f*
history in, 41–45, 42*t*
retinal detachment/retinal detachment repair and, 214–215, 227
science of, 5–31
wavefront aberrations after, 17–18, 18*f*, 19*f*, 20*f*
Registration, for laser centration, 98, 98*f*
Regular astigmatism
corneal topography in detection/management of, 8, 9*f*
wavefront aberration produced by, 16, 16*f*
Relaxing incisions, limbal, 68, 68*f*, 69*f*, 70*f*
instrumentation for, 69, 70*f*
ocular surgery after, 71
outcomes of, 70
technique for, 69*t*
Residual stromal bed, after LASIK, 51–52, 114–115
ectasia and, 143–144
ReSTOR intraocular lens, 180, 181, 181*f*, 193–194, 193*f*
Retinal detachment
after cataract surgery, 215
after clear lens extraction/refractive lens exchange, 174, 175, 177, 215
high myopia and, 74, 214–215, 227
intraocular lenses and, 169, 171, 215
after LASIK, 214
after posterior chamber phakic IOL insertion, 171
refractive surgery and, 214–215, 227
surgery for
after LASIK, 227
refractive surgery after, 215–216
Retinal disease, refractive surgery in patient with, 214–216
Retinal nerve fibers, refractive surgery and, 212
Retrobulbar anesthesia, for phakic IOL insertion, 162
ReZoom intraocular lens, 180, 181, 181*f*
Rheumatoid arthritis, refractive surgery contraindicated in, 222
Rigid gas-permeable contact lenses
after LASIK, 231
for myopia reduction (orthokeratology), 86–87

after radial keratotomy, 229
refractive surgery and, 229
after surface ablation, 231
RK. *See* Radial keratotomy
Root-mean-square (RMS) errors, magnitude of wavefront deviation and, 15
RST. *See* Residual stromal bed

Sagittal curvature. *See* Axial curvature
Sands of the Sahara (diffuse lamellar keratitis/DLK), after LASIK, 137–138, 137*f*, 138*t*, 139*t*, 140*f*
femtosecond laser flap creation and, 119
glaucoma/IOP measurement and, 233
Scanning-slit systems
for pachymetry, 51
for photoablation, 29–30
Schachar theory of accommodation, 188–190, 189*f*, 190*f*
Scleral buckle, for retinal detachment, refractive surgery after, 215–216
Scleral expansion bands, for presbyopia, 197–198, 197*f*
Scleral surgery, for presbyopia, 196–198, 197*f*
Sclerotomy, anterior ciliary, for presbyopia, 197
Shallow anterior chamber. *See* Anterior chamber, flat or shallow
Single-optic intraocular lenses, 182–183. *See also* Crystalens
Smart intraocular lens (SmartLens), 183, 200
Social history, refractive surgery and, 42–43, 42*t*
SofPort AO intraocular lens, 184
Soft contact lenses. *See* Flexible (soft) contact lenses
SOS. *See* Sands of the Sahara
Specular microscopy/photomicroscopy, before phakic intraocular lens insertion, 162
Spherical aberration, 17, 18*f*
after surface ablation, 105
SRK formulas, for IOL power selection, 226
clear lens extraction/refractive lens exchange and, 176
STAAR toric IOL, 177–178, 178*f*, 179–180
Strabismus, refractive surgery and, 46, 216–219
Striae
after conductive keratoplasty, 152, 152*f*
in LASIK flaps, 132–136, 134*t*, 135*f*
classification of, 133, 134*t*
corneal haze and, 28
visual significance and, 132
Stromal bed thickness, after LASIK, 51–52, 114–115
ectasia and, 143–144
Stromal infiltrates, after surface ablation, 107–108, 107*f*
Stromal keratitis, pressure-induced, after LASIK, 138–139, 138*f*
Suction ring
for femtosecond laser flap creation, 119
filtering bleb affecting placement of, 213
of microkeratome, 110, 111–112*f*
in flap creation, 117, 117*f*
Sulcus-supported intraocular lenses, 160*t*
Sumatriptan, refractive surgery in patient taking, 43
Surface ablation, 53*t*, 92–109. *See also specific procedure*
bandage contact lenses after, 97*f*, 99, 230
calibration of excimer laser for, 93
central islands and, 104, 105*f*
centration and ablation in, 98–99, 98*f*
complications of, 103–108
contact lens use after, 230–231
corneal curvatures affected by, 223
corneal haze and, 106–107, 106*f*
corneal transplantation after, 228
corticosteroid-induced complications after, 108
decentered ablation and, 105–106, 106*f*
dry eye after, 108, 204
endothelial effects of, 108
enhancements/reoperation and, 103
epithelial debridement for, 95, 96*f*
epithelial defects and, 107
epithelial preservation techniques for, 95–97, 97*f*
glaucoma/ocular hypertension and, 108, 211–212, 213, 233
herpes simplex virus keratitis and, 205–206
infiltrates and, 107–108, 107*f*
international trends in use of, 238
laser ablation technique in, 98–100, 98*f*
for LASIK enhancement, 129
optical aberrations and, 105
outcomes of, 100–103
overcorrection and, 103–104
patient selection for, 92–93
postablation measures and
immediate, 99
operative day, 99
subsequent postoperative care, 100
preoperative planning/laser programming for, 93–94
surgical technique for, 93–97
tracking devices for, 101
undercorrection and, 104
wavefront-guided, 146–147. *See also* Wavefront-guided laser ablation
Surgical instruments
for arcuate keratotomy, 69, 70*f*
for intrastromal corneal ring segment placement, 79, 79*t*
for LASIK, 110–113, 111–112*f*
for limbal relaxing incisions, 69, 70*f*
Synchrony intraocular lens, 183, 200
Systemic lupus erythematosus, refractive surgery contraindicated in, 222

Tangential incisions, for keratorefractive surgery, corneal biomechanics affected by, 20–23, 23*f*, 68
Tangential power (instantaneous radius of curvature), 7, 7*f*
Tear breakup time, refractive surgery and, 47, 47*f*
Tear deficiency states, aqueous, refractive surgery and, 47, 47*f*
Tears (artificial), for dry eye, after LASIK, 136
Tecnis intraocular lens, 184
Terry Astigmatome, 69, 70*f*
Thermokeratoplasty, 27, 27*f*, 149
corneal transplantation, 228
laser, 27, 150
radial, 150
Tissue addition/subtraction, corneal biomechanics affected by, 23–24, 23*f*
Tono-Pen measurement, for IOP measurement after refractive surgery, 108, 232, 233
Tonometry
after refractive surgery, 232–233
LASIK, 47, 233
surface ablation, 108, 233

Topical anesthesia, for phakic IOL insertion, 162
Topography
corneal, 5–6, 6–14, 49–50, 50*f*. *See also* Cornea, topography of
computerized, 6–14, 49–50, 50*f*
refractive surgery and, 5–6, 6–14, 49–50, 50*f*, 93
Toric intraocular lenses, 177–180, 178*f*
Toric LASIK ablations, 125
Toric photorefractive keratectomy (photoastigmatic keratectomy), 101–102
Tracking devices (excimer laser)
for LASIK, 122, 123
for surface ablation, 101
Transepithelial ablation, 95
Transverse keratotomy, 67
Trauma, LASIK flap dislocation and, 136
Trefoil, 18, 19*f*
Tropias, refractive surgery and, 46

Ultrasound/ultrasonography, for pachymetry
for intrastromal corneal ring segment placement, 80
before refractive surgery, 50–51
Ultraviolet light, corneal haze after surface ablation and, 106–107
Undercorrection, with surface ablation, 104

Vertex distance measurement, before refractive surgery, 45
Vision, diurnal variation in, after radial keratotomy, 64
Visual acuity
after bioptics, 172, 173*t*
after clear lens extraction/refractive lens exchange, 177
after conductive keratoplasty, 153
for presbyopia, 192
after intrastromal corneal ring segment placement
for keratoconus, 81–82, 84–85
for myopia, 80–81
after LASIK, 124
in diabetic patients, 221
for high myopia, 125
for hyperopia, 126
for hyperopic astigmatism, 126
for low myopia, 124
for mixed astigmatism, 126
for moderate myopia, 124–125
for myopia with astigmatism, 125
striae and, 132
with monovision, 192
after multifocal IOL insertion, 181
after phakic intraocular lens implantation, 165, 166*t*
after PRK
hyperopic, 102
hyperopic astigmatic, 102
mixed astigmatic, 102
myopic spherical, 101
toric (photoastigmatic keratectomy), 102
after radial keratotomy, 64, 65
testing
in amblyopia, refractive surgery and, 217
before refractive surgery, 45
after toric IOL implantation, 179
after wavefront-guided ablation, 31, 127, 146
Visual axis, incisional effect on corneal biomechanics and, 20–23, 23*f*
Vitamin C, corneal wound healing and, 28
Vitrectomy, for retinal detachment, refractive surgery after, 215–216

Wavefront aberrations. *See also* Wavefront analysis
coma, 17, 18*f*
higher-order, 17–18, 18*f*, 19*f*, 20*f*
wavefront-optimized/wavefront-guided ablation and, 17, 30–31
hyperopia producing (negative defocus), 16
irregular astigmatism producing, 14
lower-order, 16, 16*f*, 17*f*
measurement of, 14–16, 15*f*
before LASIK, 115–116
myopia producing (positive defocus), 16, 16*f*
piston, 16
prisms, 16, 17*f*
quadrafoil, 18, 20*f*
regular astigmatism producing, 16, 16*f*
representation of, 15–16, 15*f*
three-dimensional, 15
secondary astigmatism, 18, 19*f*
spherical, 17, 18*f*
trefoil, 18, 19*f*
Wavefront analysis/wavefront visual analysis, 14–18, 15*f*, 16*f*, 17*f*, 18*f*, 19*f*, 20*f*, 51. *See also* Wavefront aberrations
irregular astigmatism and, 14
before LASIK, 115–116
before wavefront-guided ablation, 147
Wavefront-designed intraocular lenses, 184
Wavefront-guided laser ablation, 30–31, 51, 146–147
centration for, 98
higher-order aberrations and, 17, 30–31, 146–147
instrumentation for, 147
international trends in use of, 238
LASIK, 115–116, 127, 146–147
for LASIK enhancement, 129
preoperative preparation for, 147
surface ablation, 146–147
Wavefront-optimized laser ablation, 30. *See also* Wavefront-guided laser ablation
higher-order aberrations and, 17, 30
Wound healing/repair, of cornea, 27–28
delay in after surface ablation, 107

z-height, 7–8, 8*f*
z-maps, 8, 8*f*
Zernicke polynomials, for wavefront aberrations, 15, 16*f*, 17*f*, 18*f*, 19*f*, 20*f*
Zonular fibers, lens (zonules of Zinn), in accommodation, 187–190, 188*f*, 189*f*, 190*f*